Diagnostic Ultrasound in Dermatology

Huixiong Xu • Lehang Guo
Qiao Wang
Editors

Diagnostic Ultrasound in Dermatology

SSTP

Springer

Editors
Huixiong Xu
Department of Medical Ultrasound
Shanghai Skin Disease Hospital
Shanghai, China

Lehang Guo
Department of Medical Ultrasound
Shanghai Skin Disease Hospital
Shanghai, China

Qiao Wang
Department of Medical Ultrasound
Shanghai Tenth People's Hospital
Shanghai, China

ISBN 978-981-16-7344-3 ISBN 978-981-16-7345-0 (eBook)
https://doi.org/10.1007/978-981-16-7345-0

Jointly published with Shanghai Scientific and Technical Publishers
The print edition is not for sale in China (Mainland). Customers from China (Mainland) please order the print book from: Shanghai Scientific and Technical Publishers.

This Springer imprint is published by the registered company Springer Nature Singapore Pte Ltd.
The registered company address is: 152 Beach Road, #21-01/04 Gateway East, Singapore 189721, Singapore

Foreword I

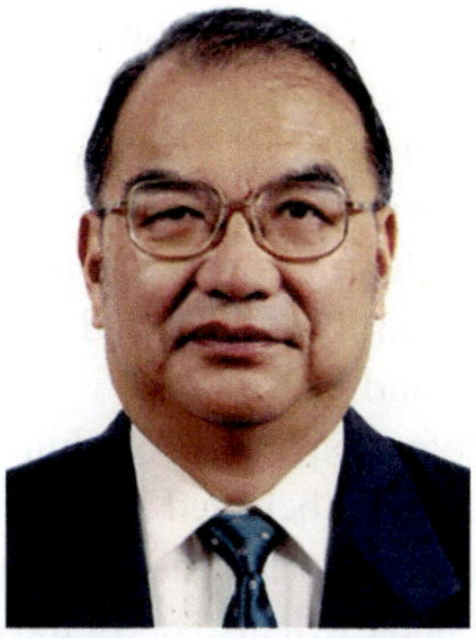

With the improvement of people's living standards and changes in the disease spectrum, the diagnosis and treatment of skin diseases have attracted more and more attention. Skin is the largest organ of the human body, and it is also the organ with the highest incidence of diseases. People suffer from skin diseases of various degrees throughout their lives, and more than a quarter of the population is afflicted with at least one skin disease. Although most skin diseases have mild symptoms, skin disease has become a heavy medical burden and even an important cause of disability due to the increasing human life span and the recurrence of skin diseases. Skin is not only a physiological organ, but also has an important social attribute. Skin diseases have a significant impact on both the psychological and the social adaptability of patients. In addition, the intrinsic physiological and pathological information of the human body will also be reflected on the skin, so the detection and imaging of the skin are also helpful for the noninvasive diagnosis of internal organs.

The types and manifestations of skin diseases are complex and various, which are easily miss-diagnosed and misdiagnosed. Therefore, accurate and quick diagnosis of skin diseases becomes the key to the management of skin diseases. At present, there are two main categories of diagnostic methods for skin diseases: observation with the naked eye, and histopathological examination by invasive skin biopsy. Both of them are hard to balance accuracy and cost-effectiveness. Therefore, dermoscopy, optical coherence tomography, high-frequency ultrasound, and other noninvasive diagnostic techniques have emerged, filling the gap between the naked eye and pathological diagnosis.

Among many noninvasive diagnostic techniques, ultrasound is one of the techniques that can realize multi-scale imaging. It can not only show deep structures, but also superficial structures. With the development of ultrasound imaging technology, ultrasound can provide more detailed information of the skin. It has unique advantages in the current skin imaging technologies. However, to display the superficial structures, it is necessary to overcome the fluctuation of the incident wave intensity in the ultrasound near-field area. In addition, skin ultrasound is a new interdisciplinary area. Conventionally, due to the defects in engineering technology (fluctuation of incident wave intensity in the near-field area of ultrasound), the two disciplines of "dermatology" and "ultrasound medicine" rarely intersect in the past. As a result, the lack of relevant research, the shortage of skin ultrasound imaging talents, and the lack of teaching system, are the current status. Therefore, there is an urgent need for a professional book on skin ultrasound to guide clinical practice.

I have been familiar with Professor Huixiong Xu, the editor-in-chief of this book, for almost ten years. Professor Xu is rigorous, pragmatic, diligent, and steady. I have witnessed his endeavors and achievements in this emerging field for many years. Therefore, I am pleased to be invited as the honorary editor-in-chief of this book and preface it.

The book is the first professional book on skin ultrasound in China. It is a meaningful reference book. It is believed that the book can play a role as a good tool for physicians in ultrasound medicine and dermatology. I believe that the publication of the book will also boost the development of skin ultrasound, and ultimately benefit human being!

Weiqi Wang
Academician, Chinese Academy of Engineering
Beijing, China

Biomedical Engineering Institute
Fudan University
Shanghai, China

Foreword II

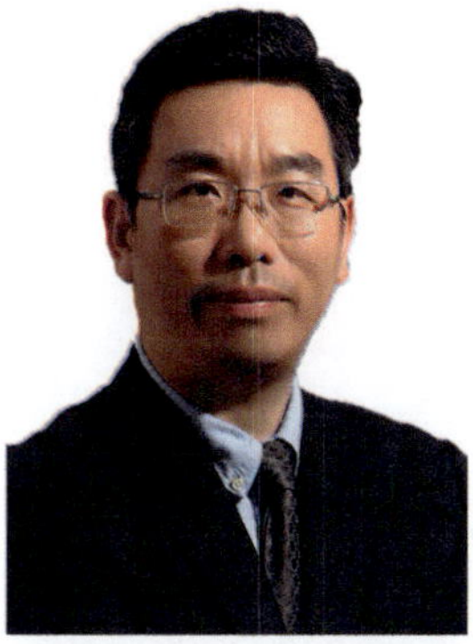

Skin is the first line of defense against various external injuries such as trauma, infection, radiation, and environmental pollution, and it is the organ of the human body most susceptible to external damage. Skin has a complex neurohumoral regulatory system, which is closely related to the functional status of various systems throughout the body. It is also one of the most commonly involved organs in various diseases. In addition, skin is one of the organs of the human body with the most vigorous metabolism and active cell proliferation. The above factors determine the high incidence and complexity of skin diseases, resulting in a great social burden and medical cost.

In the face of the complex disease spectrum and large patient population, how to quickly and accurately diagnose skin diseases has become one of the hotspots in clinical practice. Pathological diagnosis is still the gold standard for most skin diseases. However, biopsy is invasive and is restricted by factors such as high cost, long procedure, high technical requirements, and limited sampling site.

The emerging of noninvasive skin diagnosis has gradually developed. By means of visible light, ultrasound wave, laser, and electromagnetic wave, noninvasive skin diagnosis can obtain the diagnostic information of skin diseases in vivo and visually. These methods have been rapidly popularized and promoted in recent years.

High-frequency ultrasound is an important imaging technique in the field of skin diagnosis. Thanks to the development of technology, its spatial resolution has been improved from millimeter level to submillimeter level, which can display detailed structures such as epidermis and skin appendages. High-frequency ultrasound will undoubtedly become a useful tool for skin diagnosis.

It should be pointed out that although ultrasound is a mature medical imaging technology, skin is a relatively new application scenario for ultrasound. Therefore, a professional textbook is necessary.

Thank all the editors for their sincere dedication and hard work, this book is expected to help readers quickly master skin ultrasound. It is hoped that noninvasive skin diagnosis technologies, including high-frequency ultrasound, can greatly improve the diagnosis and treatment level of skin diseases.

Yong Cui
China-Japan Friendship Hospital
Beijing, China

Foreword III

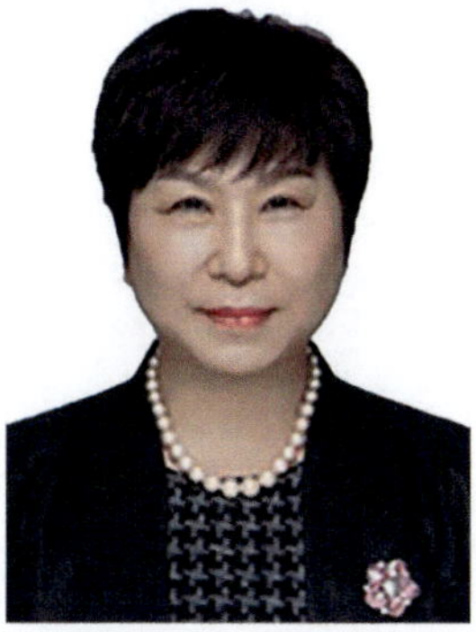

The techniques such as dermoscopy, CLSM, skin ultrasound, and OCT have been gradually applied in clinical practice. In the past, dermatologists can only rely on naked eyes and invasive pathology for diagnosis. Although pathology is the "gold standard" for diagnosis, its invasiveness limits its ability to examine and evaluate skin lesions comprehensively. Nowadays, the development of the above noninvasive technologies makes the diagnosis of skin diseases enter a new stage, and also promotes the birth of a new noninvasive modality of diagnosis and treatment of skin diseases.

In recent years, the frequency of ultrasound transducers has been increasing, which makes it possible to clearly display superficial skin lesions. For ultrasound physicians, it is still necessary to learn comprehensively to meet the needs of clinical diagnosis and treatment. For dermatologists, ultrasound is a new technology and they require to learn new knowledge in order to serve patients better. This book is the first professional book on skin ultrasound diagnosis in China. From the view of ultrasound physicians, the book integrates a large number of efforts of dermatologists and skin pathologists, with abundant contents and pictures. This book will open a new horizon for both ultrasound physicians and dermatologists engaged in noninvasive diagnosis.

My team has cooperated closely with Professor Huixiong Xu and Dr. Lehang Guo. In the photodynamic noninvasive therapy of skin tumors and port wine stains, skin ultrasound diagnosis and our existing dermoscopy and fluorescence diagnosis are complementary to each other, making an important contribution to the noninvasive diagnosis and treatment.

Finally, thank the editors for their hard work and dedication! I believed that in the future, skin ultrasound will provide broader ideas and more diverse methods for disease diagnosis and treatment, and ultimately benefit all mankind.

Xiuli Wang
Shanghai Skin Disease Hospital
Shanghai, China

Outline

With the increase of ultrasound transducer frequency, the use of ultrasound gradually expands to the more superficial organs or tissues, which greatly promotes the application of ultrasound in skin diseases. In recent years, our team has carried out a lot of clinical research in the field of skin ultrasound. The results are innovative and valuable and this book presents the clinical research and practice results in the latest several years.

This book introduces the basic knowledge of skin ultrasound, including the imaging principle, methodology, observation items, image interpretation, and so on. The ultrasound manifestation of normal skin and various skin diseases are described and the diagnostic criteria are proposed. In addition, the brand new mode of diagnosis and treatment for skin diseases is introduced.

The content of this book is concise, illustrated, informative, and easy to understand. It is a rare and excellent tool book for ultrasound doctors and dermatologists who are interested in carrying out skin ultrasound diagnosis.

The Shanghai Engineering Technology Research Center is an important part of Shanghai's science and technology innovation system. It is established to carry out engineering research and development, breakthrough industry commonality and key technologies, accelerate the transfer, promotion, and distribution of scientific and technological achievements, and lead the industry's technological progress. It is an important base for enhancing the city's technological innovation capability of strategic emerging industries. It also plays a fundamental role in promoting the innovation-driven development of this city.

The Shanghai Engineering Technology Research Center of Ultrasound Diagnosis and Treatment is an important part of Shanghai's acceleration of the construction of a scientific and technological innovation center with global influence. The center is aimed to promote the basic R&D and clinical development of ultrasound engineering technology. At the same time, it is also an important base for technology promotion, cultivating leading talents, and academic cooperation and exchanges. The center is established with the approval of Science and Technology Commission of Shanghai Municipality in 2019.

This book is organized by the Shanghai Engineering Technology Research Center of Ultrasound Diagnosis and Treatment.

Preface

Skin disease has gradually become a major public health problem due to a large number of patients and impact on their physical and mental health. There are more than 6000 kinds of skin diseases, and the prevalence rate of the population is nearly 100%. In the United States, the annual medical expenses caused by skin diseases are as high as $75 billion. Facing the huge medical demand, although the traditional diagnostic method based on naked eye is easy to perform, it is difficult to meet the requirements of accurate diagnosis. Although skin biopsy is the gold standard for the diagnosis of skin diseases, it is invasive, time-consuming, and expensive, which increases the cost and is difficult to apply on a large scale.

Noninvasive skin imaging technologies, such as dermoscopy, confocal laser scanning microscope, and high-frequency ultrasound, have emerged one after another, making up for the shortcomings of naked eye and skin biopsy. Among them, skin ultrasound has not attracted extensive attention. The reason is that the frequency of the traditional ultrasound transducer is relatively low (<15 MHz), which is difficult to display the superficial and tiny structures of the skin. In recent years, the transducer frequency has developed from 20 MHz, 30 MHz to 50 MHz or even 70 MHz, and it gradually has the ability to display the tiny structures of skin. Therefore, it has become a hotspot in the skin imaging technology. Compared with dermoscopy, high-frequency ultrasound can evaluate skin diseases on the vertical scale, providing important information below the skin surface.

Based on our experience in skin high-frequency ultrasound diagnosis for several years, we deeply realize the difficulty to master this technique, especially for the beginners. Skin ultrasound is closely associated with two disciplines: dermatology and ultrasound medicine. The long-term lack of intersection between the two has increased the difficulty of getting started with skin ultrasound. And a professional textbook is lack at present.

Skin Disease Hospital of Tongji University is a well-known tertiary dermatology hospital in China, attracting a large number of patients with various skin diseases. Based on this, we have accumulated thousands of complete ultrasound image data of skin diseases confirmed by pathology. Therefore, we summarized our cases into this book, so as to achieve a close combination of dermatology, pathology, and ultrasound images.

This book was organized by the Shanghai Engineering Technology Research Center of Ultrasound Diagnosis and Treatment. Many doctors have devoted a lot of time to the publication of this book. At the same time, many experts have given help and guidance to our work. We would like to express my heartfelt thanks. We hope this book will support the beginners to carry out skin ultrasound examinations, and further delivering high-quality service to patients. As the ultrasound diagnostic standards for many skin diseases have not been established, some common skin diseases are not included because it is difficult to obtain pathological diagnosis. Because the level of editors is limited, omissions are inevitable, the criticism and correction from readers and experts will help us to improve in future editions.

Shanghai, China Huixiong Xu
Shanghai, China Lehang Guo
Shanghai, China Qiao Wang
August 2021

Department of Medical Ultrasound, Shanghai Skin Disease Hospital
Department of Medical Ultrasound, Shanghai Tenth People's Hospital
Shanghai Engineering Technology Research Center of Ultrasound Diagnosis and Treatment
Ultrasound Research and Education Institute, School of Medicine
Tongji University

Contents

List of Editors and Contributors

Honorary Editor-in-Chief

Weiqi Wang Biomedical Engineering Institute, Fudan University, Shanghai, China

Lianfang Du Department of Medical Ultrasound, Shanghai General Hospital, Shanghai Jiao Tong University School of Medicine, Shanghai, China

Editor-in-Chief

Huixiong Xu Department of Medical Ultrasound, Shanghai Skin Disease Hospital, Ultrasound Research and Education Institute, School of Medicine, Tongji University, Shanghai, China

Department of Medical Ultrasound, Shanghai Tenth People's Hospital, Ultrasound Research and Education Institute, School of Medicine, Tongji University, Shanghai, China

Lehang Guo Department of Medical Ultrasound, Shanghai Skin Disease Hospital, Ultrasound Research and Education Institute, School of Medicine, Tongji University, Shanghai, China

Qiao Wang Department of Medical Ultrasound, Shanghai Skin Disease Hospital, Ultrasound Research and Education Institute, School of Medicine, Tongji University, Shanghai, China

Department of Medical Ultrasound, Shanghai Tenth People's Hospital, Ultrasound Research and Education Institute, School of Medicine, Tongji University, Shanghai, China

Associate Editor

Anqi Zhu Department of Medical Ultrasound, Shanghai Tenth People's Hospital, Ultrasound Research and Education Institute, School of Medicine, Tongji University, Shanghai, China

Weiwei Ren Department of Medical Ultrasound, Shanghai Tenth People's Hospital, Ultrasound Research and Education Institute, School of Medicine, Tongji University, Shanghai, China

Xiaolong Li Department of Medical Ultrasound, Shanghai Tenth People's Hospital, Ultrasound Research and Education Institute, School of Medicine, Tongji University, Shanghai, China

Yeqiang Liu Department of Pathology, Shanghai Skin Disease Hospital, School of Medicine, Tongji University, Shanghai, China

Editor-in-Chief

Huixiong Xu, MD, PhD

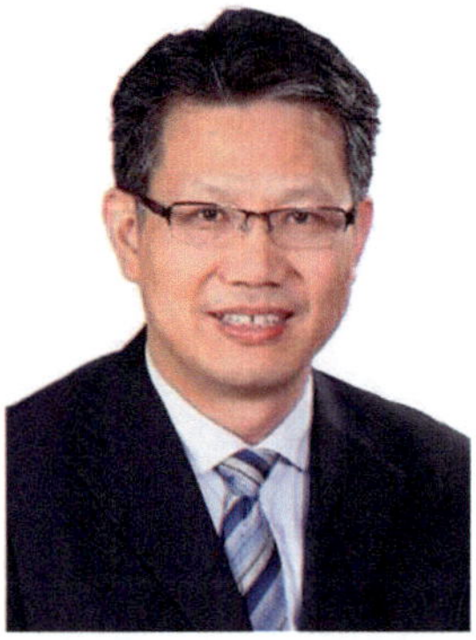

Shanghai Tenth People's Hospital, School of Medicine, Tongji University, Shanghai, China

Shanghai Engineering Technology Research Center of Ultrasound Diagnosis and Treatment, Shanghai, China

Ultrasound Research and Education Institute, School of Medicine, Tongji University, Shanghai, China

Clinical Research Center for Interventional Medicine, Tongji University, Shanghai, China

Department of Medical Ultrasound, Shanghai Skin Disease Hospital, School of Medicine, Tongji University, Shanghai, China

Department of Medical Ultrasound, Shanghai Tenth People's Hospital, School of Medicine, Tongji University, Shanghai, China

Center of Minimal Invasive Treatment for Tumor, Tongji University Cancer Center, Shanghai, China

Lehang Guo, MD, PhD

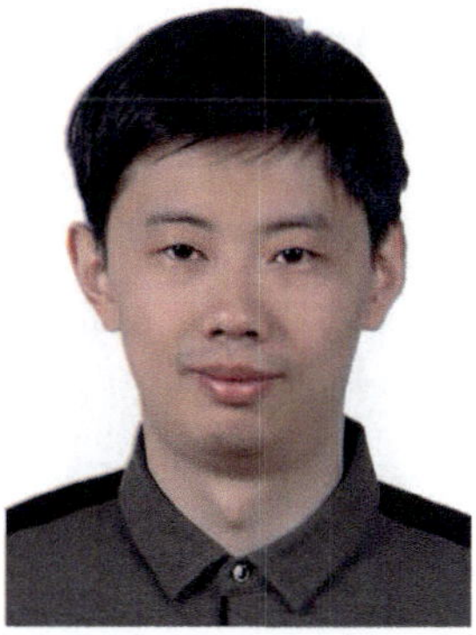

Department of Medical Ultrasound, Shanghai Skin Disease Hospital, Ultrasound Research and Education Institute, School of Medicine, Tongji University, Shanghai, China

Department of Medical Ultrasound, Shanghai Tenth People's Hospital, Ultrasound Research and Education Institute, School of Medicine, Tongji University, Shanghai, China

Qiao Wang, MD

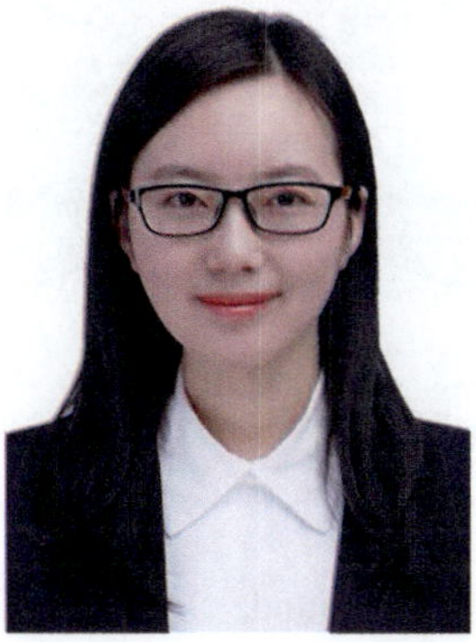

Department of Medical Ultrasound, Shanghai Skin Disease Hospital, Ultrasound Research and Education Institute, School of Medicine, Tongji University, Shanghai, China

Department of Medical Ultrasound, Shanghai Tenth People's Hospital, Ultrasound Research and Education Institute, School of Medicine, Tongji University, Shanghai, China

Associated Editor

Anqi Zhu, MD

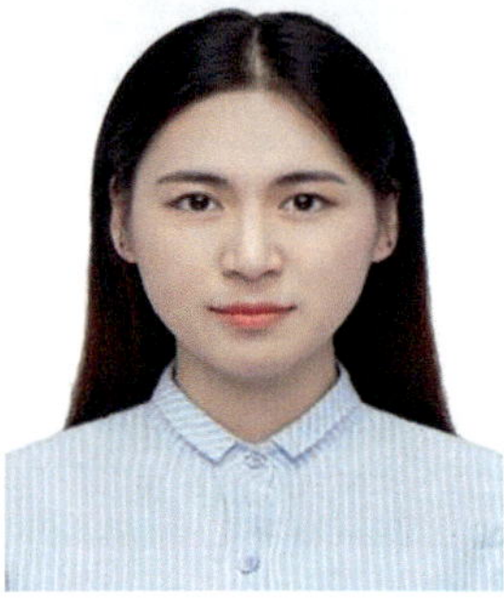

Department of Medical Ultrasound, Shanghai Tenth People's Hospital, Ultrasound Research and Education Institute, School of Medicine, Tongji University, Shanghai, China

Weiwei Ren, MD

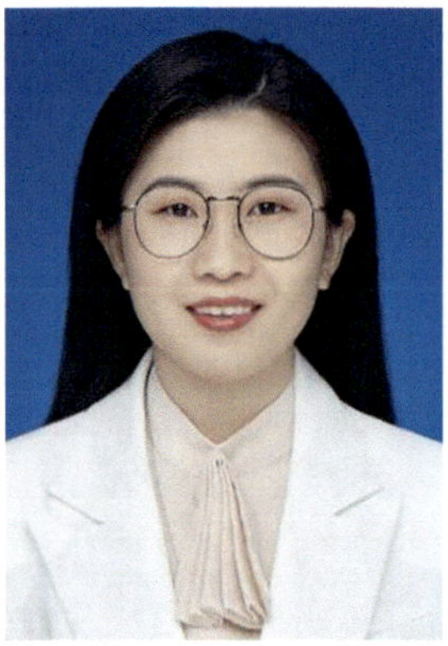

Department of Medical Ultrasound, Shanghai Tenth People's Hospital, Ultrasound Research and Education Institute, School of Medicine, Tongji University, Shanghai, China

Xiaolong Li, MD, PhD

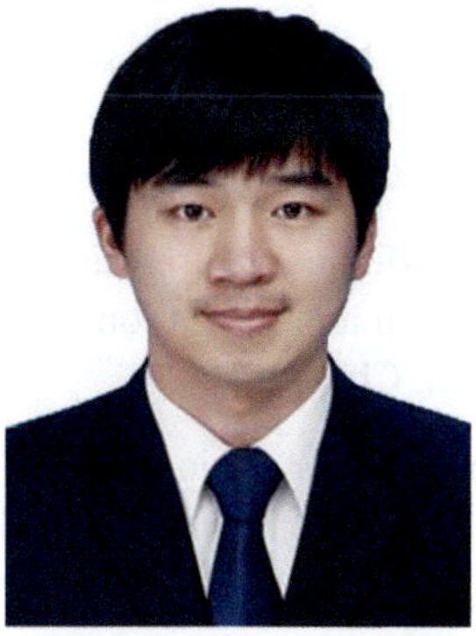

Department of Medical Ultrasound, Shanghai Tenth People's Hospital, Ultrasound Research and Education Institute, School of Medicine, Tongji University, Shanghai, China

Yeqiang Liu, MD, PhD

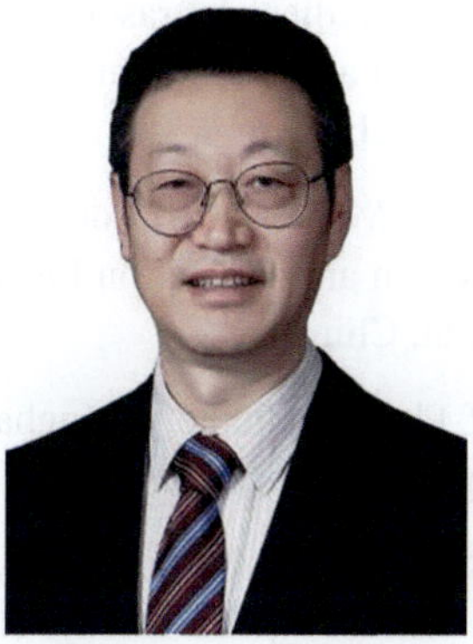

Department of Pathology, Shanghai Skin Disease Hospital, School of Medicine, Tongji University, Shanghai, China

Contributors

Hongyan Chen Department of Ultrasound, Shanghai Minhang District Central Hospital, Fudan University, Shanghai, China

Jia Chen Department of Pathology, Shanghai Skin Disease Hospital, School of Medicine, Tongji University, Shanghai, China

Yunchao Chen Department of Medical Ultrasound, Xiang'an Hospital, Xiamen University, Xiamen, China

Zitong Chen Department of Medical Ultrasound, Shanghai Tenth People's Hospital, Ultrasound Research and Education Institute, School of Medicine, Tongji University, Shanghai, China

Qian Cheng School of Physics Science and Engineering, Tongji University, Shanghai, China

Fengshan Jin Department of Medical Ultrasound, Shanghai Tenth People's Hospital, Ultrasound Research and Education Institute, School of Medicine, Tongji University, Shanghai, China

Jiaxin Li Department of Medical Ultrasound, Shanghai Tenth People's Hospital, Ultrasound Research and Education Institute, School of Medicine, Tongji University, Shanghai, China

Liang Li Department of Dermatologic Surgery, Shanghai Skin Disease Hospital, School of Medicine, Tongji University, Shanghai, China

Dandan Shan Department of Medical Ultrasound, Shanghai Tenth People's Hospital, Ultrasound Research and Education Institute, School of Medicine, Tongji University, Shanghai, China

Hui Shi Department of Medical Ultrasound, Shanghai Tenth People's Hospital, Ultrasound Research and Education Institute, School of Medicine, Tongji University, Shanghai, China

Liping Sun Department of Medical Ultrasound, Shanghai Tenth People's Hospital, Ultrasound Research and Education Institute, School of Medicine, Tongji University, Shanghai, China

Lifan Wang Department of Medical Ultrasound, Shanghai Tenth People's Hospital, Ultrasound Research and Education Institute, School of Medicine, Tongji University, Shanghai, China

Peiru Wang Institute of Photomedicine, Shanghai Skin Disease Hospital, School of Medicine, Tongji University, Shanghai, China

Jianna Yan Department of Dermatologic Surgery, Shanghai Skin Disease Hospital, School of Medicine, Tongji University, Shanghai, China

Kun Zhang Department of Medical Ultrasound, Shanghai Tenth People's Hospital, Ultrasound Research and Education Institute, School of Medicine, Tongji University, Shanghai, China

Yifeng Zhang Department of Medical Ultrasound, Shanghai Tenth People's Hospital, Ultrasound Research and Education Institute, School of Medicine, Tongji University, Shanghai, China

Chongke Zhao Department of Medical Ultrasound, Shanghai Tenth People's Hospital, Ultrasound Research and Education Institute, School of Medicine, Tongji University, Shanghai, China

Overview of Skin Ultrasound

1

Hui-Xiong Xu, Le-Hang Guo, Xiao-Long Li, Qiao Wang, Feng-Shan Jin, Zi-Tong Chen, and Kun Zhang

1.1 Development and Overview of Skin Ultrasound

As one of the conventional imaging techniques, ultrasound has been widely applied in the fields of abdomen, obstetrics and gynecology, urinary tract, cardiovascular system, thyroid, breast, and other organs, and its effectiveness and safety have been well recognized. As early as 1979, Alexander et al. first applied ultrasound to the measurement of human skin thickness, pioneering the application of ultrasound in the field of dermatology. However, due to the limitation of the resolution of conventional high-frequency ultrasound (Frequency < 15 MHz), it was difficult to display the details of human skin. It was only used for the measurement of skin thickness or the observation of deeper lesions, limiting its application in the diagnosis of skin diseases.

In recent years, with the increase of the frequency of transducer (Frequency ≥ 20 MHz), the application of ultrasound has gradually expanded to the superficial layers, from skeletal muscle and fascia, to subcutaneous tissue, gradually to dermis and epidermis. Higher frequency ultrasound provides more details of skin, making it possible to diagnose skin diseases accurately. Based on this, several application scenarios have been derived, such as the differentiation of benign and malignant skin tumors, the localization and detection of subcutaneous implants, trauma evaluation, foreign body detection, the evaluation of skin changes in systemic diseases, preoperative evaluation, intraoperative guidance, and follow-up. Therefore, the clinical application of skin ultrasound has attracted more and more attention from dermatologists.

Key Points

- Conventional high-frequency ultrasound has limited value in skin diseases diagnosis.
- Ultrasound diagnosis of skin diseases requires a higher frequency transducer (≥ 20 MHz).

H.-X. Xu (✉) · L.-H. Guo
Department of Medical Ultrasound, Shanghai Skin Disease Hospital, Ultrasound Research and Education Institute, School of Medicine, Tongji University, Shanghai, China

X.-L. Li · F.-S. Jin · Z.-T. Chen · K. Zhang
Department of Medical Ultrasound, Shanghai Tenth People's Hospital, Ultrasound Research and Education Institute, School of Medicine, Tongji University, Shanghai, China

Q. Wang
Department of Medical Ultrasound, Shanghai Skin Disease Hospital, Ultrasound Research and Education Institute, School of Medicine, Tongji University, Shanghai, China

Department of Medical Ultrasound, Shanghai Tenth People's Hospital, Ultrasound Research and Education Institute, School of Medicine, Tongji University, Shanghai, China

H. Xu et al. (eds.), *Diagnostic Ultrasound in Dermatology*,
https://doi.org/10.1007/978-981-16-7345-0_1

1.2 Ultrasound Wave and Ultrasound Imaging

1.2.1 Ultrasound Wave

1.2.1.1 Basic Concepts

Ultrasound wave is a kind of mechanical wave with vibrational frequency higher than 20,000 Hz, exceeding the frequency of acoustic wave (20 ~ 20,000 Hz) that can be perceived by the human ear.

1.2.1.2 Physical Properties

Ultrasound wave is a longitudinal wave, that is, the direction of particle vibration is consistent with the direction of acoustic wave propagation, when propagating in the mediums (Fig. 1.1). The maximum distance away from the equilibrium position when a particle vibrates is called amplitude which represents the intensity or energy of the acoustic wave. The distance between two adjacent particles with the phase difference of 2π in the same direction during acoustic wave propagation is the wavelength (λ), that is, the length of a complete wave. The time required to form a wavelength is called the Time (T). The times of periodic change are completed in a unit time, that is, the number of complete waves called frequency (f), and the unit is Hertz (Hz).

The speed of acoustic waves propagating in the mediums is the velocity of sound (c). When ultrasound waves propagate in the mediums, the speed in solid > liquid > air, the speed of its propagation in human soft tissue is generally 1540 m/s (Fig. 1.2). In a specific medium, the velocity of

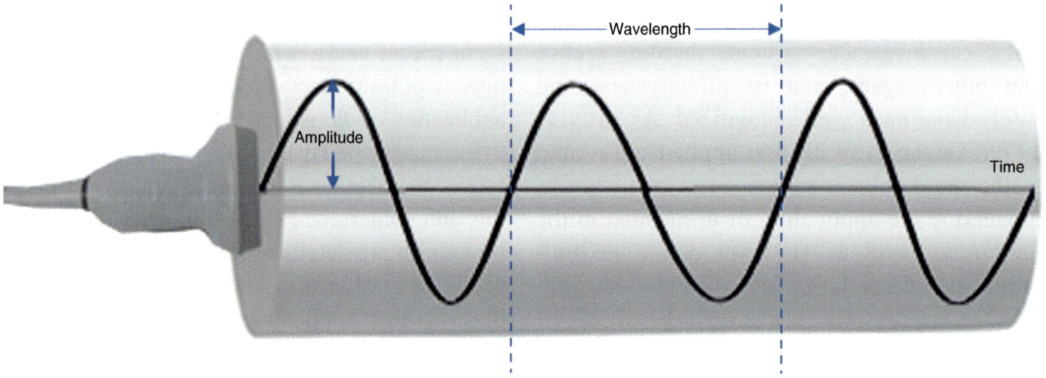

Fig. 1.1 Schematic diagram of ultrasound wave propagation

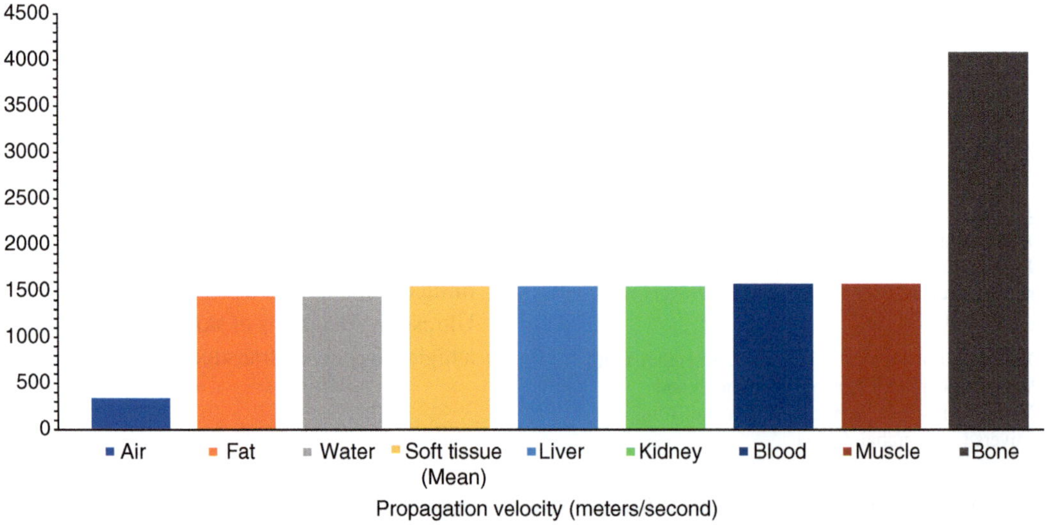

Fig. 1.2 Acoustic velocity in different media

sound (c), wavelength (λ), and frequency (f) meet the following formula (1.1):

$$c = f \cdot \lambda \quad (1.1)$$

1.2.2 Propagation Properties

1.2.2.1 Acoustic Impedance (*Z*)

Acoustic impedance, also known as acoustic impedance rate, is referred to as the plural ratio of the acoustic pressure of a medium on an area to the volume velocity passing through that area. Its unit is Rayl.

Acoustic impedance is the acoustic property of a medium to characterize the energy loss of acoustic wave propagation, which is closely related to the medium density (ρ) and the medium velocity of sound (c). Their relationship meets the formula ((1.2) as follows:

$$Z = \rho \cdot c \quad (1.2)$$

The acoustic impedance value of human soft tissue is similar, about 1.524×10^5 Rayl, but the acoustic impedance value varies significantly between soft tissue and bone or air. When ultrasound waves propagate in different media, the contact surface between different media constitutes the acoustic interface.

When the acoustic impedance difference is greater than 0.1%, the incident acoustic wave can be reflected. If the linearity of acoustic interface is less than the wavelength of acoustic wave, it is called a small interface; if it is greater than the wavelength, it is called a large interface.

1.2.2.2 Reflection, Refraction, and Scattering

When the ultrasound wave encounters a large interface in its propagation, part energy of the ultrasound wave is reflected from the interface toward another direction of the same medium, which is called reflection. Another part energy of the ultrasound wave enters another medium and continues propagation, but the direction is changed, which is called refraction (Fig. 1.3).

When the incident angle increases to a certain angle, and the refractive angle is equal to 90°, the refractive wave completely disappears, only the reflected wave left. This phenomenon is called total reflection. The reflected acoustic wave is called echo. The phenomenon of radiation in all

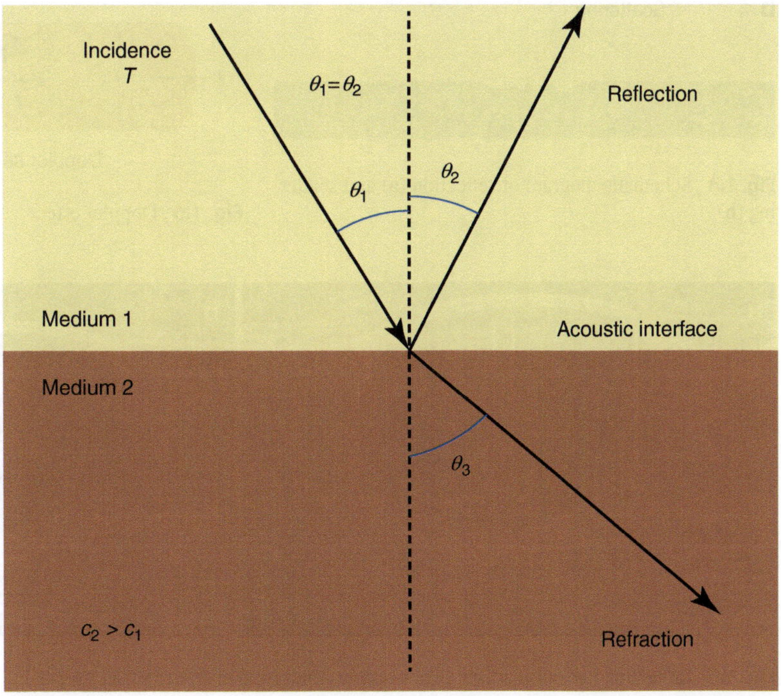

Fig. 1.3 Incidence, reflection, and refraction of ultrasound wave

directions around the small interface encountered during ultrasound propagation is called scattering (Figs. 1.4 and 1.5).

1.2.2.3 Doppler Effect

Doppler effect refers to the phenomenon that the change in frequency due to the relative motion between the sound source and the transducer (Fig. 1.6).

The frequency difference between the ultrasound frequency emitted by transducer and the ultrasound frequency reflected or scattered by moving target is called Doppler frequency shift.

The Doppler frequency shift formula (1.3) is as follows:

$$f_d = \pm \frac{2v\cos\theta}{c} f_0 \quad (1.3)$$

In the formula, f_d is the Doppler frequency shift; v is the velocity of moving target, i.e., the velocity of blood flow; θ is the included angle between the ultrasound beam and the movement direction of transducer, i.e., the included angle between the ultrasound beam and the blood flow direction. The cosθ in the formula is used to obtain the true velocity of blood flow through component velocity. In the clinic, θ must be less than 60°; c is the propagation velocity of ultrasound waves in the medium; f_0 is the frequency of ultrasound waves emitted by the transducer; the positive sign indicates that the moving target moves toward the transducer, while the negative sign indicates that the moving target moves backward the transducer.

1.2.2.4 Attenuation

The phenomenon that the acoustic wave energy reduction due to medium absorption, scattering, and heat conductivity with the increase of distance, is called acoustic attenuation. It is

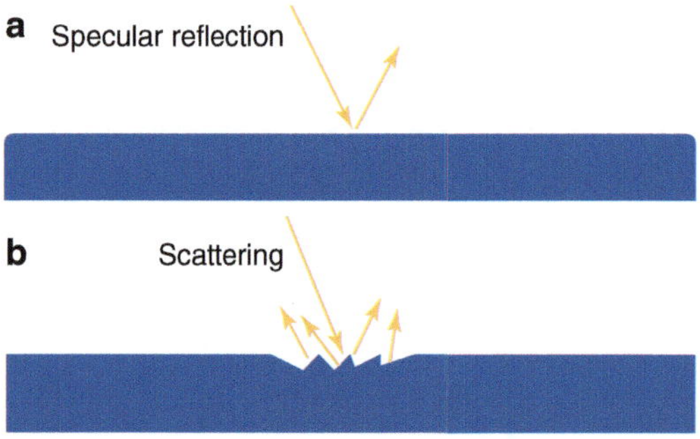

Fig. 1.4 Schematic diagram of reflection (**a**) and scattering (**b**)

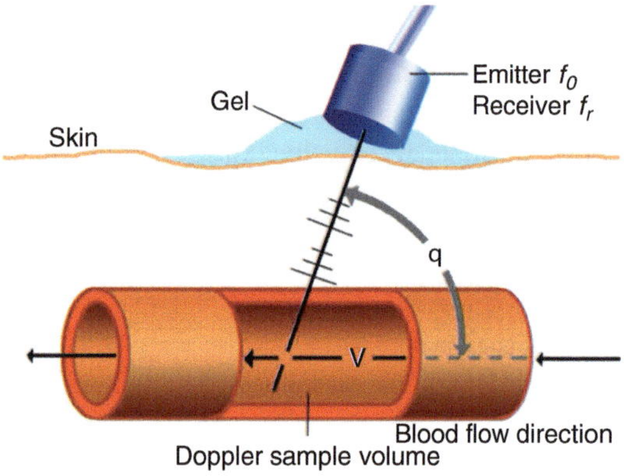

Fig. 1.6 Doppler effect

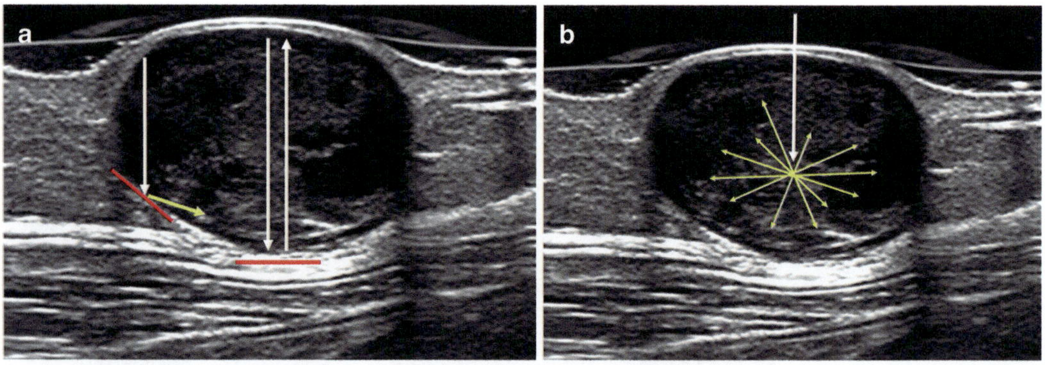

Fig. 1.5 Reflection (**a**) and scattering (**b**) of ultrasound wave in epidermoid cyst

mainly caused by reflection, scattering, and absorption, and shows acoustic shadowing on ultrasound images. The acoustic attenuation coefficient of human tissue is shown in Fig. 1.7, which is related to the ultrasound frequency and propagation distance. The formula (1.4) is as follows:

$$\text{Attenuation}\left(dB\right) = \alpha \cdot d \cdot f \qquad (1.4)$$

In the equation, α is the attenuation coefficient in dB / (cm · MHz), which refers to the sound intensity reduced along with the acoustic wave propagating the medium at unit distance; d is the propagation distance; f is the frequency.

According to formula (1.4), in skin ultrasound, attenuation increases and the penetration decreases significantly with the increase of frequency. Abnormal keratinization, scar, and crust on the surface of skin lesions are the common pathological changes that cause acoustic attenuation (Fig. 1.8).

1.2.3 Generation and Reception of Ultrasound Waves

1.2.3.1 Ultrasound Transducer

The ultrasound transducer (Fig. 1.9) is an essential device to transmit and receive ultrasound

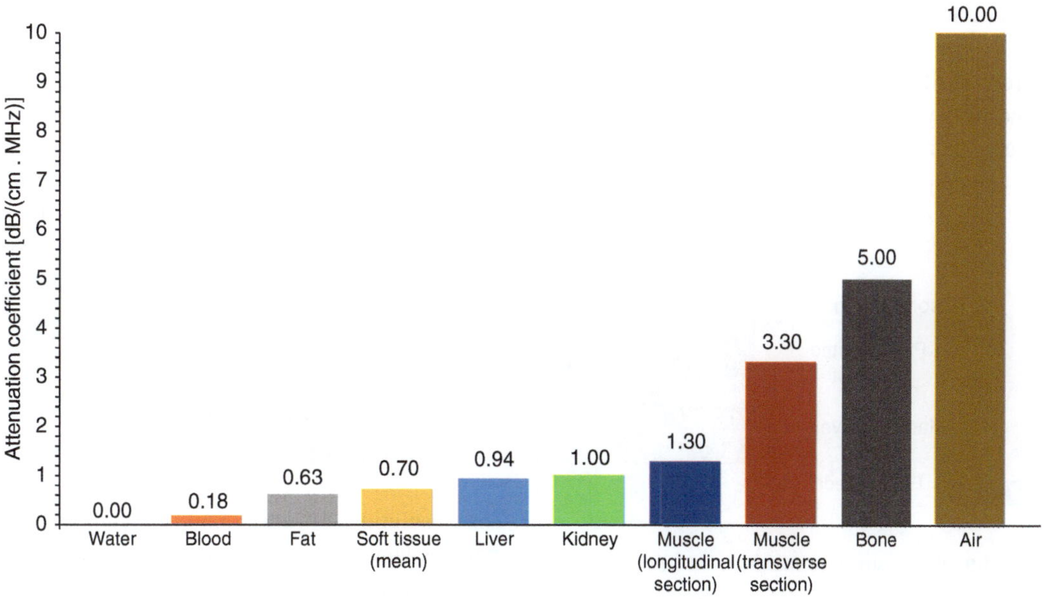

Fig. 1.7 Acoustic attenuation coefficient of human tissue

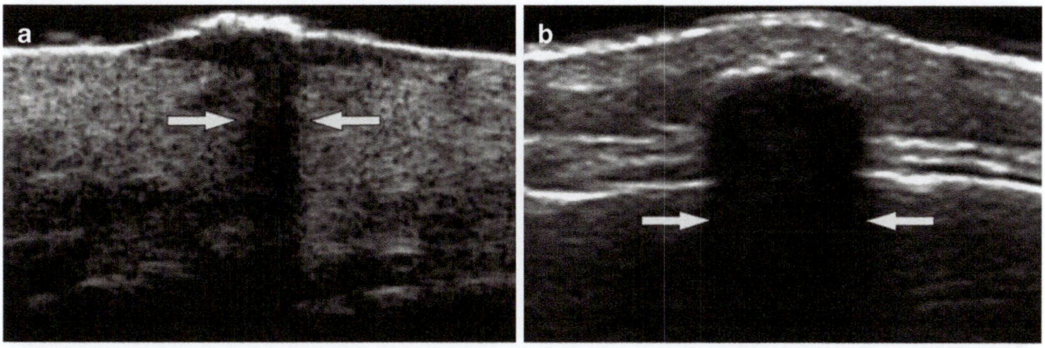

Fig. 1.8 Attenuation. (**a**) Posterior acoustic attenuation is caused by abnormal keratinization of the lesion surface (arrows). (**b**) Posterior acoustic attenuation is caused by calcification within the dermis (arrows)

waves. The key component in the transducer is the piezoelectric materials. The materials can generate a charge on the surface when compressed and generate deformation under alternating voltages, enabling the interconversion of mechanical and electrical energy, which is called the piezoelectric effect. The process of converting electrical energy into mechanical energy is called converse piezoelectric effect, which is the process of emitting ultrasound waves. The process of converting mechanical energy into electrical energy is called the direct piezoelectric effect, which is the process of receiving ultrasound waves.

The ultrasound transducer emits the ultrasound wave, the echo signals from the superficial tissue to the deepest tissue arrive at the transducer in turn and are converted into the electrical signals carrying the acoustic characteristics of different media interfaces. After the signals are received by the ultrasound device, it is demodulated, filtered, computed, analog-to-digital converted, amplified, and then imaged (Fig. 1.10).

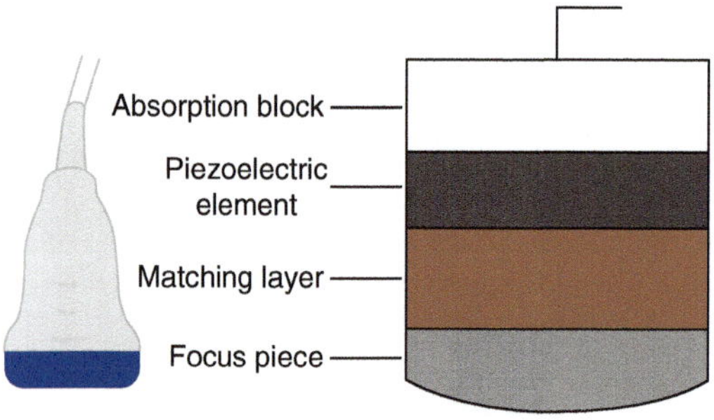

Fig. 1.9 Basic structure diagram of the ultrasound transducer

1.2.3.2 Acoustic Field

Acoustic field refers to the area where acoustic waves exist in the medium during propagation. The central axis of the transducer emitting ultrasound waves is called the acoustic axis, which is the main direction of acoustic beam propagation. The transducer emits non-focused beams continuously, and the beam diameter decreases slowly to a certain point and then widens rapidly with the increase of propagation distance. There is a near field between this point and the transducer, while a far-field area is far away from this point (Fig. 1.11).

1.2.3.3 Focusing of Acoustic Beam

The non-focused acoustic beam is difficult to use in ultrasound diagnosis because its energy distribution is confused due to the side lobe effect in the near field and diffusion in the far field. Therefore, the scanning acoustic beam is tapered by using the acoustic lens focusing, variable aperture focusing and electronic dynamic focusing, and the effect of side lobe is eliminated as much as possible. This process is called focusing of the acoustic beam (Fig. 1.11).

1.2.4 Resolution of Ultrasound Imaging

The resolution of ultrasound imaging mainly includes spatial resolution, temporal resolution, and contrast resolution.

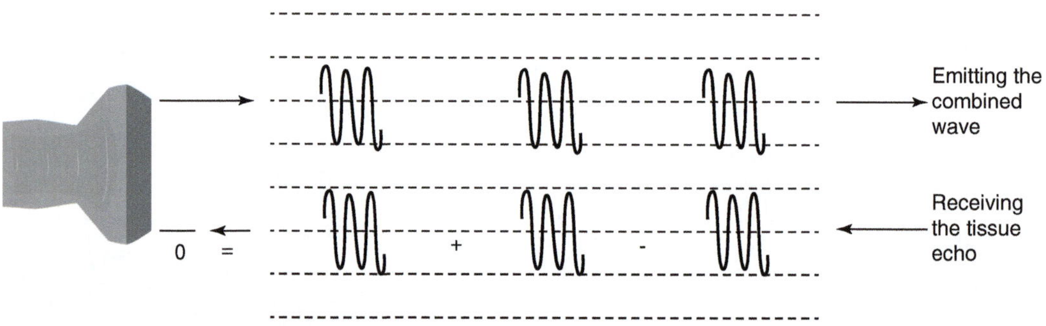

Fig. 1.10 Emission and reception of ultrasound wave

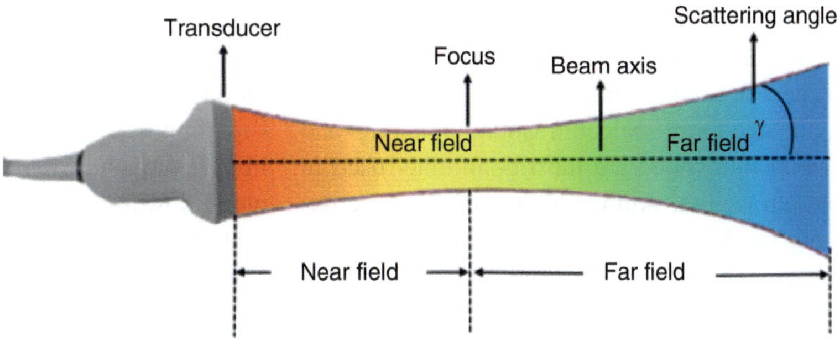

Fig. 1.11 Acoustic field and focusing of acoustic beam

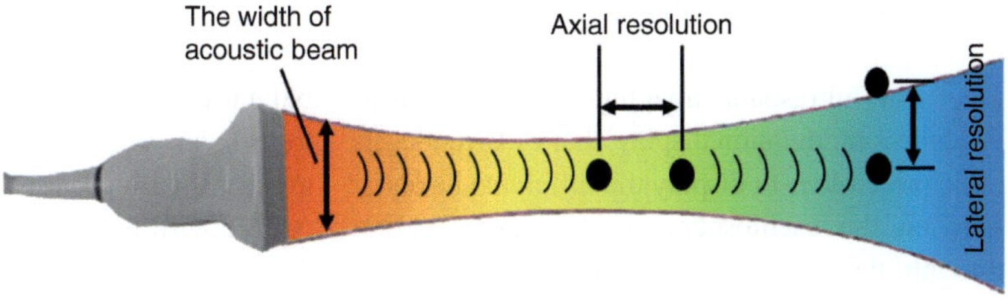

Fig. 1.12 Axial resolution and lateral resolution

1.2.4.1 Spatial Resolution

Spatial resolution refers to the ability to distinguish the minimum distance between two adjacent reflectors on screen, including axial resolution and lateral resolution (Fig. 1.12). Axial resolution refers to the ability of the ultrasound device to distinguish the minimum distance of two adjacent reflectors along the direction of acoustic beam. Lateral resolution refers to the ability to distinguish the minimum distance of two reflectors perpendicular to the direction of acoustic beam and parallel to the transducer.

In the skin ultrasound examination, since the lesions are mostly located in the epidermis and dermis, the resolution is particularly important to clearly show the internal structure of the lesion. The transducer frequency is an important parameter in ultrasound and determines the image quality. The higher the ultrasound frequency, the worse penetration but the higher resolution. The lower the frequency, the stronger penetration but the lower resolution.

The ultrasound frequency used for the diagnosis of abdominal and superficial organs is generally 1 ~ 12 MHz. The high-frequency ultrasound frequency used for skin ultrasound can reach 20 ~ 50 MHz, or even more than 70 MHz.

1.2.4.2 Temporal Resolution

Temporal resolution refers to the minimum time of image frame change and is very important for detecting the motion function of the reflector and the subtle changes in hemodynamics.

1.2.4.3 Contrast Resolution

Contrast resolution refers to the ability to display and distinguish different shades of gray (i.e., gray scale), and is an important parameter for evaluating image quality.

1.2.5 Basic Principle of Ultrasound Imaging

Ultrasound wave is widely used in medical imaging because of its good directionality and penetrability, and it is safe. The basic principle of ultrasound imaging is that there are differences in acoustic impedance between organs and tissues in the human body. Therefore, when the ultrasound wave is emitted to the human body, different tissues will generate different reflected signals. The reflected signals are received and displayed on the screen with different shades of gray by a series of bioengineering processes such as beam forming, so as to generate ultrasound images for medical observation and diagnosis.

There are many imaging modalities for ultrasound, and gray-scale ultrasound imaging and Doppler ultrasound are most commonly used in skin ultrasound. Among them, the most commonly used Doppler ultrasound imaging in the skin are color Doppler flow imaging, pulsed Doppler imaging, and power Doppler imaging.

1.2.6 Gray-Scale Ultrasound

Gray-scale ultrasound imaging is also known as brightness modulation display, that is, B-mode. Its basic principle is to display the different shades of gray on the oscilloscope of the tissue section through the echo generated by each interface encountered by a rapidly swept single sound beam or simultaneously swept multiple sound beams in its propagation. Then the two-dimensional image of the echogenicity is generated.

The change in brightness from none to saturation is divided into different levels, that is gray scale (Fig. 1.13).

1.2.7 Color Doppler Flow Imaging

For the detection of blood flow signals in skin diseases, color Doppler flow imaging is commonly used. It is based on the principle of Doppler effect. The process is realized by multiple sound beams rapid sampling, and the obtained blood flow information is subject to phase detection, autocorrelation processing, color coding. It identifies the blood flow direction by different colors, and then superimposes the color image on the B-mode images. In clinical practice, red represents the blood flow toward the transducer, and blue represents the blood flow backward the transducer. Color saturation indicates the variable velocity of blood flow (Fig. 1.14). Color Doppler flow imaging can only qualitatively detect the blood flow velocity without quantitative evaluation.

The laminar blood flow is pure red or blue, and green indicates turbulent blood flow. In turbulent blood flow, the blood flow toward the transducer is red with yellow (mixture of red and green); the blood flow away from the transducer is blue with purple (mixture of blue and green). Attention should be paid to the differentiation

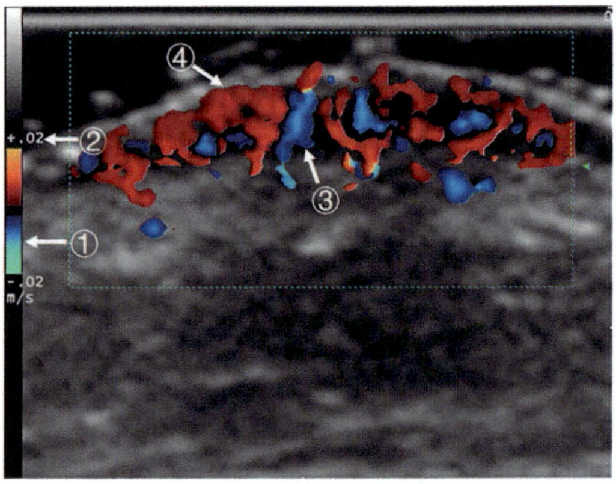

Fig. 1.14 Color Doppler flow imaging. ① Color scale, ② Nyquist speed, ③ Blood flow backward transducer, and ④ Blood flow toward the transducer

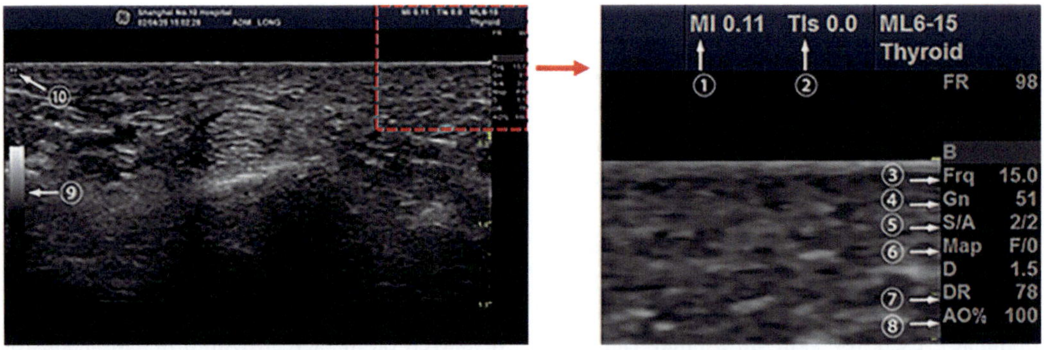

Fig. 1.13 Gray-scale ultrasound imaging. ① Mechanical index, ② Thermal index, ③ Frequency, ④ Gain, ⑤ Speckle reduction imaging/frame average, ⑥ Gray map, ⑦ Dynamic range, ⑧ Acoustic power output, ⑨ Gray scale, and ⑩ Machine Vendor Logo

from the aliasing phenomenon when analyzing the images of color Doppler flow imaging.

1.2.8 Pulse Doppler Imaging

Pulse Doppler imaging is used for quantitative detection of blood flow. It analyzes the Doppler frequency shift of the blood flow signal by means of pulse sampling, and the Doppler frequency shift signal is processed by an ultrasound device and displayed on the screen in the form of a spectrum waveform. The principle of pulse Doppler imaging for detecting blood flow is that the ultrasound transducer emits pulsed ultrasound waves into the tissue based on the Doppler frequency shift (assuming a frequency of f_0). Scatter is generated when the ultrasound wave encounters flowing red blood cells (RBC) (assuming a Doppler angle of θ) and the backscattered signal from the RBC (assuming a frequency of f_r) is received by the ultrasound transducer. Since the RBC has been moving all the time, the Doppler frequency shift is generated between the f_r and the f_0 (assume a frequency shift of f_d). According to the Doppler formula, when detecting the blood flow velocity (assume it of v), the formula (1.5) is as follows:

$$f_d = f_r = f_0 = \pm \frac{2v\cos\theta}{c} f_0$$
$$\downarrow \qquad (1.5)$$
$$v = \frac{c(\pm f_d)}{2f_0\cos\theta}$$

In the formula, v is the blood flow velocity, c is the sound velocity (1540 m/s), f_0 is the transducer frequency, f_d is the Doppler frequency shift, and θ is the angle between acoustic beam and blood flow.

The factors that determine the value of flow velocity include the transducer frequency, frequency shift, and the Doppler angle. The smaller f_0 is, the greater the blood flow velocity is. For high-velocity blood flow, low transducer frequency is recommended. Blood flow velocity is directly proportional to f_d.

The difference between the frequency shift and the real blood flow velocity depends on the Doppler angle. (1) $\theta = 0°$, $\cos\theta = 1$: at this point, the acoustic beam is parallel to the blood flow, and the detection value is closest to the real blood flow velocity. (2) $\theta = 90°$, $\cos\theta = 0$: at this time, the acoustic beam is perpendicular to the blood flow, and the detection value is 0. The Doppler angle shall be adjusted to the minimum and corrected. The detection angle must be less than 60° to control the measurement error within 20%.

In addition, when the flow velocity measured by pulsed Doppler exceeds the Nyquist frequency limit, color aliasing occurs. Pulse repetition frequency (PRF) is the number of pulse waves emitted per second. Nyquist frequency limit = 1/2 PRF. If the Doppler frequency shift exceeds 1/2 PRF, the part beyond the threshold limit is reversed, and aliasing occurs, and it is manifested as color inversion at the peak value of color Doppler blood flow velocity, with red changing to blue or blue changing to red. And the peak value of spectrum waveform is broken, and the broken part moves to the other side of baseline.

In Doppler ultrasound, the frequency shift signal received by the transducer is processed by an ultrasound device and displayed on the screen by means of Doppler spectrum waveform (Fig. 1.15).

1.2.8.1 Baseline

The baseline indicates the level at which the flow velocity is zero and is used to distinguish the direction of blood flow, with the waveform above indicating blood flow toward the transducer and the waveform below indicating blood flow backward the transducer.

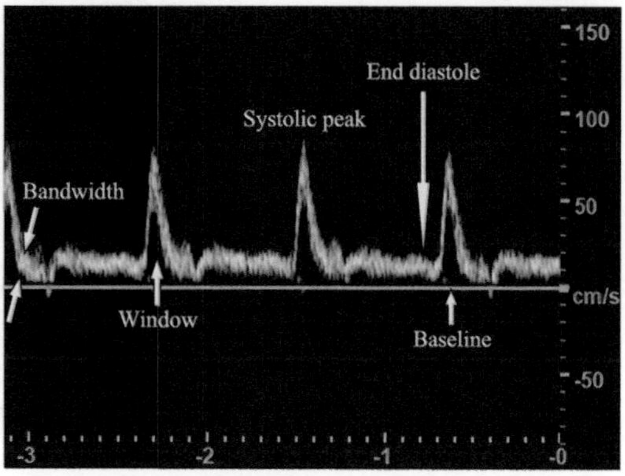

Fig. 1.15 Pulse Doppler spectrum waveform

1.2.8.2 "Window"

"Window" indicates the area without spectrum waveform.

1.2.8.3 Frequency Spectrum Bandwidth

Frequency spectrum bandwidth represents the distribution range of RBC movement velocity. When the range is large, the frequency band is wide. Conversely, it is narrow.

1.2.8.4 Systolic Peak

Systolic peak represents the peak systolic velocity achieved during the cardiac cycle.

1.2.8.5 End Diastole

End diastole refers to the last point of diastole, which is about to enter the next systole.

1.2.9 Power Doppler Ultrasound

Power Doppler ultrasound has the ability to show the distribution of small blood vessels sensitively, and it has been applied in skin ultrasound. Power Doppler ultrasound uses the signal formed by the scattered energy of RBCs to detect slow blood flow and remove the frequency shift signal. The principle of power Doppler ultrasound is to extract the energy intensity of returned Doppler signal to display the existence of blood flow, but does not display its velocity and direction. It can obtain omni-directional blood flow signal without the dependence of incident angle. It has a high signal-to-noise ratio (SNR) and improves the sensitivity of blood flow detection, especially for detecting low-velocity blood flow.

In addition, power Doppler ultrasound can show the blood perfusion area with the average velocity of zero, without Nyquist frequency limit or the color aliasing, but it is easy to appear the twinkling artifact. Images of gray-scale and Doppler ultrasound are shown in Fig. 1.16.

Key Points

- The acoustic impedance difference between different organs or tissues is the theoretical basis of ultrasound imaging.

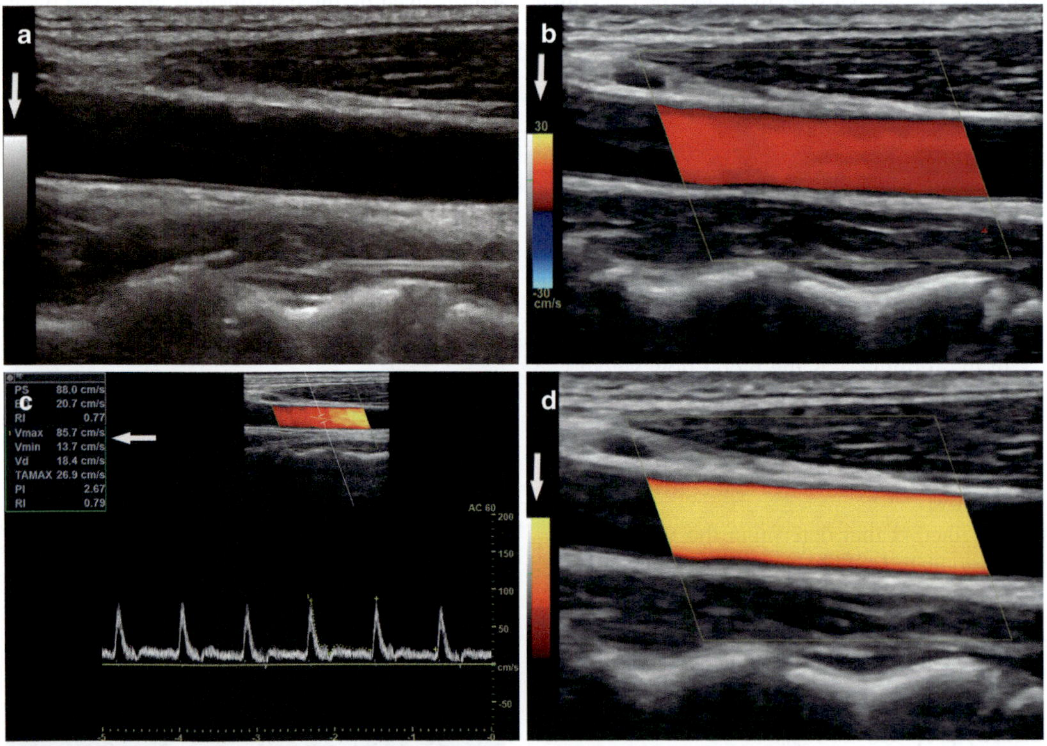

Fig. 1.16 Gray-scale and Doppler ultrasound. (**a**) Gray-scale ultrasound (Frequency: 9 MHz; arrow: gray scale). (**b**) Color Doppler flow imaging (Frequency: 9 MHz; arrow: color scale). (**c**) Quantitative measurement of pulse Doppler blood flow velocity: Vs, V_d, RI, and PI (Frequency: 9 MHz; arrow: the hemodynamic value). (**d**) Power Doppler ultrasound (Frequency: 9 MHz; arrow: color scale)

- Color Doppler flow imaging and power Doppler ultrasound can be used to detect small blood vessels in skin.

1.3 Layout of Examination Room

The facilities for the skin ultrasound examination room are as follows.

1.3.1 Room Requirement

The room area is recommended to be greater than 18 m^2. A window is required to facilitate ventilation, and a door with a big size is required to facilitate the access of sickbeds and wheelchairs.

1.3.2 Equipment

It is equipped with color Doppler ultrasound device, transducers with various frequencies, examination bed, ultrasound report system (including computer, printer, and writing desk), and image collector.

1.3.3 Materials

There shall be garbage cans and sink in the room, and if necessary, a movable trolley for placing gel, alcohol, medical gloves, paper tissues, and hand sanitizing gel will be equipped. In addition, it is particularly important to protect the privacy of patients during the examination, so there must be screens or isolation curtains in the ultrasound room.

1.3.4 Disinfection Equipment

In order to protect various ultrasound equipment and keep the examination room dry and clean, the room needs to be ventilated and avoid light, and it is recommended to install sterilization and disinfection equipment such as ultraviolet lamps.

The layout in the examination room is equally important. Generally, the examination bed is placed on the right side of the ultrasound device, and the computer and writing desk are placed on the left side. When the operator is left-handed, the above orientations are changed from left to right. Figure 1.17 shows the equipment and layout of the ultrasound examination room.

1.4 Preparation for Examination

1.4.1 Preparation

Ultrasound examination of the skin is convenient and easy to perform. Patients do not need special preparations such as fasting or holding back urine. They only need to fully expose the lesion. If the lesion is ulcerated, simple hemostasis and

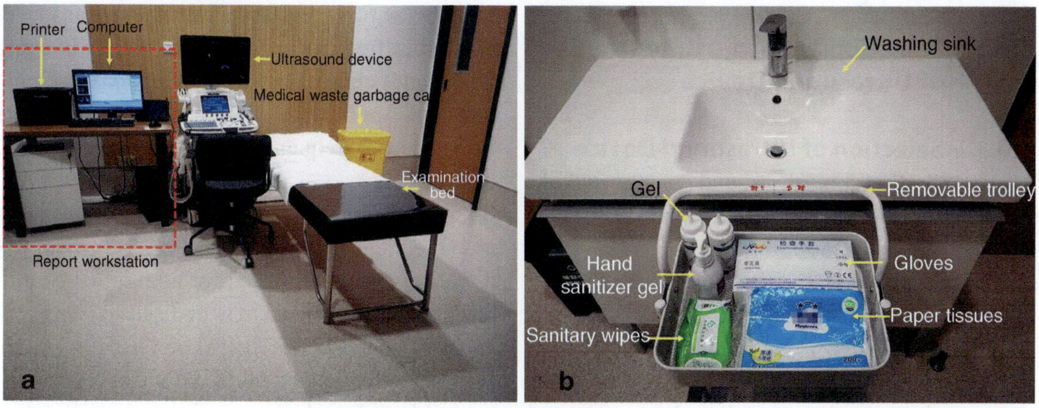

Fig. 1.17 The equipment and layout of the ultrasound examination room. (**a**) Layout of skin ultrasound examination room. (**b**) Washing sink, removable trolley, and other materials placement

debridement should be performed first, and the hand of the examiner, ultrasound transducer and normal skin around the lesion should be protected and isolated. It is not recommended to examine immediately when there is active bleeding.

Physicians should carefully inquire about the patient's medical history before the examination, including the time of the initial presentation, the growth speed of the lesion, number of lesions, symptoms (pain, itching, etc.), history of trauma, history of infectious diseases and history of treatment and other clinical information. After the examination, attention should be paid to cleaning the transducer and discarding the waste according to relative regulations.

1.4.2 Position

Sitting position can be selected when the lesion is located on the scalp, dorsum of the hands, and dorsum of the feet. Supine position can be selected when the lesion is located on the frontal face, anterior chest wall or abdominal wall, upper and lower extremities. Prone position can be selected when the lesion is located on the back and buttocks. Lateral position can be selected when the lesion is located on the lateral waist. Lithotomy or lateral position can be selected when the lesion is located on the perineum. In general, the appropriate position should be flexibly selected based on the location of the lesion (Fig. 1.18).

1.4.3 Selection and Adjustment of Ultrasound Device

1.4.3.1 Selection of Ultrasound Device

The devices for skin ultrasound mainly include conventional ultrasound devices and ultrasound biomicroscopy (UBM).

The conventional ultrasound device is equipped with an ultrasound transducer with a frequency ≤ 20 MHz to carry out skin ultrasound. The function is similar to that of a conventional ultrasound device. It can realize the imaging of multi-modal imaging such as gray-scale, color Doppler, power Doppler, and elastography.

The UBM is equipped with an ultrasound transducer with a frequency ≥ 50 MHz. At present, most UBM only have a single gray-scale imaging function, but can clearly display very superficial structures of skin layers (especially for the epidermis and superficial dermis).

In addition, laptop and hand-held ultrasound devices are increasingly used to meet bedside needs (Fig. 1.19).

1.4.3.2 Selection, Application of Ultrasound Transducer, and Image Interpretation

Selection of Ultrasound Transducer

The ultrasound transducers are divided into low-frequency transducers (1 ~ 8 MHz), conventional high-frequency transducers (HFUS) (9 ~ 20 MHz), ultrahigh-frequency transducers (20 ~ 50 MHz), and UBM (≥ 50 MHz).

Unlike other organs, the ultrasound transducer used for skin disease has a large frequency range. The most common transducers are ultrahigh-frequency ultrasound transducers and UMB transducers.

However, when the skin lesions are too large and deep to be presented completely, it is necessary to select the low-frequency ultrasound transducer for evaluation.

In the skin ultrasound examination, it is recommended to preferentially select the transducer with the frequency of 20 ~ 25 MHz for preliminary evaluation, and then select the transducer with other frequencies according to the imaging status and clinical need. The appearance and scope of application of ultrasound transducers with different frequencies are as follows:

(1) Low-frequency ultrasound transducer (Frequency: 1 ~ 8 MHz, Fig. 1.20): convex arrays, generally used for abdominal examination, rarely used in skin diseases, only recommended when the skin lesion is large, deep or suspected of deep organs, or abdominal lymph node metastasis.

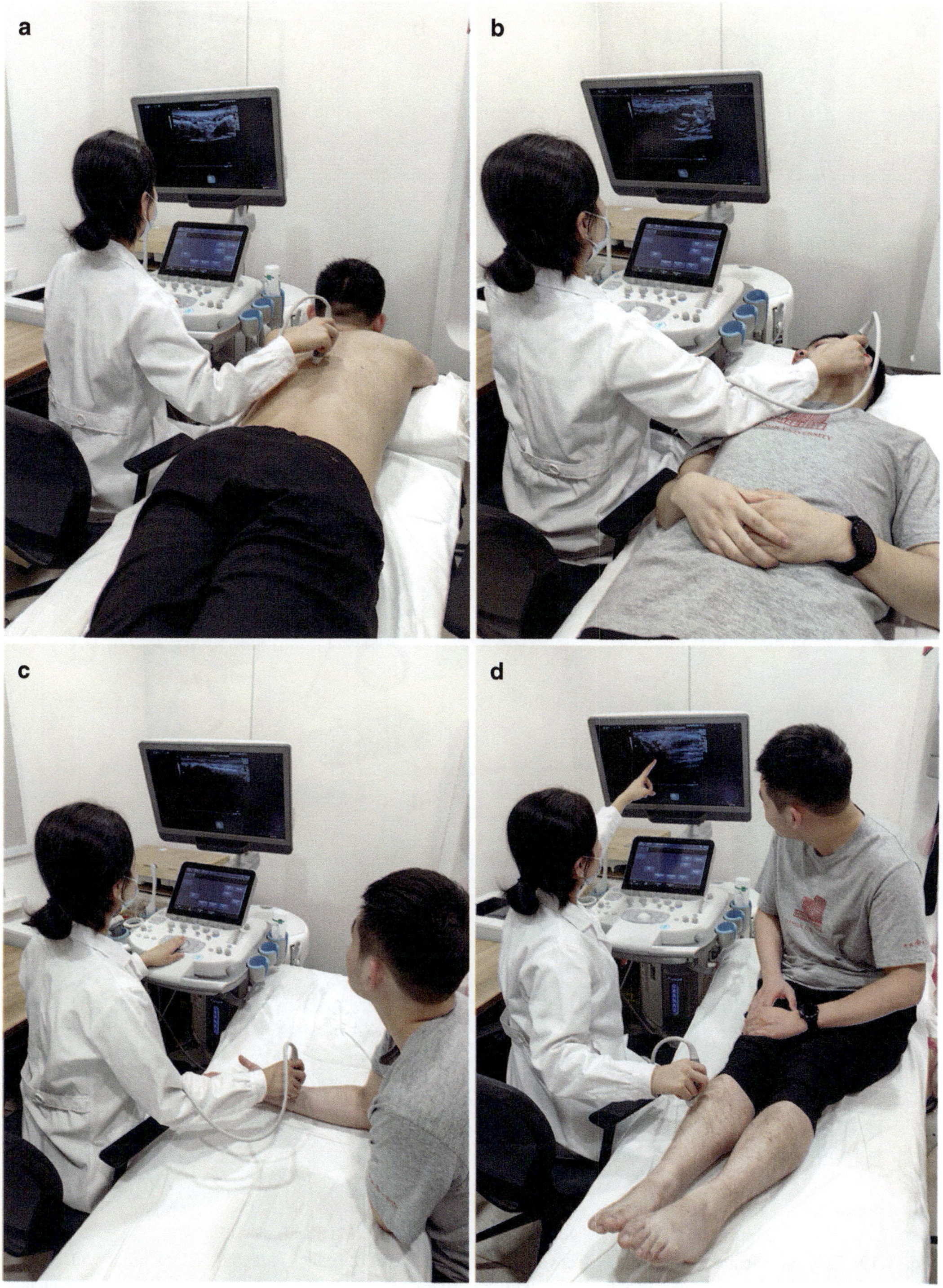

Fig. 1.18 Examination position. (**a**) The patient is examined in prone position (lesion located on the back). (**b**) The patient is examined in supine position (lesion located on the face). (**c**) The patient is examined in a sitting position, and he sits on one side of the examination bed (lesion located on the palm of the hand). (**d**) The patient is examined in sitting position (lesion located on the leg)

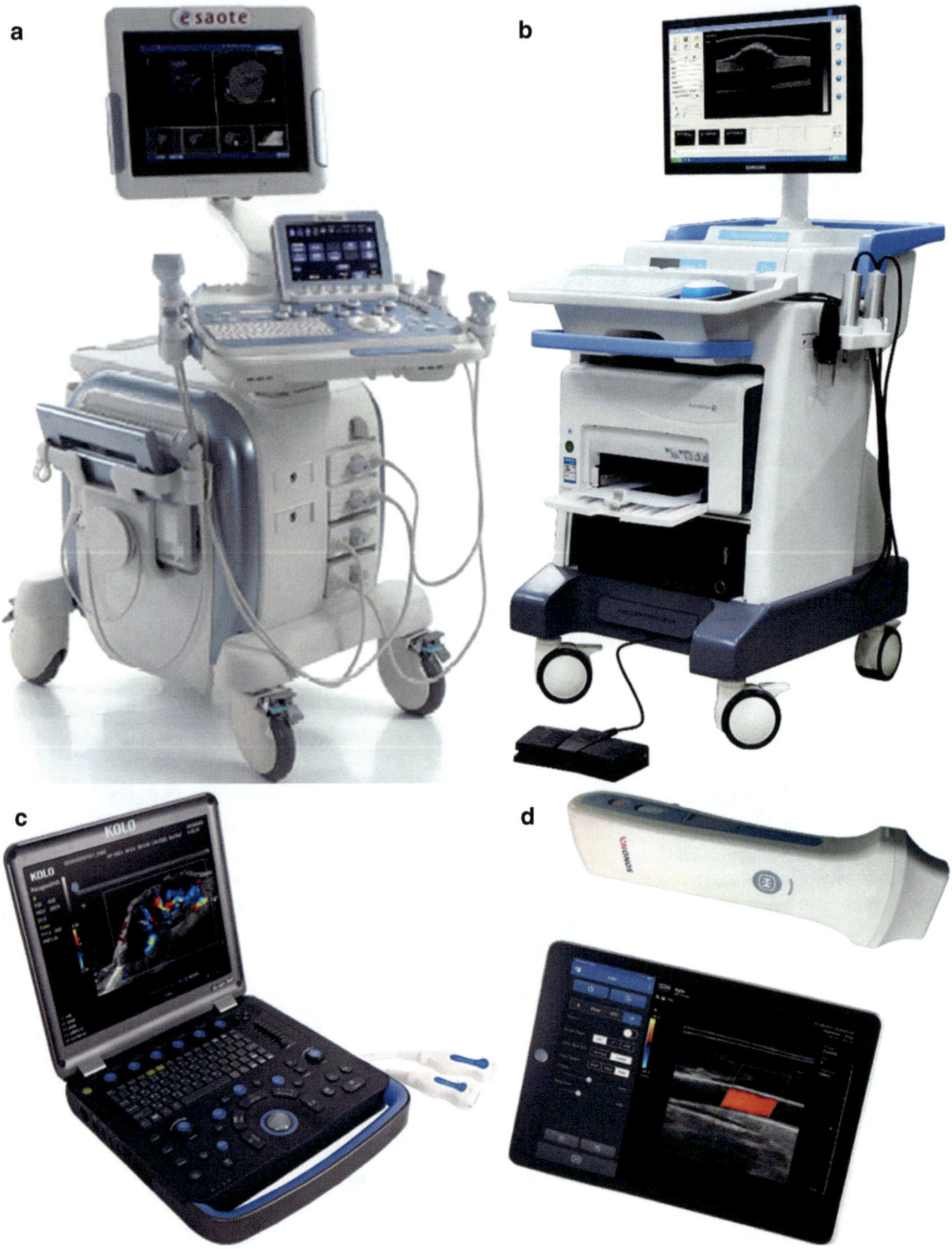

Fig. 1.19 Skin ultrasound devices. (**a**) Conventional ultrasound devices (MyLab Twice, Esaote, Italy), with a high-frequency ultrasound transducer (Frequency: 22 MHz), can realize the examination of skin diseases. (**b**) Ultrasound biomicroscopy (Frequency: 50 MHz) is dedicated to the examination of skin diseases (Tianjin Meda, model MD-310SII, China). (**c**) A laptop ultrasound device (Kolo, model Paragon XHD, China) with a high-frequency ultrasound transducer (Frequency: 22 ~ 38 MHz) can realize the examination of skin diseases. (**d**) Hand-held wireless ultrasound device (Frequency: 5/7/10 MHz) can realize the examination of skin diseases (Healcerion, model Sonon 300 L, Korea) [Image cited from Li XL et al, AUDT, 2020, 02: 050-056]

(2) Conventional HFUS transducer (Frequency: 9 ~ 20 MHz, Fig. 1.21): linear arrays, often used for examinations of superficial organs, blood vessels, and pediatric abdomen. It can also be used for skin diseases when a higher frequency ultrasound transducer is lacking.
(3) Ultrahigh-frequency ultrasound transducer with frequency ≥ 20 MHz (Fig. 1.22): linear array, mostly used for the examination of skin lesions in superficial location, which can clearly display the internal details of the lesion.
(4) Ultrasound transducer with frequency ≥ 50 MHz, known as "ultrasound biomicroscopy" (UBM), the spatial resolution reaches submillimeter level, which can display tiny structures such as epidermis and skin appendages. The preparations before examination are as follows (Fig. 1.23).

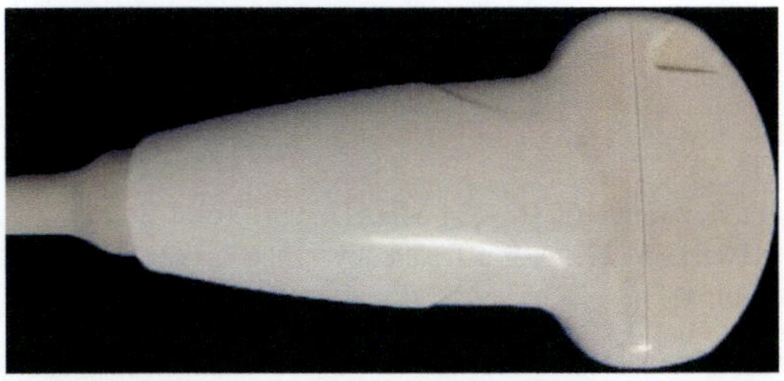

Fig. 1.20 Low-frequency convex arrays ultrasound transducer (Esaote CA431, Italy; Frequency: 1 ~ 8 MHz)

Utilization of the Ultrasound Transducer and Image Interpretation

(1) Operator posture: During the examination, the operator can sit or stand on the right side of the patient. The operator can hold the transducer with the right hand and operate the control panel with the left hand. When the transducer is small, pen-holding method can be adopted, and when the transducer is large, it can be grasped by the thumb and the remaining four fingers are opposite (Fig. 1.24). The transducer is held firmly throughout the examination. When the operator is left-handed, the above orientations are changed.
(2) Transducer placement: Before examination, the operater should observe the lesion (Fig. 1.25A), apply sufficient gel to completely embed the lesion to form an isolation zone (Fig. 1.25B), take care to eliminate large bubbles in the gel. When the lesion is in the epidermis, the operater should place the transducer on the surface of gel isolation zone to keep a gap between the transducer and the lesion surface (Fig. 1.25C). When the lesion is in the subcutaneous tissue, the transducer could touch the body surface without pressure.
(3) Image orientation: The ultrasound image shows the skin structure longitudinally with the epidermis anteriorly and the deep tissue posteriorly. All transducers have a raised

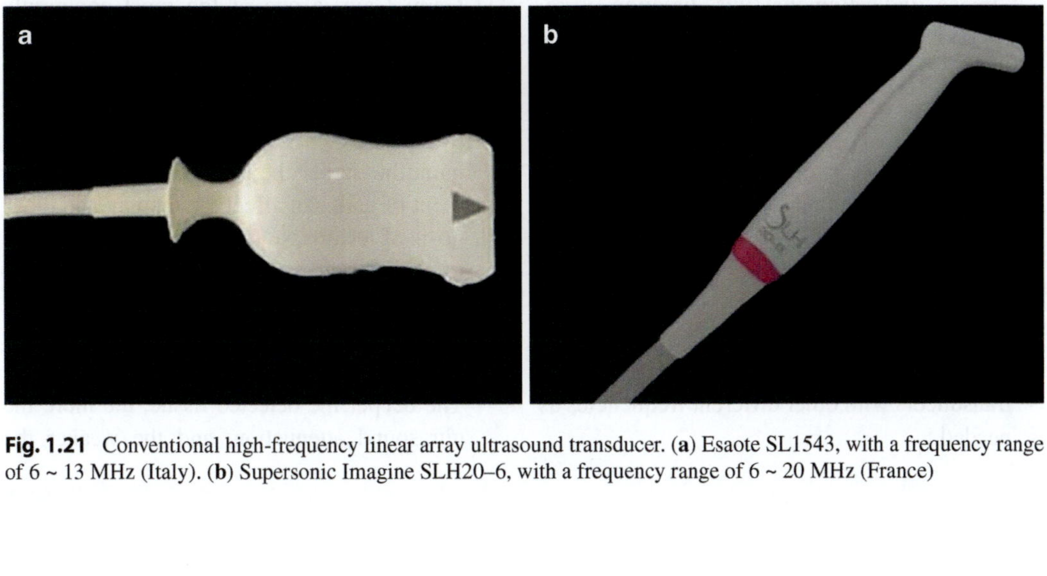

Fig. 1.21 Conventional high-frequency linear array ultrasound transducer. (**a**) Esaote SL1543, with a frequency range of 6 ~ 13 MHz (Italy). (**b**) Supersonic Imagine SLH20–6, with a frequency range of 6 ~ 20 MHz (France)

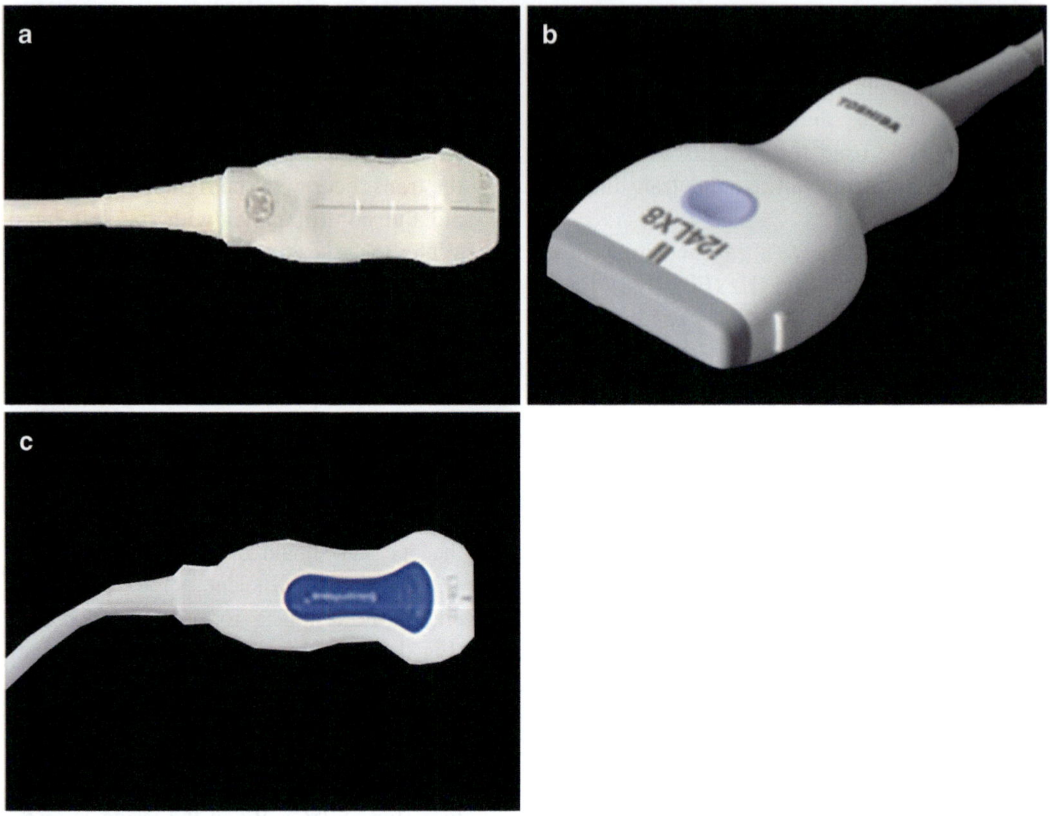

Fig. 1.22 High-frequency linear array ultrasound transducer. (**a**) GE L10–22-RS, with a frequency range of 10 ~ 22 MHz (USA). (**b**) TOSHIBA i24LX8, with a frequency range of 16 ~ 24 MHz (Japan). (**c**) Kolo Paragon XHD L38–22, with a frequency range of 22 ~ 38 MHz (China)

mark at the lateral side to orient the image (arrow on Fig. 1.26). There is a mark (generally a trademark of the device manufacturer) on the upper left corner of the ultrasound image, indicating that this direction corresponds to the raised mark on the lateral side of the transducer (Fig. 1.26).

Key Points

- The devices for skin ultrasound include conventional ultrasound device and ultrasound biomicroscopy.
- In the skin ultrasound examination, it is recommended to preferentially select the transducer with a frequency of 20 ~ 25 MHz for preliminary evaluation, and then select the transducers with other different frequencies as needed.

1.4.3.3 Adjustment of Ultrasound Devices

Adjustment of Gray-Scale Ultrasound

(1) Gain: Gain is one of the most commonly used buttons on the operator panel of ultrasound devices, which mainly adjusts the brightness of the image. The higher the gain, the brighter the image, while the lower the gain, the darker the image. Improper adjustment of gain can affect the display and diagnosis of lesions, so the gain is often adjusted to obtain a clear image during the examination (Fig. 1.27).

(2) Time gain compensation (TGC): Ultrasound is attenuated as propagating deep into tissue. The deeper the detected tissue, the more the ultrasound attenuation, and the weaker the

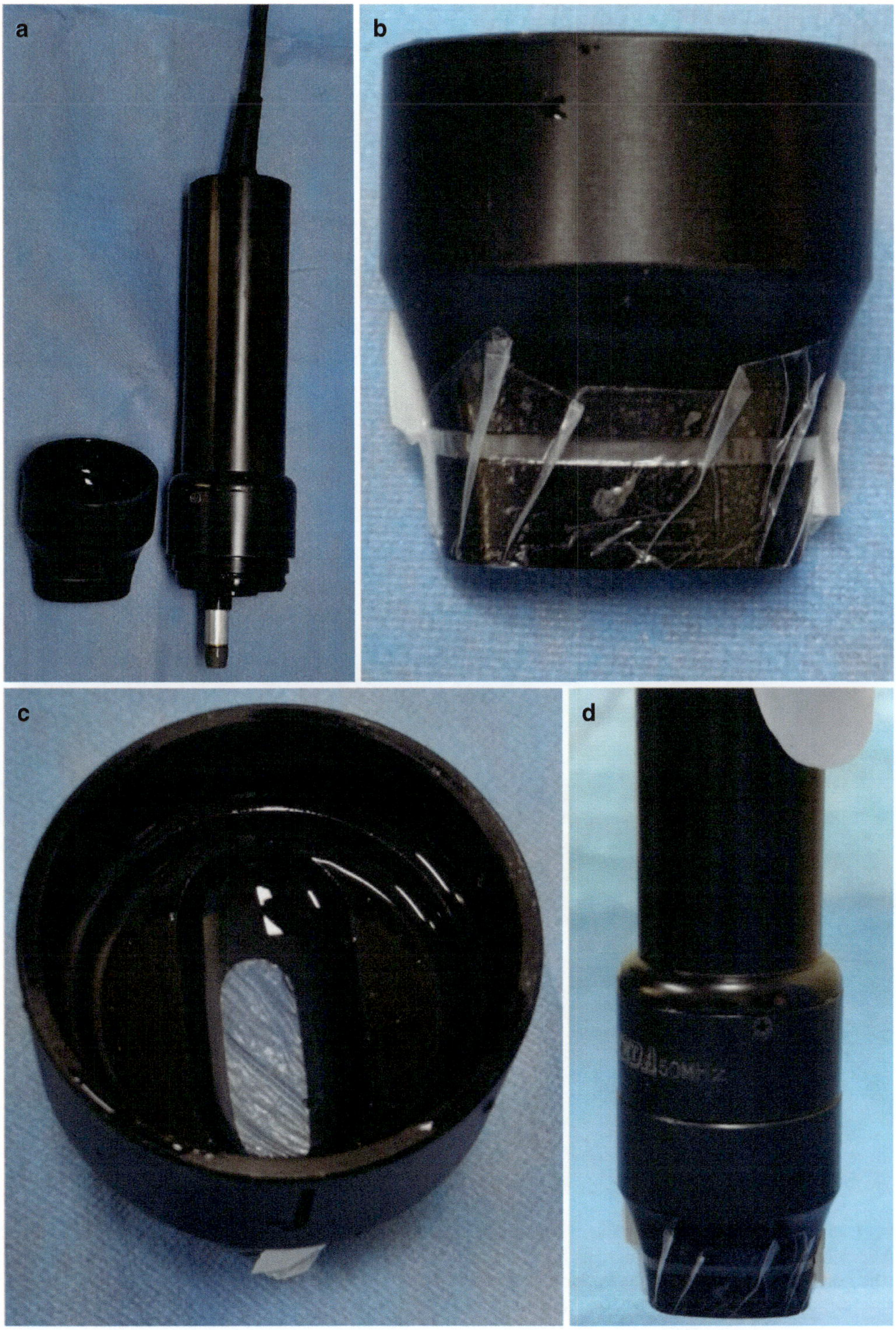

Fig. 1.23 Preparations before UBM examination. (**a**) Step 1: Transducer preparation includes a transducer and a silicone waterproof sac. (**b**) Step 2: Stick the special waterproof PU film at the front end of silicone waterproof sac tightly without water leakage. (**c**) Step 3: Inject an appropriate amount of distilled water (not normal saline) into the silicone waterproof sac, so that the transducer can be immersed. (**d**) Step 4: Install the marks on both sides of silicone waterproof sac in line with the marks on transducer handle. After the examination, remove the waterproof sac, discard the water and place the waterproof sac separately from the transducer to keep the transducer dry

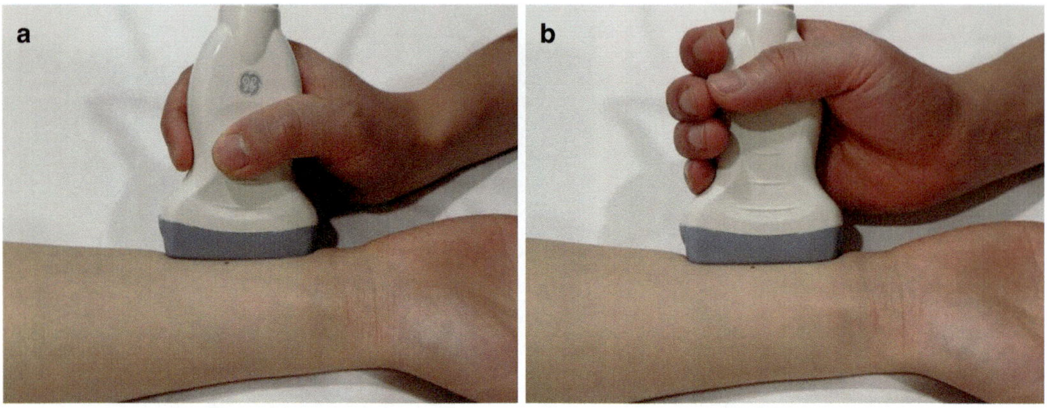

Fig. 1.24 Holding method of ultrasound transducer. (**a**) Pen-holding method. (**b**) Grip holding method

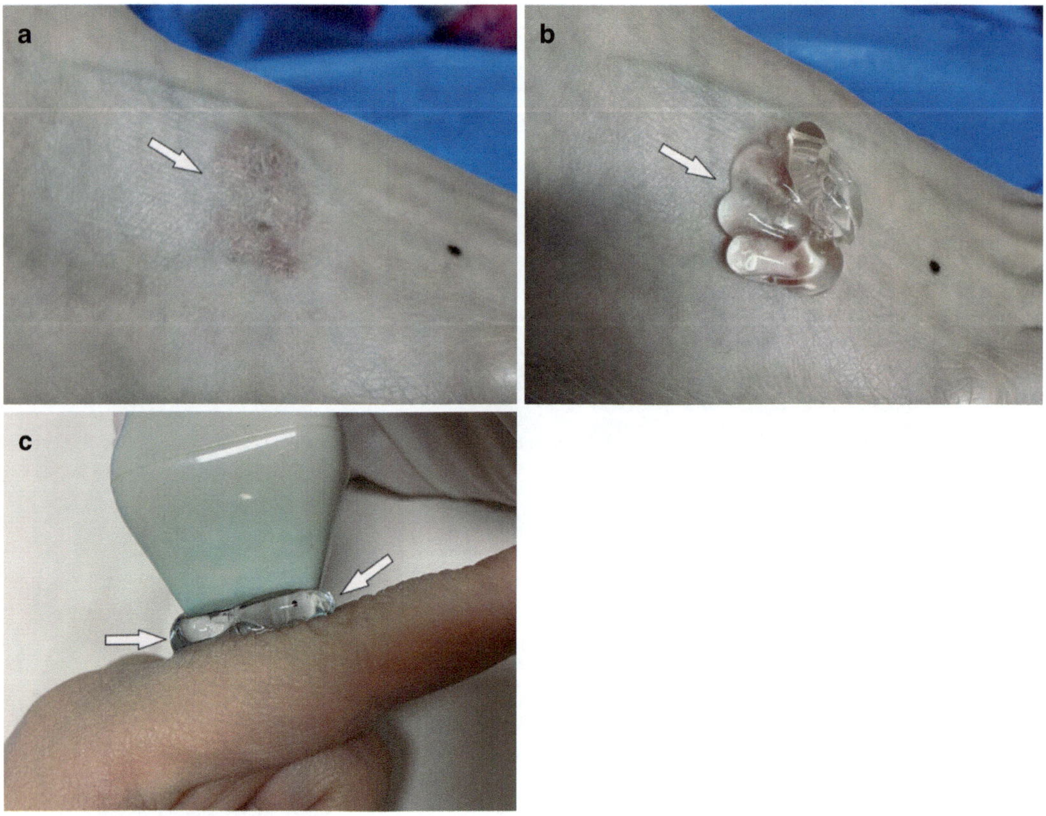

Fig. 1.25 Diagram of transducer placement. (**a**) Superficial lesion on dorsum of right foot (arrow). (**b**) The lesions are embedded with gel prior to examination to create an isolation zone (arrow). (**c**) Place the transducer over the surface of the gel and keep a distance from the lesion (take another hand lesion as an example) (arrows point to the gel)

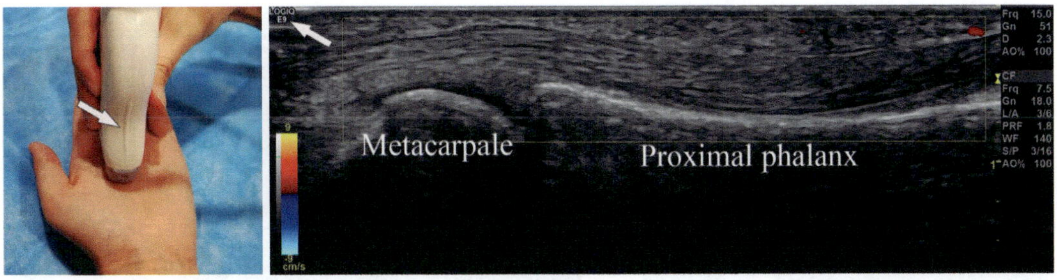

Fig. 1.26 Image orientation. The raised mark on the transducer corresponds to the orientation mark on the ultrasound image (arrow)

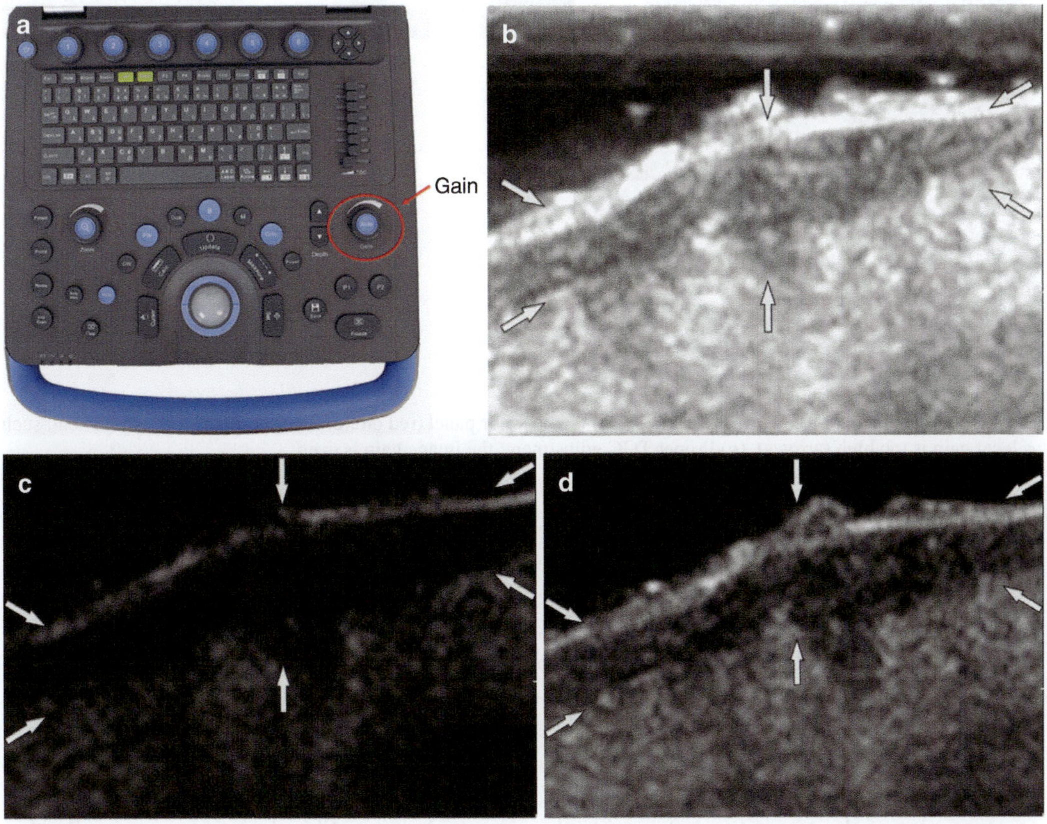

Fig. 1.27 Adjustment of gain. (**a**) Gain button on the operator panel (red circle). (**b**) Gain is too high. (**c**) Gain is too low. (**d**) Gain is proper (lesion indicated by arrows)

ultrasound wave signal received by the transducer. Therefore, the ultrasound wave signal of deep tissue is weaker than that of superficial tissue, which corresponds to deep tissue showing darker than the superficial tissue on gray-scale ultrasound image. TGC corrects and compensates for image attenuation due to increased depth, allowing the brightness of the image to be adjusted evenly from shallow to deep (Fig. 1.28). It is also feasible to adjust the image brightness of a specific depth by changing the TGC of that depth.

(3) Depth: It is adjusted by the Depth button on the operator panel. The target lesion should

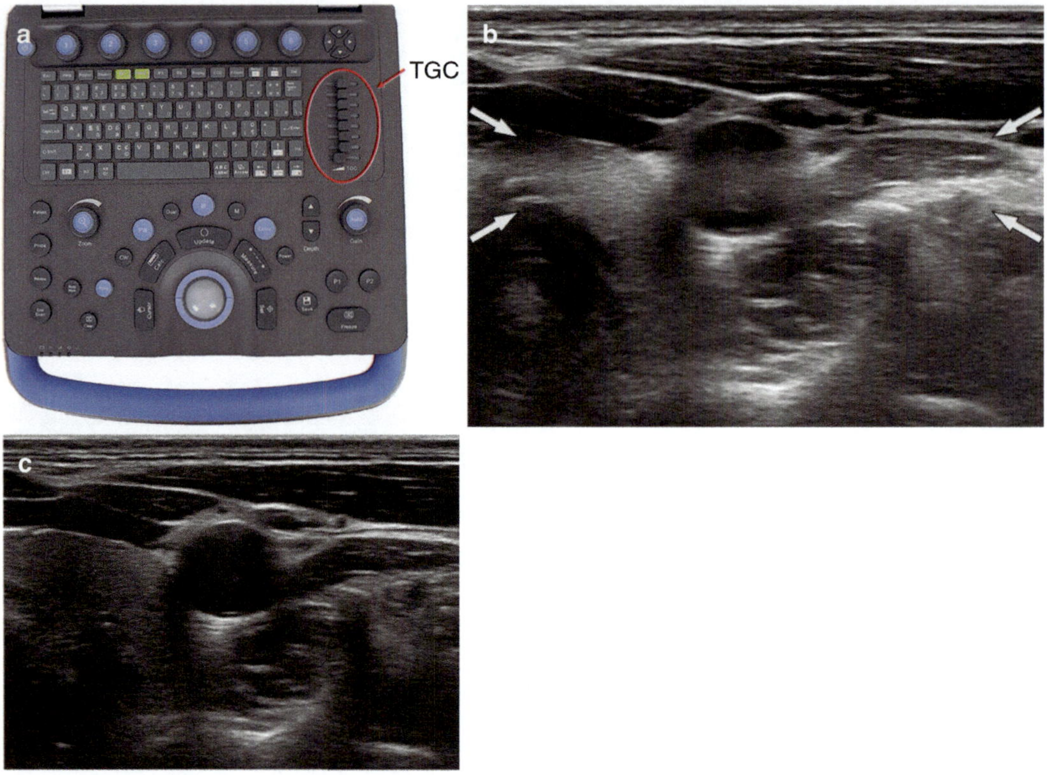

Fig. 1.28 Adjustment of TGC. (**a**) TGC buttons on the operator panel (red circle). (**b**) Improper TGC adjustment, such as local gain is too high (arrows). (**c**) Proper TGC adjustment, the image gain is even

normally be displayed in the center of the image. The depth scale is usually on the right side of the ultrasound image, and the unit is cm usually. When the depth is adjusted too deep, too much irrelevant deep tissue is incorporated, causing the reduction and off-center of the target. When the depth adjustment is too shallow, it may result in incomplete display of the target, even part of the target located outside the screen. In general, it is appropriate to take the lesion in the center of the screen (Fig. 1.29).

(4) Focus: This parameter is related to the lateral resolution, which reflects the differentiation between the lesion from its peripheral tissue at the same depth.

On most ultrasound devices, the focus is displayed as a special marker on the right side of the screen, which can be adjusted up and down with the Focus button (Fig. 1.30).

In general, the focus marker should point to the center of the lesion as possible. When the target is large, the number of foci can be increased so that the focal zone contains the lesion and its adjacent tissue as much as possible. However, it should be noted that excessive foci will lead to the reduction of image frame rate, causing the image lagging. Skin lesions are generally thin and superficial, so it is recommended to select one focus and place it at the upper side of the screen.

(5) Output: The output of ultrasound power is adjusted to optimize the image, with the adjusted range of 0 ~ 100%. The greater the output power, the stronger the ultrasound penetration and the more ambiguous the image display. On the contrary, the lower the

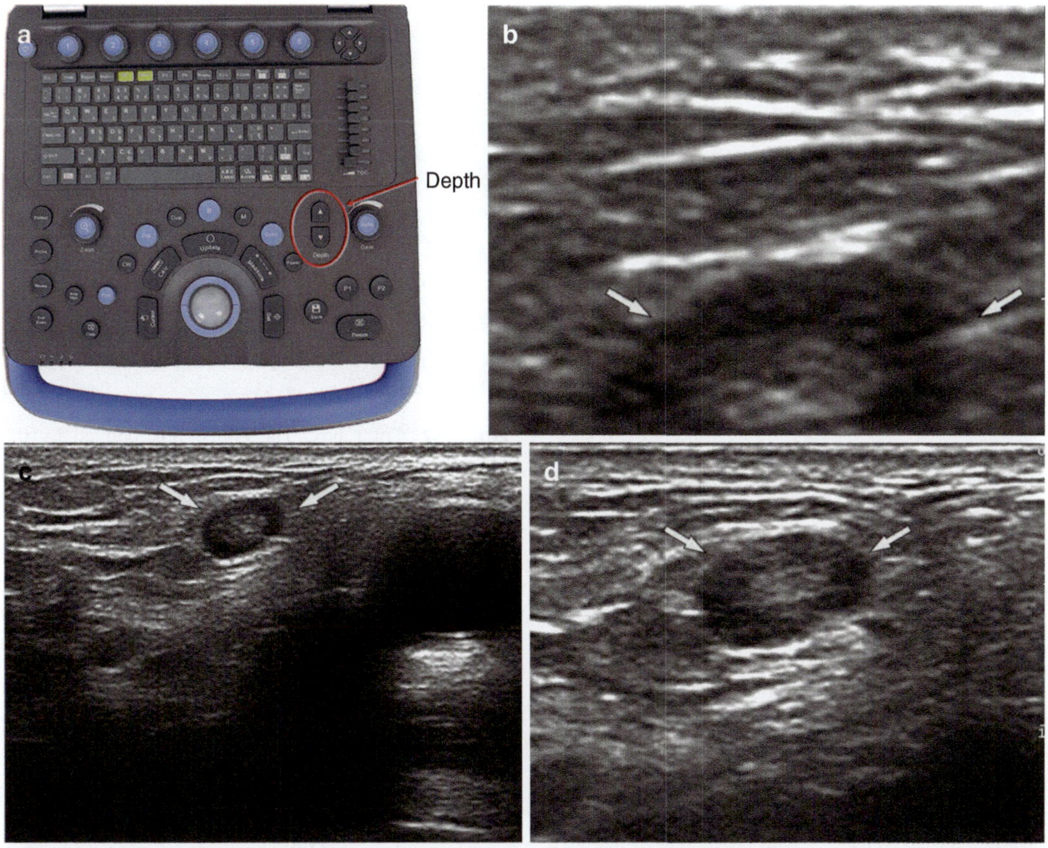

Fig. 1.29 Adjustment of depth. (**a**) Depth buttons on operator panel (red circle). (**b**) Depth is too shallow. (**c**) Depth is too deep. (**d**) Depth is proper (lesion is indicated by arrows)

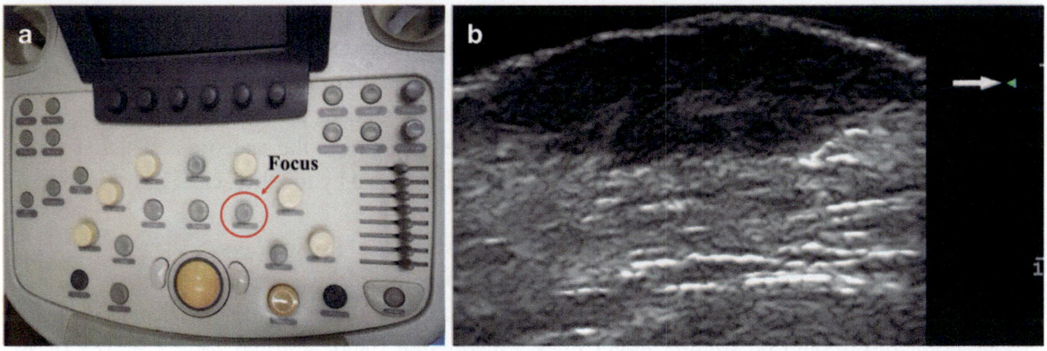

Fig. 1.30 Focus. (**a**) Focus button on the operator panel (red circle). (**b**) Focus marker on the right side of the screen (arrow)

output power, the weaker the ultrasound penetration, and the clearer the image display.

(6) Dynamic range: It is referred to the logarithm of the amplitude ratio of the maximum processed signal to the minimum processed signal, which is used to adjust the contrast resolution of the image. The wider the dynamic range, the lower the contrast resolution; conversely, the higher the contrast resolution. In general, the dynamic range of the skin ultrasound is narrower than that of the abdominal ultrasound (Fig. 1.31).

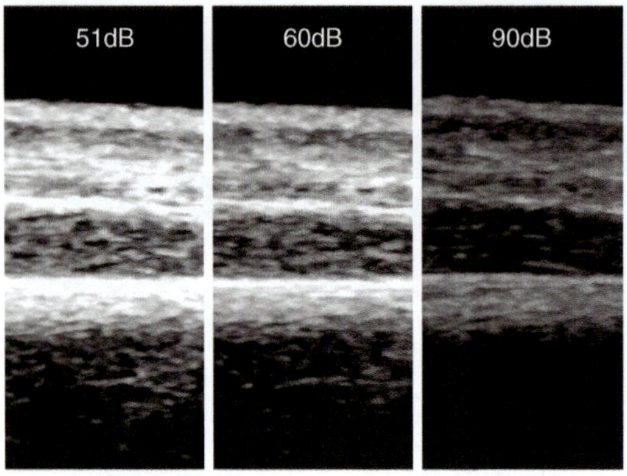

Fig. 1.31 Dynamic range. Left: The narrower the dynamic range (51 dB), the higher the contrast resolution. Right: The wider the dynamic range (90 dB), the lower the contrast resolution. Middle: the contrast resolution is optimal when the dynamic range is proper (60 dB)

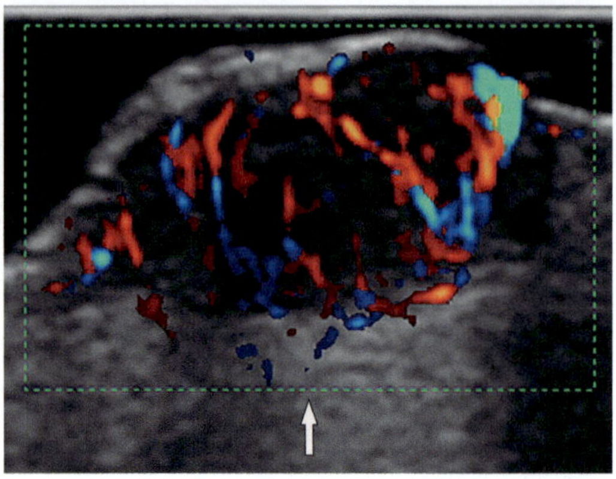

Fig. 1.32 Color box. The dotted box pointed by the arrow is the color box

Adjustment of Color Doppler Flow Imaging

(1) Preparation to establish a satisfactory blood flow display environment: (1) Selecting a transducer with appropriate frequency. Understanding the characteristics of PRF, and taking into account penetration, resolution, and real-time performance according to specific needs, (2) Optimizing the gray-scale image. Appropriately reducing the gain of the two-dimensional image. (3) Displaying the longitudinal axis of the vessel, and adjusting the Doppler angle to the minimum.

(2) Color box: Firstly, it is necessary to adjust the size of the color box on color Doppler ultrasound. If the color box is too large, the frame rate will reduce, resulting in image lagging. If the color box is too small, the blood flow of the target lesion cannot be displayed completely. Therefore, the appropriate color box should be slightly larger than the lesion, including some surrounding tissues (Fig. 1.32).

(3) Color gain: Proper gain settings are essential to accurate and reproducible Doppler measurements. When the color gain is too high, color flow signals overflow with artifacts in the perilesional area occurs; while the color gain is too low, intralesional blood flow signals cannot be completely displayed (Fig. 1.33). The proper color gain setting is firstly increasing the color gain until the extravascular noise appears, then reducing the color gain until the disappearance of extravascular noise. Also, the gray-scale gain should be appropriately reduced.

(4) Scale (pulse repetition frequency): In order to optimize the display of blood flow, it is necessary to adjust PRF, also known as scale. Frequency (Hz), average velocity value (cm/s), or velocity level (high, medium, and low) can be used to represent the magnitude of PRF in color Doppler. The general principle of regulating PRF is to make the blood flow signal as rich as possible in the color box, without aliasing artifact (that is, the blood flow signal in the same direction shows the red and blue at the same time, which is generally caused by too low scale) as optimal.

Adjustment of Pulse Wave Doppler Imaging

1. Sample volume: It should be kept as central as possible, and adjusted to 1/2 ~ 1/3 of the diameter of the target vessel in width.
2. Doppler gain: The Doppler gain is adjusted by rotating the Doppler Gain button. When Doppler flow visualization is clear and the background is clean, the Doppler gain is believed to be proper.
3. Angle correct: Angle correct refers to the adjustment of Doppler angle, which is used

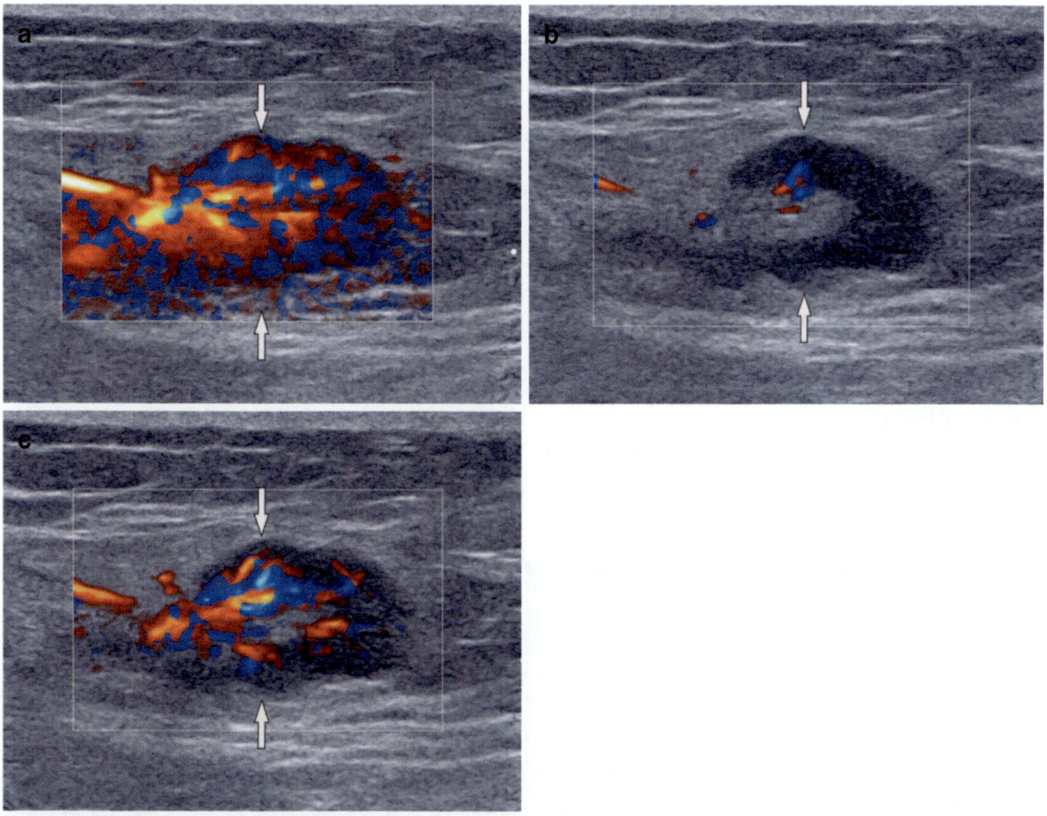

Fig. 1.33 Adjustment of color gain. (**a**) Color gain is too high (arrows). (**b**) Color gain is too low (arrows). (**c**) Color gain is proper (arrows)

to calibrate the angle between acoustic beam and blood flow direction of the target vessel, and display the actual blood flow velocity through the correction of cosine value of this angle. The acoustic beam shall be kept parallel with the direction of blood flow, and the angle between the two shall be as minimal as possible, with the maximum angle less than 60°.

4. Velocity scale: The velocity scale was selected according to the velocity of blood flow in the vessels. Lower velocity scales are generally selected for skin diseases.
5. Wall filter: By adjusting the filter button to change the wall filter value, the low-frequency and high-intensity noise caused by vessel wall or tissue motion is eliminated. The wall filter values can be set to low, medium, and high. Low-pass filter is used for low-velocity blood flow, and high-pass filter is used for high-velocity blood flow.

The adjustment of power Doppler flow imaging is similar to that of color Doppler flow imaging, so it will not be repeated here.

1.4.4 Influencing Factors for Skin Ultrasound Imaging

1.4.4.1 Pressure

Surface pressure has a great impact on high-frequency skin ultrasound imaging, and pressure may lead to deformation or blood flow imaging distortion of the lesion, even lead to the lesion or its blood flow invisible. Direct contact of the transducer with the skin should be avoided during skin ultrasound examinations, and it is recommended to fill with gel (>1 mm in thickness) to isolate the skin from the transducer, thereby eliminating the surface pressure caused by the transducer. In addition, the gel pad can also be used to isolate the skin from the transducer to improve the image quality, but the pressure of the gel pad itself on the skin still cannot be ignored.

1.4.4.2 Hairs

Small and fine hairs have no significant effect on ultrasound imaging. The thick hair may produce acoustic shadowing, while air is present among the hairs, both of which can reduce the quality of the ultrasound image (Fig. 1.34). In this regard, the image quality can be improved by hair removal or filling with more gel.

1.4.4.3 Wrinkles

There are various wrinkles formed naturally in the skin, thus the skin surface cannot be closely fitted with the transducer, affecting the quality of ultrasound imaging. At this time, the image quality can be ensured by straightening the skin, filling it with more gel, adding a gel pad, or other methods to fit the skin at the wrinkles to the transducer (Fig. 1.35).

1.4.4.4 Temperature

Temperature mainly affects the blood flow signal of color Doppler flow imaging. If the temperature is too low, the blood flow signal may be reduced. If the temperature is too high, it may cause an abnormal increase in blood flow. Examination at room temperature around 20 °C is recommended, and heated gel is not recommended.

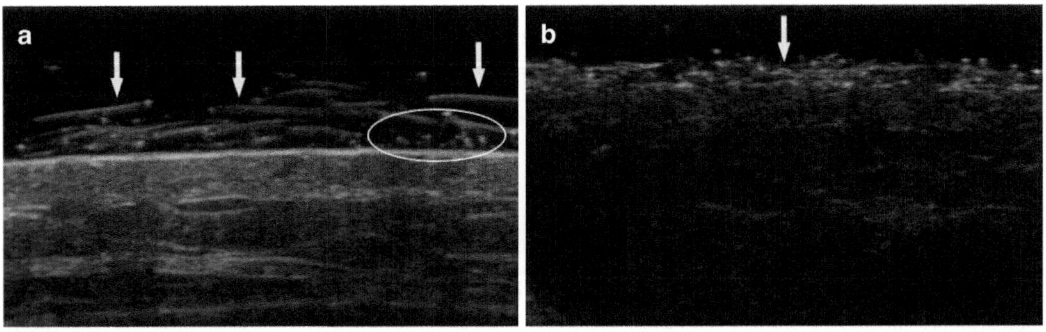

Fig. 1.34 Effect of hairs on skin ultrasound imaging. (**a**) Sparse hairs and a small amount of air are observed on the skin surface, and the image quality is not significantly affected (male, leg; transducer frequency: 30 MHz). (**b**) Dense hairs and air form acoustic shadowing, significantly reducing the image quality (male, head; transducer frequency: 30 MHz). Arrows point to the hair, circle is air among hairs

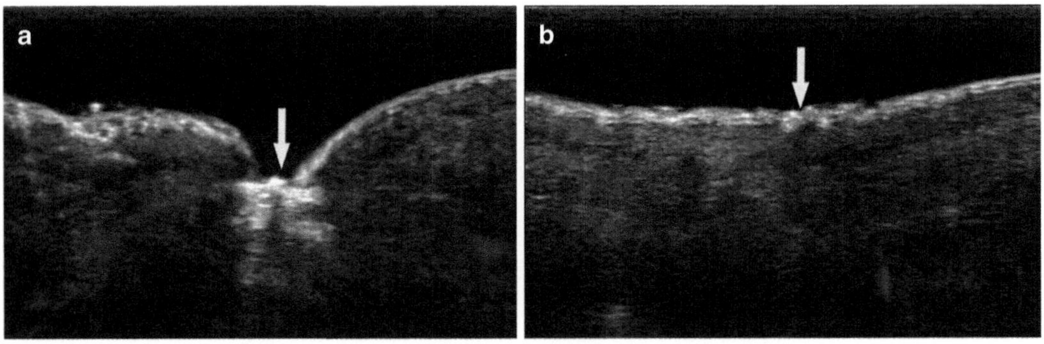

Fig. 1.35 Effect of wrinkles on skin ultrasound imaging. (**a**) Skin wrinkles contain air, forming acoustic shadowing and resulting in unclear display of skin structure and layers (male, palm; transducer frequency: 34 MHz). (**b**) The skin at this site is straightened, and then the skin structure and layers can be clearly displayed. Arrows point to skin wrinkles

1.4.4.5 Precautions

Due to the superficial location of the skin and related diseases, ultrasound images are required to have sufficient resolution to show tiny structures. At the same time, the depth involvement of skin diseases is closely related to disease progression, and ultrasound with sufficient penetration ability is needed to display the information of depth involvement of the lesion. Therefore, skin ultrasound imaging needs to take into account both resolution and depth. In addition, various pathophysiological conditions such as obesity, keratinization, scar, and edema can lead to acoustic wave attenuation, impacting the quality of ultrasound imaging.

Finally, the skin ultrasound imaging is sensitive to pressure. When the transducer is placed on the skin surface, the deformation and distortion of lesion morphology and ultrasound image may result from the weight of the transducer itself or the pressure applied during the examination.

Therefore, according to previous literatures and our clinical practice, attention should be paid to the following factors when performing skin ultrasound imaging.

1. For dermal and epidermal ultrasound imaging, the frequency of the transducer shall be at least 20 MHz. When the frequency meets this condition, it is feasible to distinguish epidermis, dermis, and subcutaneous tissue and clearly display various layers of skin. If the frequency of the transducer increases to 50 MHz, the internal structure of the epidermis can be further visualized, but the structures below the papillary dermis may not be visualized due to decreased penetration. As the frequency increases further (e.g., ≥100 MHz), the penetration of ultrasound will decrease significantly and cannot show the whole lesion, which is not clinically practical.
2. The skin varies greatly among individuals, the lesion is complex, and the size may span multiple scales from nm, μm, mm to cm, so the frequency of the transducer needs to be frequently switched to meet the imaging requirements of lesions with different sizes. In clinical practice, it is necessary to take into account the imaging resolution and depth at the same time according to specific circumstances, so as to obtain the optimal images.
3. In case of poor contact due to the presence of hairs and wrinkles on the surface of the lesion, more gel or gel pad should be used. The transducer should not be pressed to avoid deformation of the lesion.
4. It is necessary to pay attention to the disinfection and isolation of ultrasound transducers, so as to avoid cross infection. The transducer must be disconnected from the ultrasound device and cleaned with running water or soap solution after each patient examination. For lesions with open wounds, it is recommended to use a protective sleeve to isolate the transducer prior to examination to protect the transducer from blood, tissue debris, secretions, or other body fluids.

Key Points

- Before the ultrasound examination, a detailed history of the patient and careful observation for the appearance of the lesion are required.
- Multiple factors should be avoided in skin ultrasound examinations.
- Skin ultrasound imaging needs to take into account both resolution and depth.
- Protecting throughout the examination to avoid cross infection.

1.5 Cleaning of Ultrasound Device and Personnel Protection

1.5.1 Cleaning of Ultrasound Device

1. Ultrasound devices should be avoided to contact the patient during the whole examination.
2. It is recommended to cover the operator panel with transparent plastic film to prevent dust and water, and to wipe the film with a medical disinfectant wipe after a daily examination.

3. Wiping the screen of the ultrasound device daily with a non-woven cloth to remove stains.
4. After daily check, the device is disinfected by ultraviolet irradiation, and the screen is protected by drape during irradiation.
5. The above maintenance and cleaning shall be carried out under power-off status. Other precautions can refer to the instructions for use or consult the engineer.

1.5.2 Cleaning of Transducer

1. At the end of the daily work, the transducer and cable are wiped with medical sterile towels.
2. If the surface of the lesion is without rupture and ulceration, the transducer does not require special protection and cleaning, and the examination can be continued after wiping the residual gel on the transducer.
3. When there is an open wound on the skin surface or there is blood or exudates, the transducer should be isolated to avoid cross infection as following.

1) Prior to examination, the transducer should be disconnected from the ultrasound device. It is recommended to use running water to clean the transducer, and routinely apply gel on the surface of the transducer (either sterile or conventional), and then use a special disposable protective sleeve to wrap the transducer (if not, wrap it with rubber gloves).
2) During the examination, the transducer is contacted with the wound surface by using the sterile gel, and attention should be paid to keep the transducer from the surrounding skin of the lesion and other objects.
3) After the examination, the gel on the wound surface should be wiped with sterile gauze. It is recommended to change the dressing and bandaging of the lesion according to the surgical routine disinfection. Discard the medical waste generated in the above process according to the relevant requirements.
4) Finally, the transducer is disconnected from the device. The transducer is washed again with running clean water, and is cleaned with soap solution or disinfectant wipe.
5) After using the transducer to check lesions with open wounds of patients with infectious diseases such as condyloma acuminatum, syphilis, or acquired immune deficiency syndrome (AIDS), 2% glutaraldehyde should be used for disinfection 30 min, then washed with clean water or sterilized with UV-C ultraviolet lamp. However, it should be noted that the chemical reagents may corrode the transducer material. The instructions or the engineer should be consulted before use.

1.5.3 Personnel Protection

1. For lesions without open wounds, blood, or exudates, the operator and the assistant do not need special protection.
2. For lesions with open wounds, blood, or exudates, the operator and the assistant need to wear gloves and masks during the examination and to clean the transducer after the examination. Hand disinfection is required before and after each examination (Fig. 1.36).

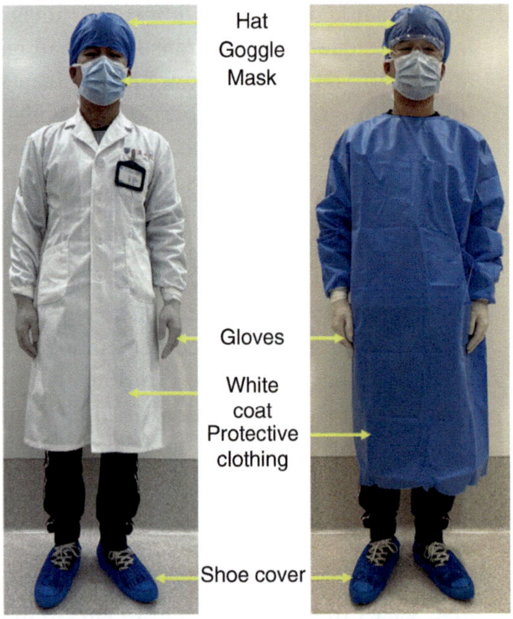

Fig. 1.36 Protection of examiner. The left figure shows level 1 protection, and the right shows level 2 protection

3. When the patient suffers from Class B or above infectious diseases, no matter whether the lesion is ulcerated or not, the operator and the assistant need to wear protective clothing, shoe covers, protective goggles for full protection (Fig. 1.36).
4. Before and after the examination, the window should be opened daily for ventilation for 30 min. If the lesion is odorous, ventilation should be performed for at least 10 min after the examination.
5. Room environment disinfection is performed regularly in a week.

Key Points

- It is necessary to clean the device and protect the operator during the ultrasound examination.
- Cleaning of ultrasound devices and protection of operator should be carried out according to relevant regulations and quality control standards.

1.6 New Ultrasound Technology in Skin Ultrasound

In recent years, a number of new ultrasound technologies have been gradually used in clinical practice. These technologies can provide more information for the diagnosis of skin diseases and further broaden the application of ultrasound in the diagnosis and treatment of skin diseases. These new technologies are mainly as follows.

1.6.1 Extended Field of View

Extended field of view (EFOV) imaging, also known as broad-view imaging, can obtain image information beyond the display range of normal ultrasound images. EFOV is suitable for large lesions. The basic principle is to obtain a series of two-dimensional ultrasound images through the unidirectional, constant speed, and stable movement of transducers on the basis of conventional ultrasound. When the transducer moves, the image moves from one frame to the next, which has a great overlap area. At this time, it is necessary to use the calculation of computer vector change to accurately estimate the movement of the transducer from one frame to another frame, register the frame by frame, and finally reconstruct and stitch this series of two-dimensional images into an image with continuous extended field of view. For larger skin lesions, complete visualization of the whole lesion on one image can be achieved using EFOV imaging (Fig. 1.37).

1.6.2 Ultrasound Elastography

Because different tissues have different stiffness, it is possible to differentiate the benign from malignant lesions by stiffness information. At present, the elastography used in clinical practice mainly includes strain elastography (SE) and shear wave elastography (SWE). SE is based on manual pressure to deform the tissue which can only provide qualitative data. SWE is based on the measurement of the transverse shear wave

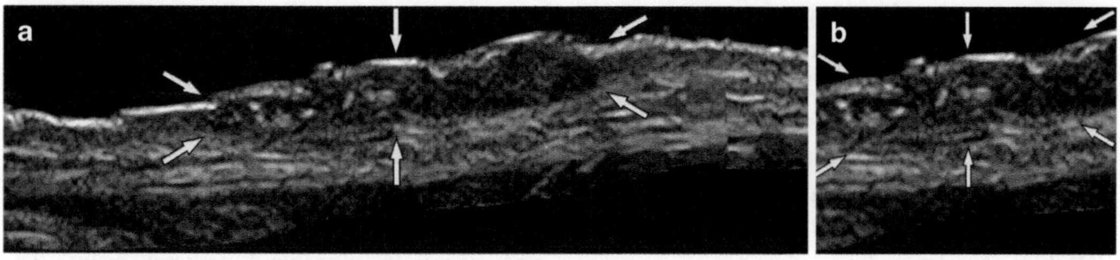

Fig. 1.37 Extended feld of view imaging of superficial basal cell carcinoma. Male, lesion located in left temporal of the face. (**a**) The examination is performed using a high-frequency ultrasound transducer with a frequency of 22 MHz, and the broad-view of the lesion (arrows) and the adjacent normal skin are displayed by extended feld of view imaging. (**b**) The lesion (arrows) is only partially displayed without extended feld of view imaging. The boundary and adjacent tissue of the lesion is invisible

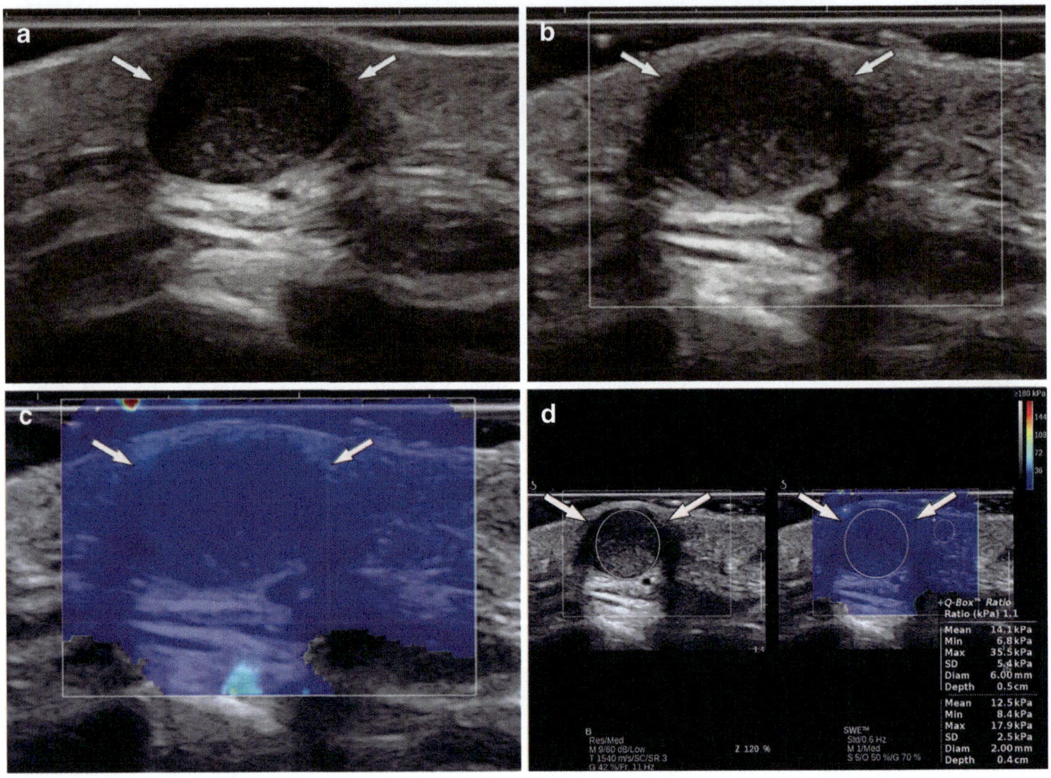

Fig. 1.38 Ultrasound elastography. (**a**) Gray-scale ultrasound shows an oval, well-defined, hypoechoic structure (arrows) in the dermis and subcutaneous tissue. The lesion is heterogeneous (Frequency: 15 MHz). (**b**) Color Doppler ultrasound shows no blood flow signal in the lesion (arrows) (Frequency: 15 MHz). (**c**) Two-dimensional shear wave elastography is conducted to assess the stiffness of the lesion qualitatively. The lesion and the surrounding tissues show homogeneous blue, indicating no significant difference in the stiffness between the lesion and surrounding tissues (arrows). (**d**) Shear wave elastography is conducted to assess the stiffness of the ROI quantitatively (arrows), with a maximum elastic modulus of 35.5 kPa, a mean elastic modulus of 14.1 kPa, and a minimum elastic modulus of 6.8 kPa

propagation speed induced by acoustic pulse from the ultrasound transducer within the tissue. Shear wave speed can be quantified as the Young's modulus in kilopascals (kPa). SWE includes point SWE and two-dimensional SWE. Among them, point SWE reflects the quantitative information of stiffness in the region of interest (ROI), and two-dimensional SWE not only can provide quantitative information, but also intuitively reflect the tissue stiffness in the ROI through color coding.

Elastography is widely used in the liver, thyroid, breast, and other organs. It is also suitable for skin lesions to differentiate benign from malignant lesions by measuring the stiffness of lesions. This technique provides stiffness information in addition to anatomical information and a new modality for the diagnosis of skin diseases (Fig. 1.38).

1.6.3 Contrast-Enhanced Ultrasound

Contrast-enhanced ultrasound is a pure blood pool imaging technology, adopting low mechanical index contrast-specific imaging technique and second-generation ultrasound contrast agent. The microcirculation perfusion of a target lesion is dynamically visualized in real time by injecting microbubble contrast agent into peripheral vein, which can reflect the blood supply and perfusion in the lesion. Contrast-enhanced ultrasound improves the diagnostic accuracy of skin diseases by obtaining morphological and functional information of the lesion through qualitative and quantitative analysis (i.e., enhancement pattern, enhancement intensity, and time intensity curve) (Fig. 1.39).

Parametric imaging technology is a post-processing mode based on the original data of contrast image. The basic principle is that each ROI on the contrast image has its corresponding time intensity curve (TIC) to reflect the amount and speed of contrast agent entering into the lesion. The technology can automatically identify and display the average arrival time and area under the curve corresponding to the intensity threshold on the TIC in each ROI, constituting the image of parametric imaging. Other quantitative parameters of TIC are also obtained such as peak intensity (i.e., the maximum intensity of the TIC), time to peak (i.e., the time from the first microbubble entering the lesion to the microbubble reaching the peak intensity), ascending slope, etc. Compared with the original contrast image analysis, the parametric imaging can more intuitively display the subtle differences in the contrast agent perfusion of the internal and peripheral of the lesion, overcoming the shortcomings of conventional qualitative diagnosis. Studies have showed that malignant tumors can achieve higher peak intensity on TIC than benign tumors, which is conducive to the differential diagnosis of benign and malignant diseases. TIC showing a rapid increase often indicates malignant perfusion characteristics (Fig. 1.40).

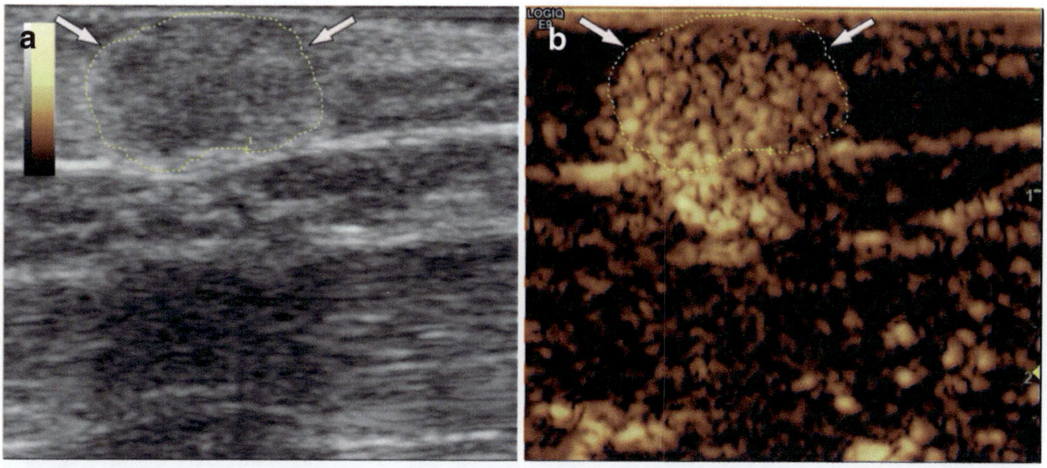

Fig. 1.39 Contrast-enhanced ultrasound. (**a**) Gray-scale ultrasound shows an oval, well defined, slightly hypoechogenic lesion (arrows and dotted line) in the dermis and subcutaneous tissue, with slight posterior acoustic shadowing (Frequency: 15 MHz). (**b**) Contrast-enhanced ultrasound shows that the lesion (arrows and dotted line) is homogeneously hyperenhanced compared with the surrounding soft tissue (Frequency: 9 MHz)

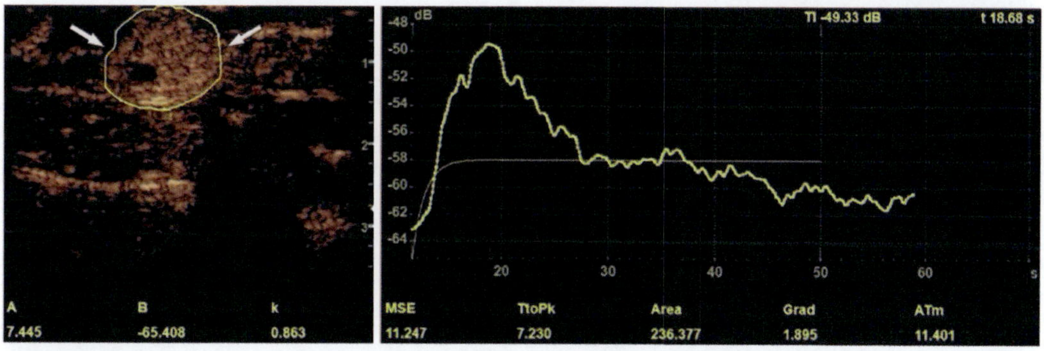

Fig. 1.40 Time intensity curve (TIC). TIC analysis of the lesion (arrows and dotted line) shows peak intensity is −65.4 (dB); time to peak, 7.230 seconds; ascending slope, 0.863, and area under the TIC is 236.377

The contrast agent SonoVue (Bracco, Italy), which is now widely used in clinical practice, is a representative of the second-generation ultrasound contrast agent (Fig. 1.41). It has high safety and good tolerance, and the probability of life-threatening allergic reaction is extremely low, about 0.001%, which can be injected repeatedly (Fig. 1.42). SonoVue is mainly composed of sulfur hexafluoride (SF6) gas and white lyophilized powder. This contrast agent stays only in the blood pool without entering into the extracellular space and is a pure-blood pool contrast agent.

Novel ultrasound contrast agents such as Sonazoid can be phagocytosed by Kupffer cells in the liver and spleen and have a special post-vascular phase beyond the vascular phase, which can provide more diagnostic information.

In addition, two new ultrasound molecular imaging contrast agents, BR55 and Multiselection, have emerged in recent years. Those agents can specifically bind to disease-related molecular markers expressed by endothelial cells and achieve molecular imaging with high sensitivity and long duration.

1.6.4 Three-Dimensional Ultrasound

Three-dimensional ultrasound is an imaging mode based on two-dimensional ultrasound. Through mechanically or electronically driven transducers, a series of two-dimensional images with equal distance or angle are obtained to form a three-dimensional database. After processing and reconstruction by computer, the three-dimensional image of ROI is obtained. It can visually and vividly display more information of

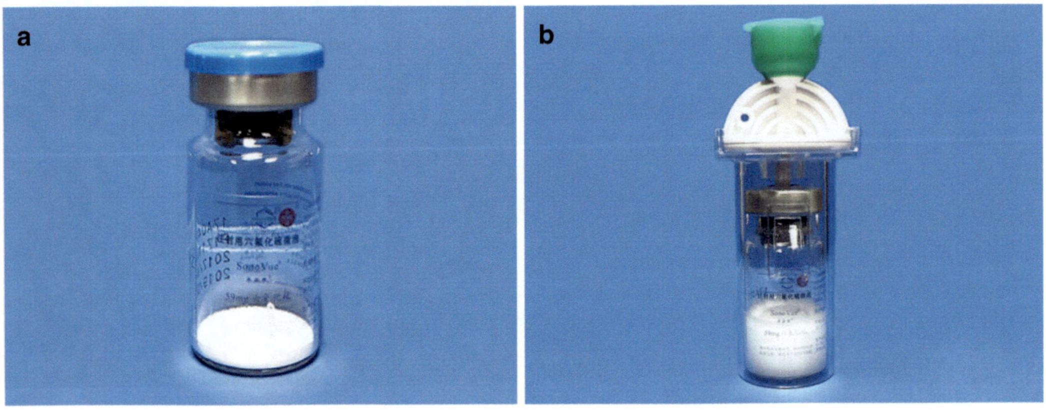

Fig. 1.41 Sample of contrast agent. (**a**) Contrast agent before use. (**b**) Contrast agent after dispersion with normal saline

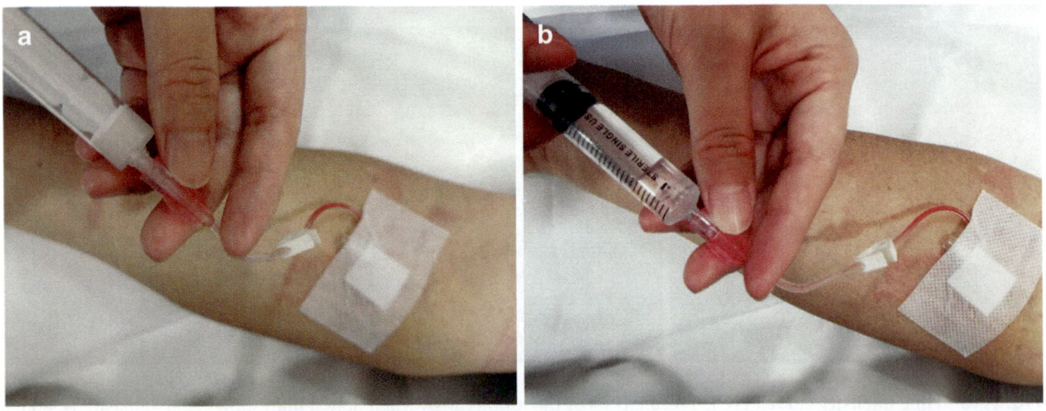

Fig. 1.42 Injection of contrast agent. (**a**) Injection of contrast agent. (**b**) Flush the tube with normal saline

the lesion from any angle, as well as the relationship between the lesion and adjacent tissue, especially the image of coronal plane parallel to the transducer that is not easy to obtain by two-dimensional ultrasound (Fig. 1.43).

1.6.5 Interventional Ultrasound

Interventional ultrasound refers to various operations such as needle biopsy, ablation, and injection under real-time ultrasound guidance or monitoring, which can effectively improve the accuracy of operation, reduce complications, and improve efficacy. The applications in interventional ultrasound to the skin are few and have a great prospect (Fig. 1.44).

The location of skin diseases is superficial, and the ultrasound-guided biopsy of skin diseases has the advantages of accuracy, no radiation and simple operation, and so on. Therefore, it has high practical value. Ultrasound-guided puncture and drainage sclerotherapy can treat cystic lesions, thus alleviating or eliminating the clinical symp-

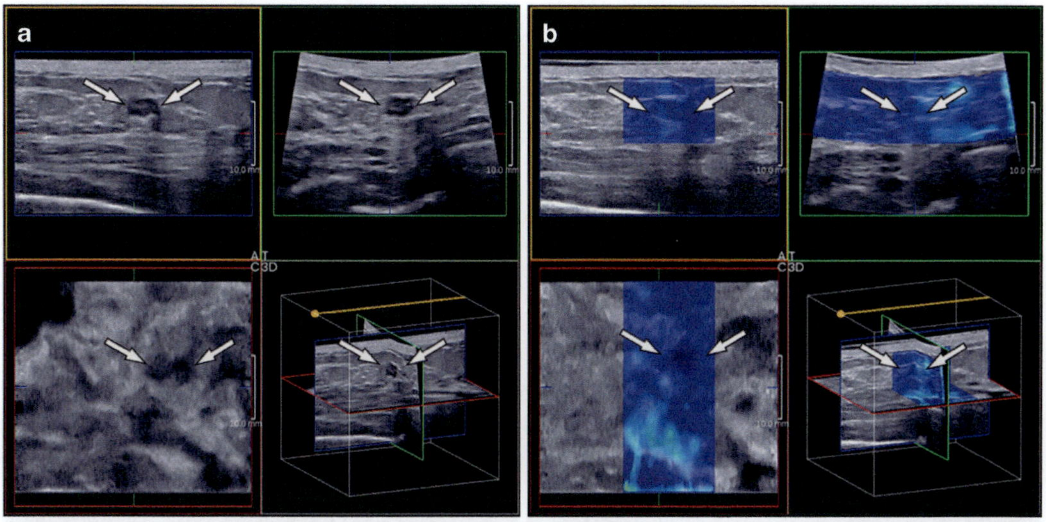

Fig. 1.43 Three-dimensional gray-scale ultrasound and three-dimensional shear wave elastography. (**a**) Gray-scale ultrasound shows an oval, well-defined, hypoechoic lesion (arrows) located in the subcutaneous tissue. The lesion is heterogeneous (Frequency 15 MHz). (**b**) Three-dimensional shear wave elastography shows the lesion (arrows) and surrounding tissues are homogeneous blue, indicating that there is no significant difference in the stiffness between the lesion and surrounding tissue (Frequency: 15 MHz)

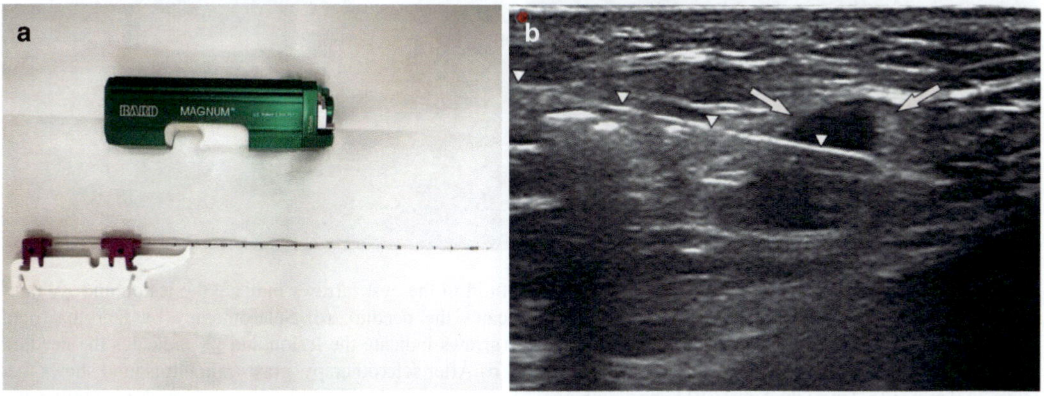

Fig. 1.44 Ultrasound-guided cervical lymph node biopsy (Frequency: 15 MHz). (**a**) Biopsy gun and disposable biopsy needle. (**b**) A disposable biopsy needle has penetrated the target lymph node. Arrows show the lymph node and △ shows the biopsy needle

toms (Fig. 1.45). For hemangioma located in deep subcutaneous tissue, the surgical procedure is difficult, and it is easy to miss the lesion since it is hard to make a distinction between hemangioma and adjacent structures by visual observation. However, the ultrasound-guided sclerotherapy has the advantage of real-time display, which can completely embolize the blood vessels in the hemangioma with clear visualization of the lesion margin on ultrasound image (Fig. 1.46).

1.6.6 Artificial Intelligence in Skin Ultrasound

Artificial intelligence (AI) is a technology used to study and develop for simulating, extending, and expanding human intelligence. With the rapid growth of image data and the maturity of basic technical conditions such as computer algorithm and computing power, medical imaging artificial intelligence has developed rapidly. Through training and learning a large number of image pictures, AI can get the same ability to accurately diagnose diseases as human beings. Moreover, it can get more information at a faster speed.

There are some studies about AI diagnosis of melanoma and nonpigmented skin cancer. A number of noninvasive, computer-assisted methods, including Raman spectroscopy, multispectral instrumentation, and AI with various algorithms have been developed for use at the bedside to obtain a timely diagnosis of mela-

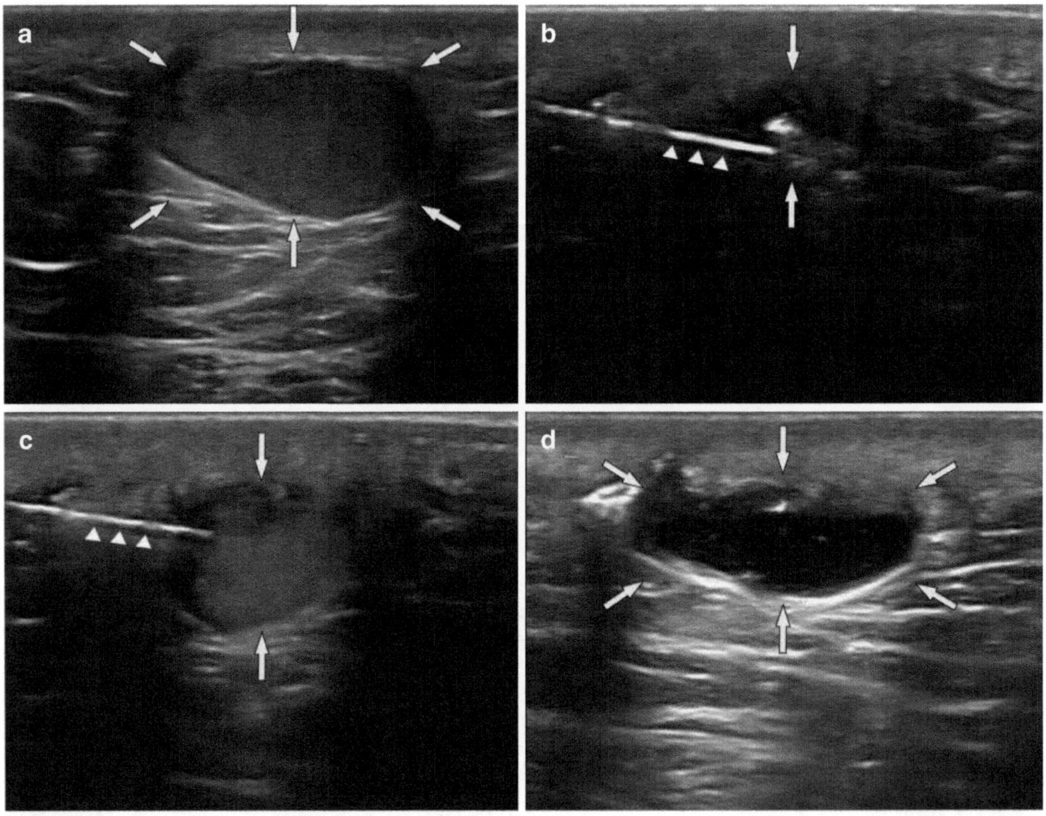

Fig. 1.45 Ultrasound-guided aspiration and sclerotherapy of an epidermoid cyst (Frequency: 15 MHz). (**a**) Gray-scale ultrasound shows an oval, well-defined hypoechogenic lesion (arrows) in the subcutaneous tissue (size: 24.0 mm × 16.2 mm; thickness: 10.8 mm) with posterior acoustic enhancement (Frequency: 15 MHz). (**b**) Ultrasound-guided puncturing and draining of the fluid in the cyst (arrows indicate the lesion and △ indicates the needle). (**c**) Sclerotherapy by lauromacrogol (arrows indicate the lesion and △ indicates the needle). (**d**) After sclerotherapy, gray-scale ultrasound shows that the volume of the cystic lesion (arrows) is significantly reduced (size: 13.2 mm × 6.8 mm; thickness: 5.4 mm)

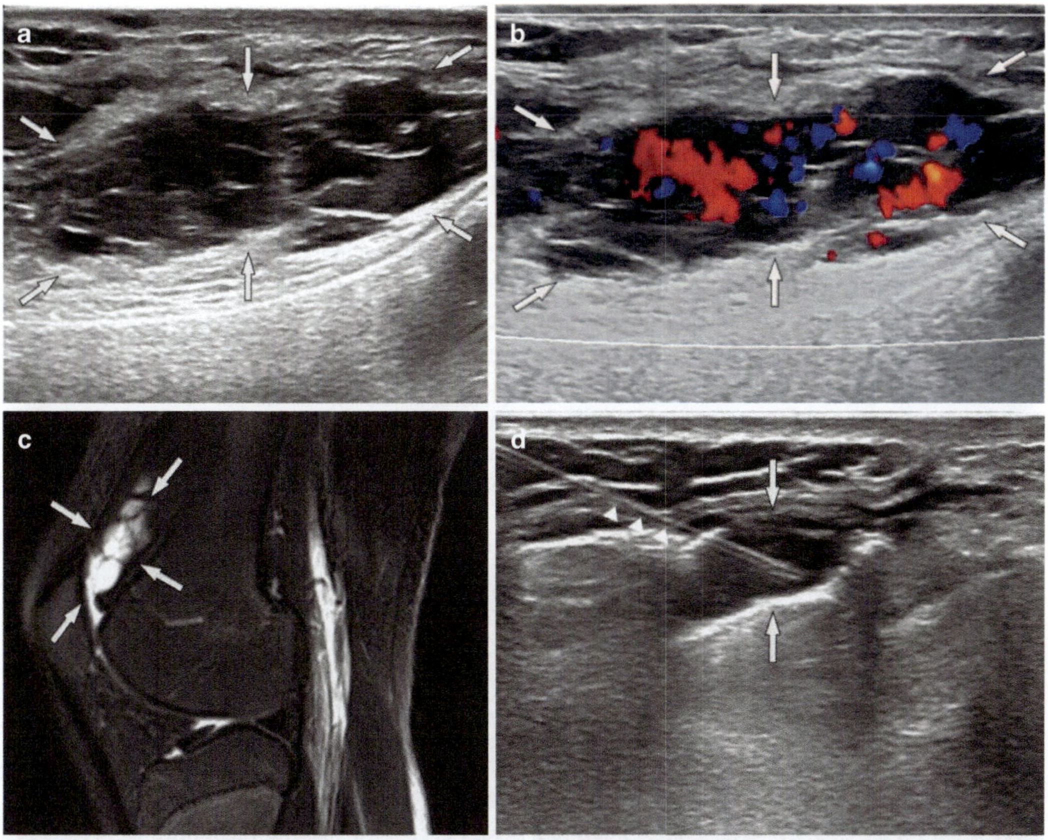

Fig. 1.46 Ultrasound-guided sclerotherapy of a hemangioma (Frequency: 11 MHz). (**a**) Gray-scale ultrasound shows an irregular, ill-defined mixed lesion (arrows) in the subcutaneous tissue (size: 26.0 mm × 19.0 mm; thickness: 10.9 mm). The lesion is heterogeneous, and honeycomb-like hypoechogenicity is visible (Frequency: 11 MHz). (**b**) Color Doppler ultrasound shows the blood flow signals increased transiently once the transducer is pressed onto the surface of the lesion (arrows) (Frequency: 11 MHz). (**c**) Contrast-enhanced magnetic resonance imaging shows that the lesion (arrows) is hyperenhanced. (**d**) Sclerotherapy by lauromacrogol (arrows indicate the lesion and △ indicates the needle)

noma. These methods have showed improved sensitivity in distinguishing melanoma from benign skin lesions. Studies showed that convolutional neural networks (CNNs) might achieve expert-level accuracy in the diagnosis of pigmented melanocytic lesions on clinical images. Meanwhile, neural networks have been shown to be able to classify dermoscopic and close-up images of nonpigmented skin lesions as accurately as experts.

Most studies on AI diagnosis of skin tumors are based on the recognition and classification of dermoscopic and clinical images. However, to our knowledge, there are few studies of AI in skin ultrasound currently. Skin ultrasound can provide information such as morphology, layer of involvement, and blood flow signals of the lesion that cannot be seen by dermoscopy. The combination of skin ultrasound and AI will play a positive role in promoting the diagnosis and treatment of skin diseases.

There is optimism that AI will result in positive clinical outcomes, which is driving research and investment in the use of AI for skin disease. However, AI for skin disease has not been widely practiced in clinical dermatology presently.

1.6.7 Superb Microvascular Imaging

Superb microvascular imaging (SMI) is an ultrasound imaging technique based on the of Doppler effect. SMI distinguishes the spectral signals generated by normal tissue movement and fine blood flow through adaptive algorithms.

SMI has the characteristics of high resolution, high sensitivity, high frame rate, and few motion artifacts. Also, it can detect low-velocity blood flow and fine blood vessels excellently. The application of SMI technology to measure blood perfusion in skin diseases has a wide application prospect (Fig. 1.47).

1.6.8 Tissue Harmonic Imaging

Tissue harmonic imaging (THI) is a kind of imaging method that uses the second or higher harmonic of echo signals from tissue. Based on the principle of nonlinear action between acoustic wave and tissue, filtering technology is used to remove the fundamental wave in the imaging process.

Tissue harmonics have the characteristics of acoustic nonlinearity, which can eliminate the reverberation caused by side lobes, and the noise and interference of fundamental waves. This can improve the SNR and the quality of far-field images, thereby improving the ability to detect lesions (Fig. 1.48).

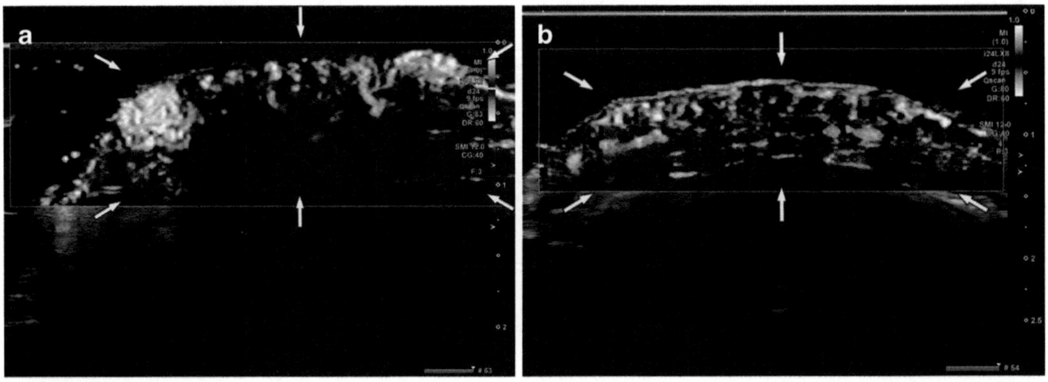

Fig. 1.47 Superb microvascular imaging (cutaneous hemangioma). (**a**) Superb microvascular imaging: the transducer is slightly placed on the surface of the lesion, and rich blood flow signals are visualized in the lesion (arrows) (Frequency: 24 MHz). (**b**) Superb microvascular imaging: When the transducer is pressed, the blood flow signals in the lesion are significantly decreased (arrows) (Frequency: 24 MHz)

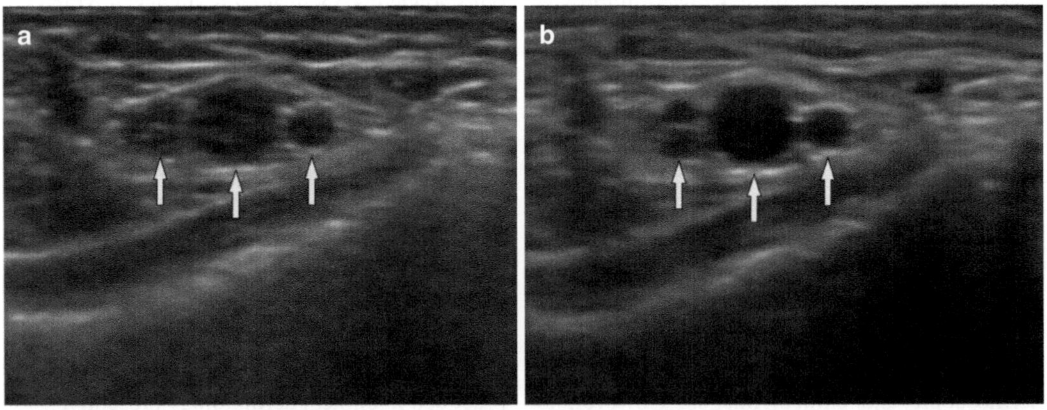

Fig. 1.48 Tissue harmonic imaging (subcutaneous vessel). (**a**) Image without THI (Frequency: 15 MHz). (**b**) Image with THI (Frequency: 15 MHz) (arrows show the vessels)

Key Points
- A variety of new ultrasound technologies are applied in the field of skin ultrasound.
- The clinical value of these new ultrasound techniques needs to be further evaluated.

1.7 Indications for Skin Ultrasound

High-frequency ultrasound realizes the visualization of the internal structure of skin diseases, and provides a variety of information inside the lesion, such as anatomical structure, involved layers, adjacent relationship, blood perfusion, and so on. It compensates for the lack of conventional visual observation and dermoscopy which can only provide information of lesion appearance. Through adjusting parameters and selecting auxiliary function, high-frequency ultrasound can perform local focusing and extended field of view of lesions, providing information of "details → whole → adjacency" of skin diseases, which is helpful for doctors to comprehensively evaluate skin diseases.

High-frequency ultrasound has the advantages of noninvasiveness, convenience, efficiency, and high cost-effectiveness, with high patient acceptance. Skin ultrasound can be widely carried out without contraindications. The commonly used indications are as follows.

1. Examination of subcutaneous mass (including palpable mass, changed appearance, and paresthesia).
2. Skin wound examination (including the evaluation of damage extend examination of residual foreign body, and scar and repair evaluation).
3. Differentiation between benign and malignant skin tumor.
4. To assess the involved layers and classification and staging of skin malignancies (including tumor thickness, peripheral tissue invasion, skin appendage involvement, deep tissue involvement, lymph node metastasis, and organ metastasis).
5. To assess the degree of involvement by skin inflammatory diseases, sinus formation, and effusion.
6. Used for formulating a plan before treatment.
7. Used for efficacy evaluation and follow-up monitoring after treatment.
8. Ultrasound-guided precise interventional diagnosis and treatment of skin diseases.

Key Points
- High-frequency ultrasound can provide a variety of information inside the lesion, such as anatomical structure, involved layers, adjacent relationship, blood perfusion, and so on.
- Skin ultrasound is widely used without contraindications.

Suggested Reading

1. Harald L, Elisabetta B. WHO manual of diagnostic ultrasound[M]. 2nd. ed. Malta: Gutenberg Press Ltd; 2011.
2. Kremkau FW. Sonography principles and instruments[M]. 8th ed. St. Louis: W.B. Saunders company; 2010.
3. Rukavina B, Mohar N. An approach of ultrasound diagnostic techniques of the skin and subcutaneous tissue [J]. Dermatologica. 1979;158(2):81–92.
4. Wortsman X, Wortsman J. Clinical usefulness of variable-frequency ultrasound in localized lesions of the skin [J]. J Am Acad Dermatol. 2010;62(2):247–56.
5. Fujimura T, Osanai O, Moriwaki S, et al. Development of a novel method to measure the elastic properties of skin including subcutaneous tissue: new age-related parameters and scope of application [J]. Skin Res Technol. 2008;14(4):504–11.
6. MacFarlane D, Shah K, Wysong A, et al. The role of imaging in the management of patients with nonmelanoma skin cancer: diagnostic modalities and applications [J]. J Am Acad Dermatol. 2017;76(4): 579–88.
7. Karimkhani C, Dellavalle RP, Coffeng LE, et al. Global skin disease morbidity and mortality: an update from the global burden of disease study 2013 [J]. JAMA Dermatol. 2017;153(5):406–12.
8. Rallan D, Harland CC. Ultrasound in dermatology-basic principles and applications [J]. Clin Exp Dermatol. 2003;28(6):632–8.
9. Song H, Robinson SN, Huang JT. Outpatient dermatology consultation impacts the diagnosis and management of pediatric oncology patients: a retrospective study [J]. J Am Acad Dermatol. 2017;77(5): 879–85.

10. Schmid-Wendtner MH, Burgdorf W. Ultrasound scanning in dermatology [J]. Arch Dermatol. 2005;141(2):217–24.
11. El-Zawahry MB, Abdel EEHM, Abd-El-Rahman RS, et al. Ultrasound biomicroscopy in the diagnosis of skin diseases [J]. Eur J Dermatol. 2007;17(6):469–75.
12. Piscaglia F, Bolondi L. Italian Society for Ultrasound in medicine and biology (SIUMB) study group on ultrasound contrast agents. The safety of Sonovue in abdominal applications: retrospective analysis of 23188 investigations [J]. Ultrasound Med Biol. 2006;32(9):1369–75.
13. Claudon M, Cosgrove D, Albrecht T, et al. Guidelines and good clinical practice recommendations for contrast enhanced ultrasound (CEUS) – update 2008 [J]. Ultraschall Med. 2008;29(1):28-44.
14. Sigrist RMS, Liau J, Kaffas AE, et al. Ultrasound elastography: review of techniques and clinical applications [J]. Theranostics. 2017;7(5):1303–29.
15. Alfageme F, Salgüero I, Nájera L, et al. Increased marginal stiffness differentiates infiltrative from non-infiltrative cutaneous basal cell carcinomas in the facial area: a prospective study [J]. J Ultrasound Med. 2019;38(7):1841–5.
16. Wang L, Yan F, Yang Y, et al. Quantitative assessment of skin stiffness in localized scleroderma using ultrasound shear-wave elastography [J]. Ultrasound Med Biol. 2017;43(7):1339–47.
17. Liu H, Hou Y, Zhu QL, et al. A preliminary study of skin ultrasound in diffuse cutaneous systemic sclerosis: does skin echogenicity matter? [J]. PLoS One. 2017;12(3):e0174481.

Anatomy and Ultrasound Manifestation of Normal Skin

2

Wei-Wei Ren, Li-Fan Wang, An-Qi Zhu, Chong-Ke Zhao, and Yi-Feng Zhang

2.1 Normal Skin Anatomy

The skin is the largest organ of the human body, which is the first barrier to the hostile external damage and environment. Skin is composed of epidermis, dermis, subcutaneous tissue, and skin appendages.

The epidermis mainly includes corneum, granulosum, spinosum and basale, and lamina lucida on the palms and soles.

The dermis mainly includes the papillary and reticular layers, containing structures such as blood vessels, lymphatic vessels, nerves, and sweat glands.

The skin appendages include blood vessels, lymphatic vessels, nerves, hair follicles, sebaceous glands, sweat glands and nails, etc. Among them, the texture of the nail is very hard, also known as nail plate, divided into two layers: dorsal nail plate and ventral nail plate.

Subcutaneous tissue mainly includes adipose tissue (Fig. 2.1). The thickness of normal human skin varies greatly according to age, gender, and location, with the approximate thickness range of 0.5 ~ 4.0 mm.

W.-W. Ren (✉) · L.-F. Wang · A.-Q. Zhu
C.-K. Zhao · Y.-F. Zhang
Department of Medical Ultrasound, Shanghai Tenth People's Hospital, Ultrasound Research and Education Institute, School of Medicine, Tongji University, Shanghai, China

2.2 Ultrasound Manifestation of Normal Skin

2.2.1 Epidermis and Dermis

When the ultrasound transducer with a frequency of 50 MHz is used to examine the normal skin, from shallow to deep, it showed three echo bands: high-echo, hyper-echo, and hypo-echo, representing the epidermis, dermis, and subcutaneous soft tissues, respectively. Among the above three echo bands, there are approximately two parallel demarcation lines, which are: the demarcation between high-echo epidermis and hyper-echo dermis, and the demarcation between hyper-echo dermis and hypo-echo subcutaneous soft tissue.

The hyperechogenicity of the epidermis is caused by the reflection of the acoustic beam due to the smooth surface and the dense stratum corneum. The thickness of the epidermis is thin, generally ranges from 1.0 mm to 2.0 mm. Discontinuous oblique hyperechogenicity is visible in the surface, representing hair. Due to the presence of the hypoechoic lamina lucida on the palms and soles, the epidermis shows a special "double line sign", that is, two parallel hyperechoic thin lines.

The dermal tissue is relatively loose and shows hyperechogenicity, with scattered punctate or linear hypoechoic or anechoic areas, representing skin appendages and blood vessels in the dermis.

H. Xu et al. (eds.), *Diagnostic Ultrasound in Dermatology*,
https://doi.org/10.1007/978-981-16-7345-0_2

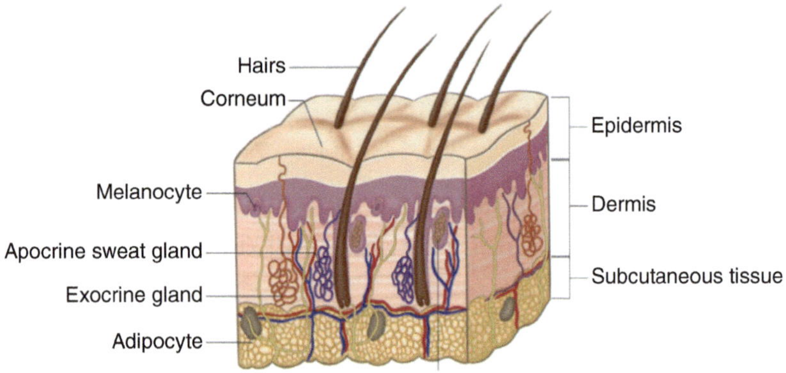

Fig. 2.1 Schematic diagram of skin anatomy

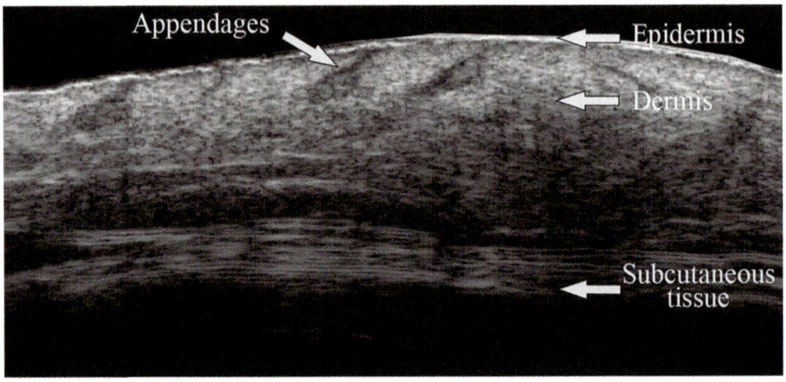

Fig. 2.2 High-frequency ultrasound of normal skin (Frequency: 50 MHz)

The adipose tissue in subcutaneous tissue layer is hypoechoic, and the fibrous connective tissue shows hyperechoic strip or reticular septa (Fig. 2.2).

When normal skin is examined by an ultrasound transducer with a frequency of <20 MHz, the demarcation between hyperechoic dermis and hypoechoic subcutaneous tissue can still be visible. However, the demarcation between hyperechoic epidermis and hyperechoic dermis is often invisible, and it is also difficult to show tiny structures such as skin appendages. When lesions appear in these layers, they are visible using a transducer with a frequency of >20 MHz (Fig. 2.3).

It should be emphasized that the thickness of skin layers varies in different parts of the human body, and there are significant differences between individuals. Overall, the thickness of all layers of skin: male > female, adult > child, dorsal > ventral, trunk > extremities > face (Fig. 2.4).

In addition, the lips, anus, and glans are mucosal tissues. Although they show layer-like structures similar to the skin, they are completely different from the layers of the skin, and there are no appendages. Therefore, the anatomical terms of the skin cannot be applied. Generally, the superficial mucosa and deep mucosa are used to express the location and depth of the lesions.

2.2.2 Skin Appendages

2.2.2.1 Nails

The dorsal and ventral nail plates of the nails show isometric linear hyperechogenicity on ultrasound, with anechoic interdeck space between them. The nail matrix is located in the proximal nail plate and is the germinal area of the nail plate. The ventral nail matrix may be hypoechoic in some people. The nail bed is located in the deep part of the nail plate and adjacent to the nail plate, and appears as a hypoechoic

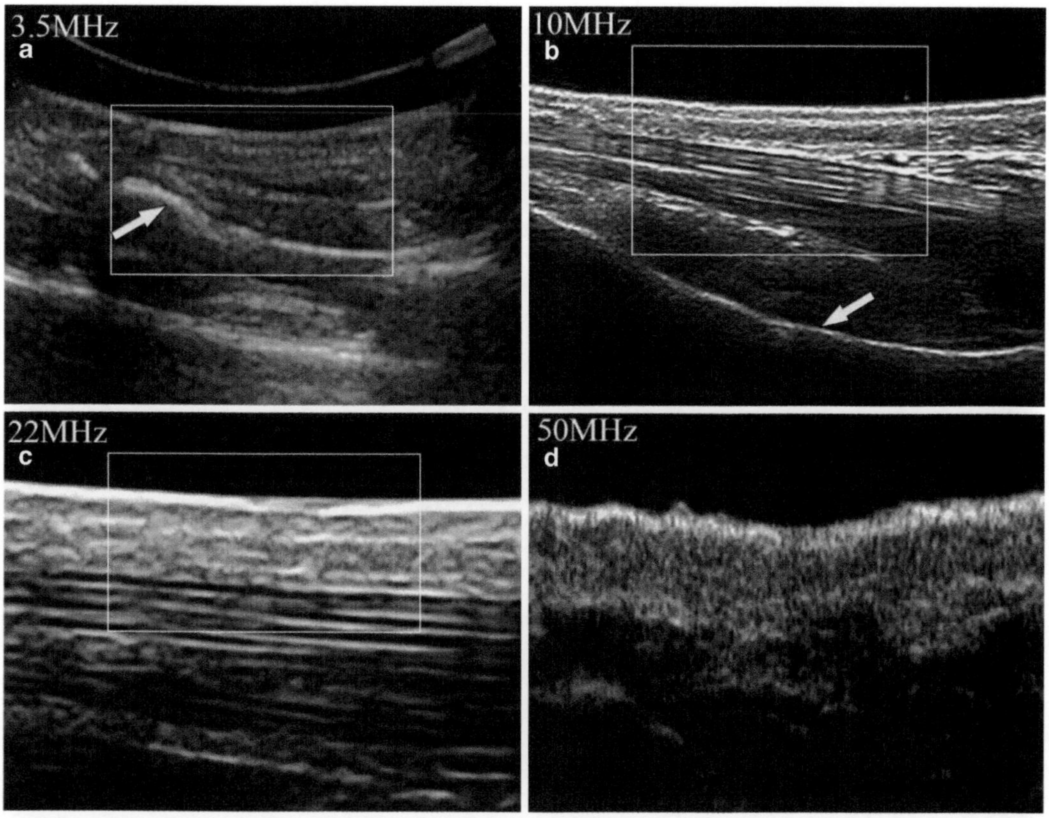

Fig. 2.3 High-frequency ultrasound of normal skin in the same part of human body (palm) at different frequencies. Fig. b is the part inside the white box in Fig. a, Fig. c is the part inside the white box in Fig. b, and Fig. d is the part inside the white box in Fig. c. With the frequency of the ultrasound transducer increases, the skin structure is more clearly displayed. The arrow indicates the metacarpal bone

structure on ultrasound. The thickness of the nail bed should be measured in the middle of the distal phalanx. The distal phalanx is located deep in the nail bed and appears as a linear hyperechogenicity on ultrasound (Fig. 2.5).

2.2.2.2 Nerves

The basic constituent units of peripheral nerves are nerve fibers, which are composed of axons and myelin sheaths (Schwann cells) of neurons. The connective tissue surrounding the myelin sheath is the endoneurium. Several nerve fibers make up the nerve bundle, which is surrounded by the fascia. Several nerve bundles make up the nerve trunk, which is surrounded by the epineurium.

On high-frequency ultrasound, the nerve bundles are hypoechoic, and the perineurium and epineurium are hyperechoic. In the transverse section, the nerve bundles show oval or round hypoechogenicity in different sizes, and formed a "mesh like" structure with the hyperechoic nerve bundles. In the longitudinal section, the nerve bundles show hypoechogenicity arranged in parallel strips, with several hyperechoic perineurium in the middle (Fig. 2.6).

2.2.2.3 Blood Vessels

Blood vessels refer to a series of tubes through which blood flows. Except epidermis, hair, cornea, and dentin, blood vessels are spread throughout the human body. The dermis, subcutaneous tissues, and skin appendages are distributed with blood vessels, including arteries, veins, and capillaries that supply the sweat glands, nerves, and muscles (Fig. 2.7).

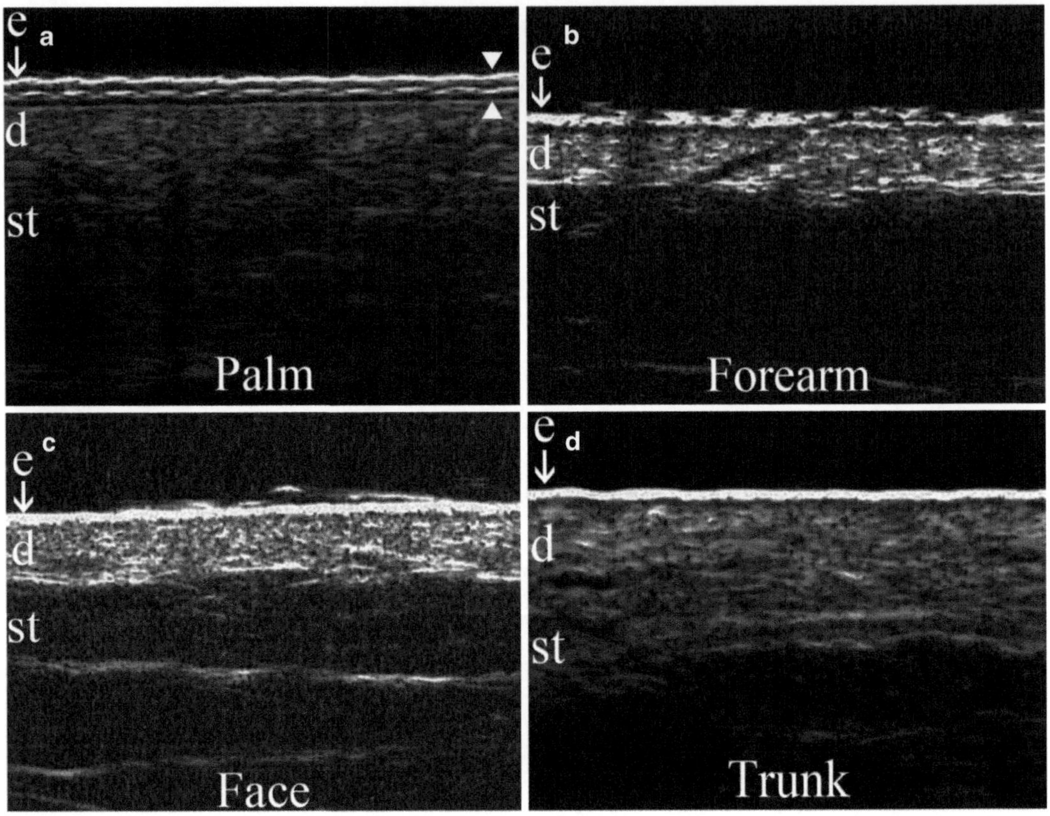

Fig. 2.4 High-frequency ultrasound of normal skin at different positions of human body (Frequency: 50 MHz). (**a**) High-frequency ultrasound of skin in the palm. (**b**) High-frequency ultrasound of skin in the forearm. (**c**) High-frequency ultrasound of skin in the face. (**d**) High-frequency ultrasound of skin in the trunk. e indicates the epidermis, d indicates the dermis, st indicates the subcutaneous tissue; △ indicates the "double line sign" at the palm

2.2.3 Subcutaneous Tissue

The subcutaneous tissue is located deep in the dermis, and mainly includes adipose tissue. Adipose tissue not only stores energy, but also buffers external pressure. The subcutaneous tissue also includes rich blood vessels, nerves, lymphatic vessels, and hair follicles (Fig. 2.8).

Key Points

- For skin ultrasound, it is recommended to select the transducer with frequency of >20 MHz. The ultrasound biomicroscope can display more details.
- On high-frequency ultrasound with frequency of >20 MHz, the skin can show "three echo bands" and "two demarcations," providing an important reference for the diagnosis of skin diseases.
- The thickness of skin layer varies from site to site, and there are also significant differences between individuals.

2.3 Training and Suggestions

For the centers that carry out skin high-frequency ultrasound for the first time, standardized personnel training shall be carried out and sufficient assistance shall be provided.

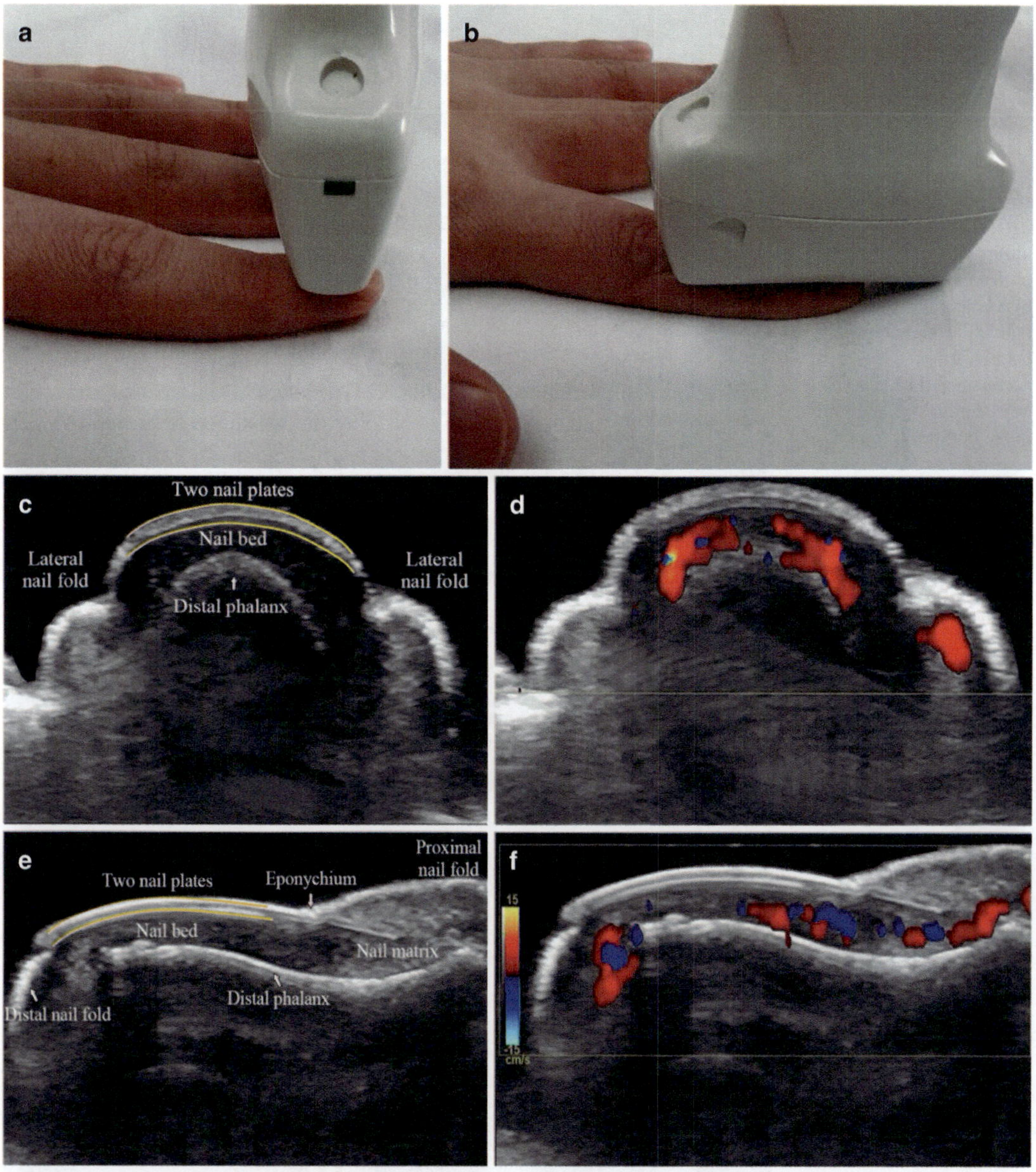

Fig. 2.5 High-frequency ultrasound of nail (Frequency: 15 MHz). (**a**) Schematic diagram of short-axis ultrasound of nails. (**b**) Schematic diagram of long-axis ultrasound of nails. (**c**) Gray-scale ultrasound of short-axis of nails. (**d**) Color Doppler ultrasound of short-axis of nails shows blood flow signals inside the nail bed. (**e**) Gray-scale ultrasound of long-axis of nails. (**f**) Color Doppler ultrasound of long-axis of nails shows blood flow signals inside the nail bed

2.3.1 Personnel Training

It is recommended to select and cultivate specialized skin ultrasound doctors from physicians with a background in dermatology or ultrasound medicine. Before making independent diagnosis, ultrasound diagnosis of skin diseases with gold standard reference shall be completed at a minimum of 200 cases and the doctors should pass the relevant national competence accreditation test.

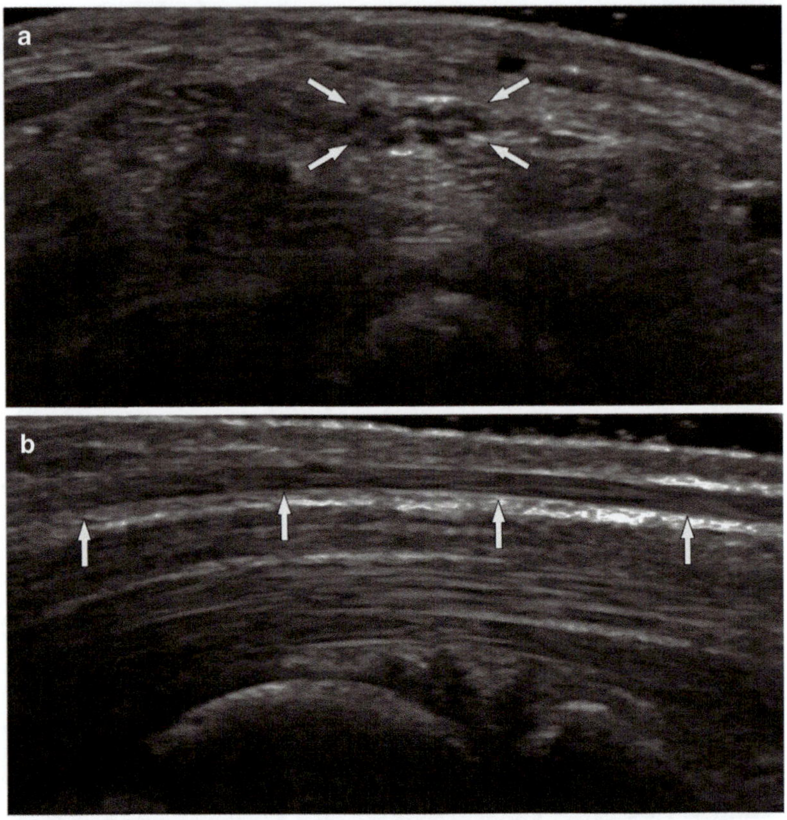

Fig. 2.6 High-frequency ultrasound of nerves (Frequency: 15 MHz). (**a**) The short-axis gray-scale ultrasound of the nerve with a "mesh like" structure (arrows). (**b**) Gray-scale ultrasound of long-axis of nerves shows hypoechogenic nerve bundles arranged in parallel strips, accompanied by several hyperechoic perineurium in the middle (arrows)

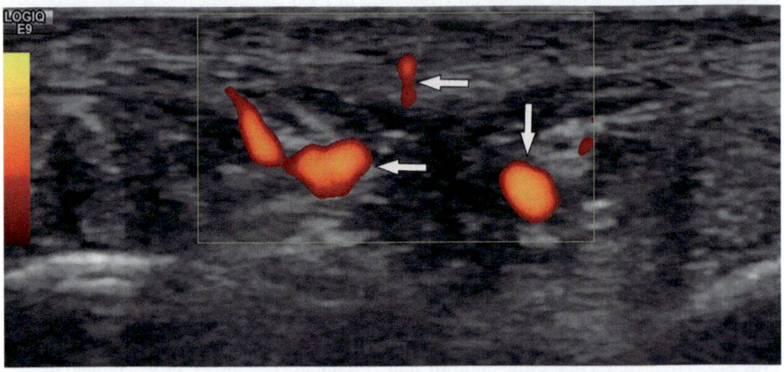

Fig. 2.7 Power Doppler ultrasound of small subcutaneous vessels (arrows) (Frequency: 15 MHz)

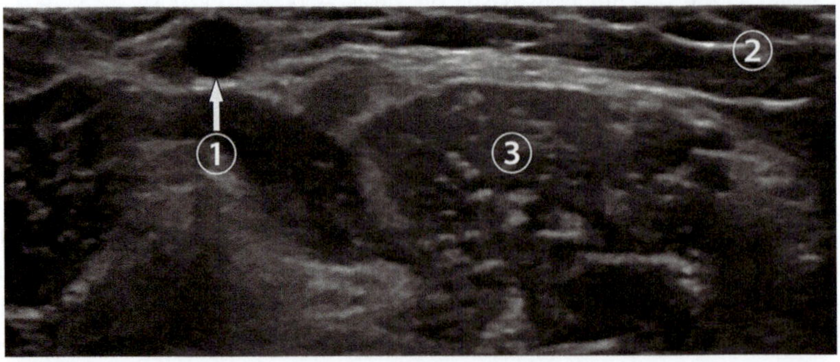

Fig. 2.8 Subcutaneous tissue. ① Blood vessel; ② Adipose tissue; ③ Muscle

A standardized report of the US examination is recommended and images should be provided together with the report.

2.3.2 Ultrasound Device

The frequency of skin ultrasound transducer should be ≥20 MHz. If possible, more transducers with different frequencies are equipped, including low-frequency transducers and ultrasound biomicroscope. Desktop or portable color Doppler ultrasound devices can be selected. If the frequency is high enough, pocket ultrasound devices can also be used.

2.3.3 Disinfection Materials

Skin diseases often have open wound and secretion on the skin surface. In order to protect the transducer and prevent cross infection, it is recommended to provide the isolation sleeve, gel pad, and sterile gel. It is also equipped with medical gauze or medical wet wipe for cleaning the patient's skin and ultrasound transducer after examination. In addition, it is necessary to provide ultraviolet lamp and disinfectant for the ultrasound device and environment.

2.3.4 Image Database

The operators should develop the working habit of saving the ultrasound images of skin diseases, including gray-scale image, color Doppler ultrasound image, and appearance photograph. The operators should archive them according to certain rules, and establish a retrievable image database for future scientific research and teaching. It is recommended to use digital imaging and communication in medicine (DICOM) format for image format, so as to facilitate subsequent image analysis. At the same time, a follow-up system is also established to record the pathological results and clinical data of each case.

2.3.5 Popularization and Communication

It is recommended to fully communicate with clinicians, introduce the advantages and potential clinical benefits of high-frequency ultrasound, and provide relevant special training when necessary. At the same time, popularization can be achieved through exhibition board, electronic screen, Internet, social media, TV, and others to improve patient awareness and acceptance.

2.3.6 Skin Ultrasound Examination Reporting

It is recommended to establish a picture archiving and communication systems (PACS) workstation to form a standard report template of skin ultrasound. The report is divided into four parts. The first is the basic information of the patient for the confirmation and retrieval of the patient's identity. The second is the ultrasound description, in which the complete information of the disease is recorded through a unified ultrasound terminology. The third, all information is synthesized to give one or several (in order of priority) possible ultrasound diagnoses, and clinical suggestions are made when necessary. The last is the signature of the ultrasound doctor and the date. In addition, according to local regulations and clinical needs, figures can be attached.

2.3.7 Other Suggestions

In principle, each lesion should be described in detail. If multiple lesions have similar manifestations, representative lesions can be selected for description. When the ultrasound features or the final diagnosis of different lesions varies, the lesions need to be described separately. If malignancy is suspected, the draining lymph nodes need to be examined.

Suggested Reading

1. Ran ML, Liu DH, Zhang JQ, et al. Comparative study of 20 MHz and 50 MHz ultrasound skin imaging and measurement [J] (in Chinese). Chinese J Dermatol. 2017;50(7):482–6.
2. Wortsman X. Sonography of dermatologic emergencies [J]. J Ultrasound Med. 2017;36(9):1905–14.
3. Mlosek RK, Malinowska S. Ultrasound image of the skin, apparatus and imaging basics [J]. J Ultrason. 2013;13(53):212–21.
4. Kleinerman R, Whang TB, Bard RL, et al. Ultrasound in dermatology: principles and applications [J]. J Am Acad Dermatol. 2012;67(3):478–87.
5. Schmid-Wendtner MH, Burgdorf W. Ultrasound scanning in dermatology [J]. Arch Dermatol. 2005;141(2):217–24.
6. El-Zawahry MB, Abdel EEHM, Abd-El-Rahman RS, et al. Ultrasound biomicroscopy in the diagnosis of skin diseases [J]. Eur J Dermatol. 2007;17(6):469–75.
7. Losquadro WD. Anatomy of the skin and the pathogenesis of nonmelanoma skin cancer [J]. Facial Plast Surg Clin North Am. 2017;25(3):283–9.

Other Imaging Techniques for Skin

3

An-Qi Zhu, Hui-Xiong Xu, Le-Hang Guo, Li-Fan Wang, Qiao Wang, Li-Ping Sun, Hui Shi, and Pei-Ru Wang

3.1 Dermoscopy

Dermoscopy is the most widely used non-invasive technique for the examination of skin diseases. It is essentially a skin microscope that can magnify tens of times and observe the subtle structure of the lesion by filtering polarized light and optical amplification. Using dermoscopy, the operator can visualize the fine contour and color of the surface of the lesion that is not visible to the naked eye (Fig. 3.1). Studies have showed that dermoscopy can be used as a method for pre-operative assessment of the margin of basal cell carcinoma (BCC), which can significantly increase the rate of complete resection.

Dermoscopy can be used to observe the appearance characteristics of the surface of the lesion. However, it cannot detect the internal information of the lesion, such as the depth of lesion infiltration, the relationship with the surrounding tissues, etc. In addition, many skin diseases have no obvious appearance change, such as deep mass located in subcutaneous tissue, and it is difficult for dermoscopy to provide valuable information at this time.

Studies have showed that in melanoma, dermoscopy improves sensitivity from 71% to 90% and specificity from 81% to 90% compared to macroscopic inspection. Dermoscopy has a high sensitivity for the diagnosis of cutaneous malignancies and can reduce the number of unnecessary biopsies of skin lesions. However, some skin malignancies may lack specific dermoscopic features, and the dermoscopic appearance of skin diseases may vary according to age, skin type, location, and degree of sun damage. As a result, some skin diseases cannot be directly diagnosed by dermoscopy alone.

A.-Q. Zhu (✉) · L.-F. Wang · L.-P. Sun · H. Shi
Department of Medical Ultrasound, Shanghai Tenth People's Hospital, Ultrasound Research and Education Institute, School of Medicine, Tongji University, Shanghai, China

H.-X. Xu · Q. Wang
Department of Medical Ultrasound, Shanghai Tenth People's Hospital, Ultrasound Research and Education Institute, School of Medicine, Tongji University, Shanghai, China

Department of Medical Ultrasound, Shanghai Skin Disease Hospital, Ultrasound Research and Education Institute, School of Medicine, Tongji University, Shanghai, China

L.-H. Guo
Department of Medical Ultrasound, Shanghai Skin Disease Hospital, Ultrasound Research and Education Institute, School of Medicine, Tongji University, Shanghai, China

P.-R. Wang
Shanghai Skin Disease Hospital, Institute of Photomedicine, School of Medicine, Tongji University, Shanghai, China

H. Xu et al. (eds.), *Diagnostic Ultrasound in Dermatology*,
https://doi.org/10.1007/978-981-16-7345-0_3

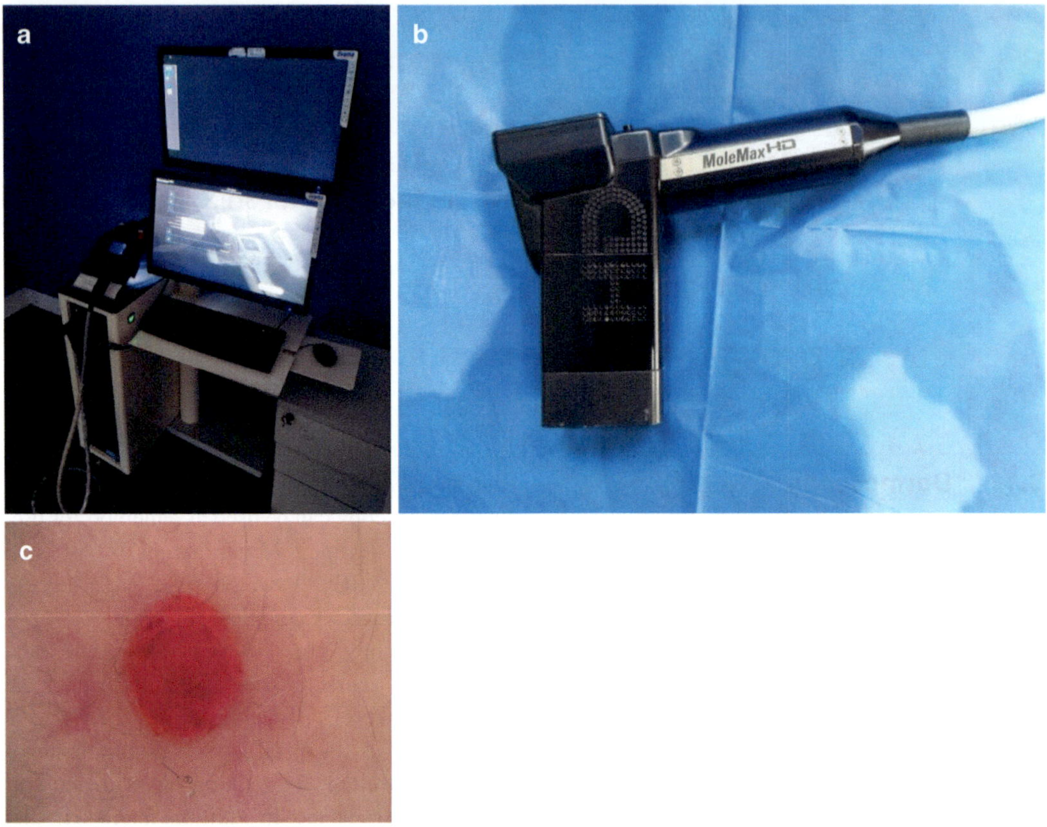

Fig. 3.1 Dermoscopic (Austria: MoleMax HD) for skin diseases (granulomatous inflammation). (**a**) Dermoscopy device. (**b**) The camera of dermoscopy. (**c**) Dermoscopic appearance of the erythematous lesion on the face shows a round well-defined erythema, with smooth surface and no scales

3.2 Optical Coherence Tomography

Optical coherence tomography (OCT) uses light in the near-infrared spectral range to irradiate the tissue and produce interference according to the coherence characteristics of the light, so as to realize tissue imaging (Fig. 3.2).

OCT is a new and high-definition tomography imaging technology integrating optics, laser, ultrasensitive detection control, and computer image process. Since its invention in 1991, OCT has been initially applied in ophthalmology in the medical field and subsequently developed in dermatology. The axial resolution of OCT is as high as 1.0 ~ 15.0 μm, and the penetration depth is as high as 1.5 ~ 2.0 mm.

The longitudinal image of skin tissue can be obtained, and the morphology of epidermis and dermis can be clearly shown (Fig. 3.3). The disadvantage is that it cannot achieve cell-level imaging, and lesions with a depth of more than 2.0 mm cannot be visualized. OCT has not been widely used in clinical practice yet.

3.3 Confocal Laser Scanning Microscope

Confocal laser scanning microscope (CLSM) is a new non-invasive light microscope, also known as skin CT, which is a cellular biological image analyzer (Fig. 3.4). The imaging principle is based on the different reflection and refraction coefficients of different cells and tissues to the laser, and it achieves cell-level imaging and clearly shows the subtle structure of cells.

CLSM can perform layer-by-layer cellular imaging, which can obtain coronal images of tissues, and its images are comparable to histological sections (Fig. 3.5). In addition, CLSM can also perform multiple imaging of the lesion site, which has the advantages of real-time and dynamic scanning, facilitating the operator to observe the cellular and histological characteristics of the lesion site.

The limitation of CLSM is that its detection range is limited by the depth of laser penetra-

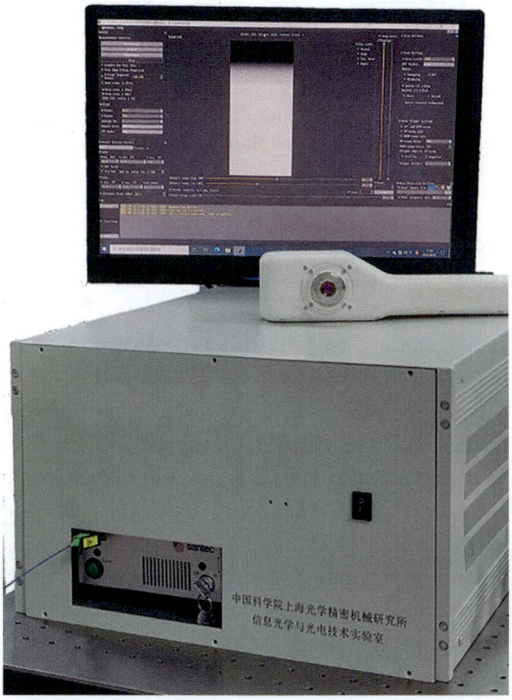

Fig. 3.2 Optical coherence tomography (Shanghai Institute of Optics and Fine Mechanics, Chinese Academy of Sciences)

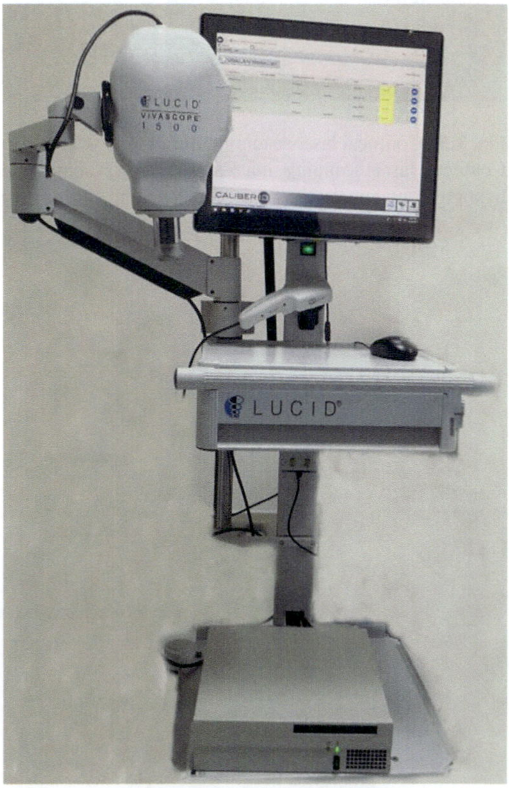

Fig. 3.4 Confocal laser scanning microscope (LUCID: VivaScope®)

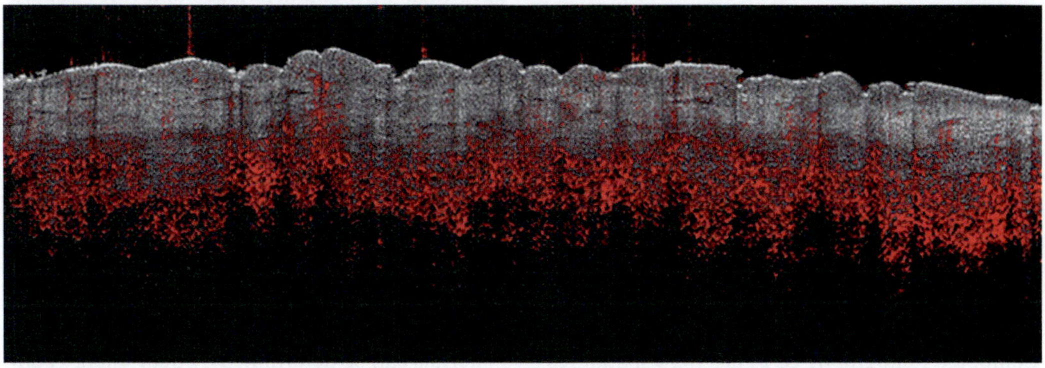

Fig. 3.3 Optical coherence tomography image of normal skin (male, dorsum of hand). Full-field thickness = 3.0 mm, display thickness = 1.5 mm

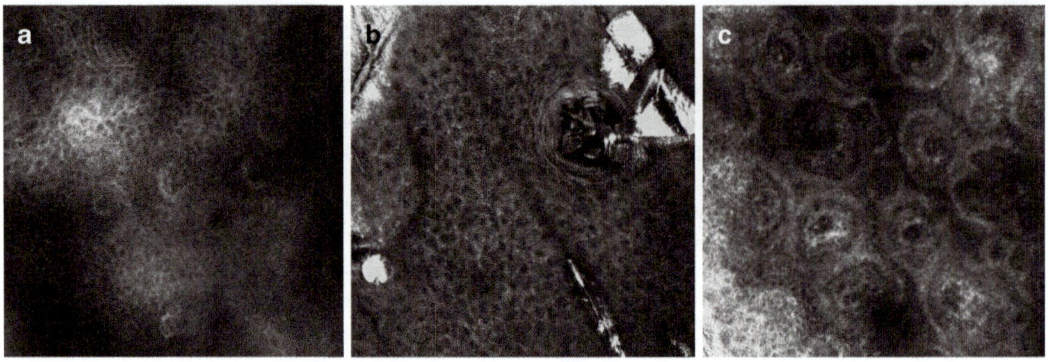

Fig. 3.5 Confocal laser scanning microscope images. (**a**) Confocal laser scanning microscope shows significant hypopigmentation in the basal cell layer in vitiligo. (**b**) Confocal laser scanning microscope shows Demodex mites in rosacea. (**c**) Confocal laser scanning microscope shows papillomatous hyperplasia in psoriasis

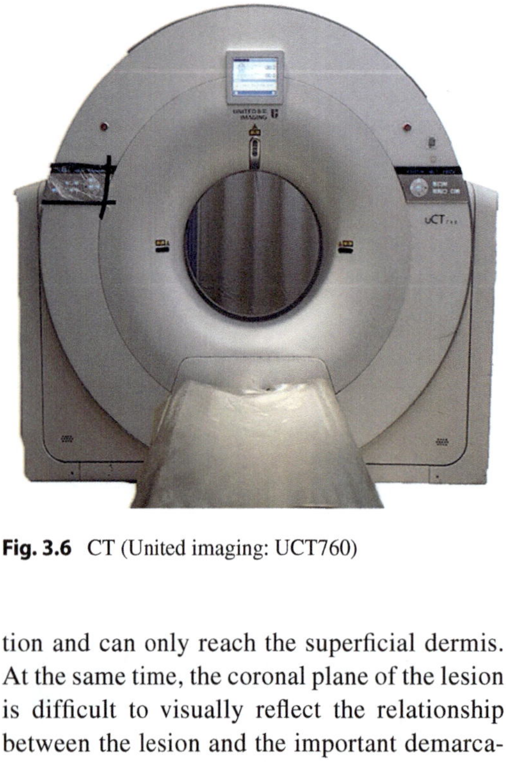

Fig. 3.6 CT (United imaging: UCT760)

tion and can only reach the superficial dermis. At the same time, the coronal plane of the lesion is difficult to visually reflect the relationship between the lesion and the important demarcation line of the skin, and is inconsistent with the section direction of the pathological specimen.

3.4 Computed Tomography

Computed tomography (CT) has high spatial resolution and is superior to other imaging examinations for bone. Therefore, CT is often used as a preoperative assessment method for some cutaneous malignancies with a large extent of invasion (Fig. 3.6).

CT can not only show the location, size, border, depth of invasion of the lesion, and the relationship between the lesion and the surrounding tissues, but also show the presence of bone erosion, surrounding lymph nodes and distant organ metastasis. It is frequently used for systemic assessment of more aggressive tumors such as cutaneous squamous cell carcinoma and melanoma.

During CT scan, when the density of the lesion is close to that of normal tissue, the lesion is difficult to be visualized. Contrast-enhanced CT is emerged with the contrast agent injected. The quantity (iodine content) and distribution (iodine distribution) of contrast agent absorption have their own characteristics and rules according to different tissues and different pathological properties. In this condition, not only the image contrast is increased, the demarcation between the lesion and the normal tissue is clear, and the density, shape, and size are more distinguishable, which is also conducive to the detection and diagnosis of lesions (Fig. 3.7).

By analyzing the difference in attenuation observed in a material exposed to two different X-ray spectra simultaneously, the composition of materials can be determined by dual-energy computed tomography (DECT). It has recently been shown to reliably help identify uric acid deposi-

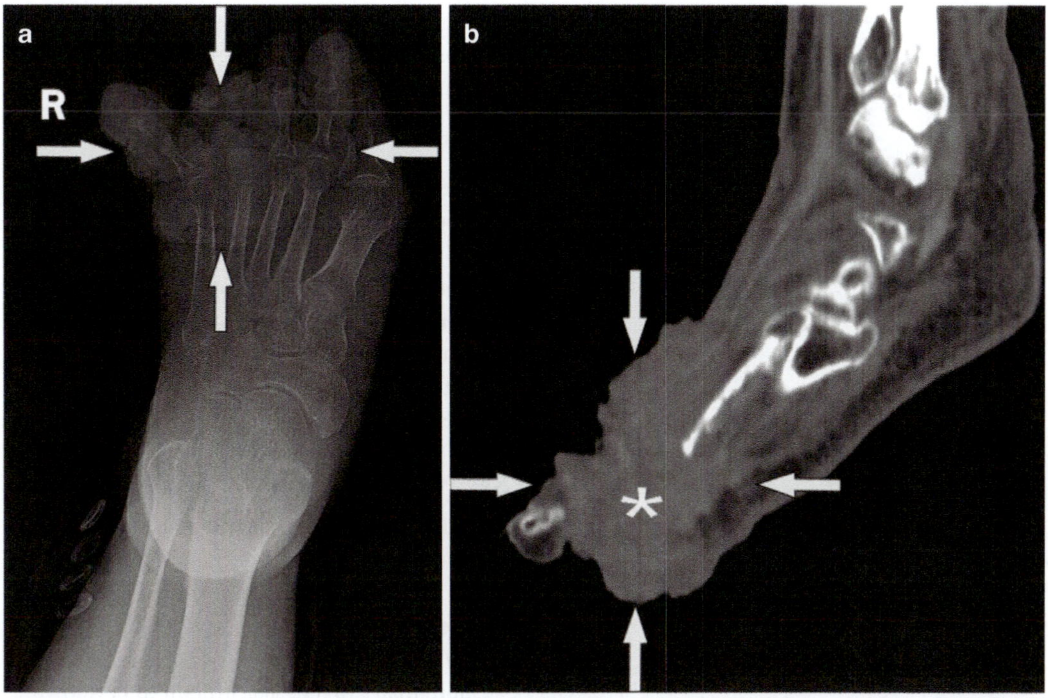

Fig. 3.7 X-ray and CT of cutaneous squamous cell carcinoma on foot. Female, 50 years of age. (**a**) X-ray shows the soft tissue in the distal part of the left foot (plantar and dorsal foot) is swollen and elevated. An irregular, ill-defined lesion is seen with uneven density (arrows). The bone resorption of the fourth and fifth phalangeal of the left foot is basically complete, and the bone resorption of the fourth metatarsal bone is partial. (**b**) CT scan shows detailed morphology of the lesion and the degree of bone destruction (arrows)

tion by exploiting the photon energy-dependent attenuation of different materials (Fig. 3.8).

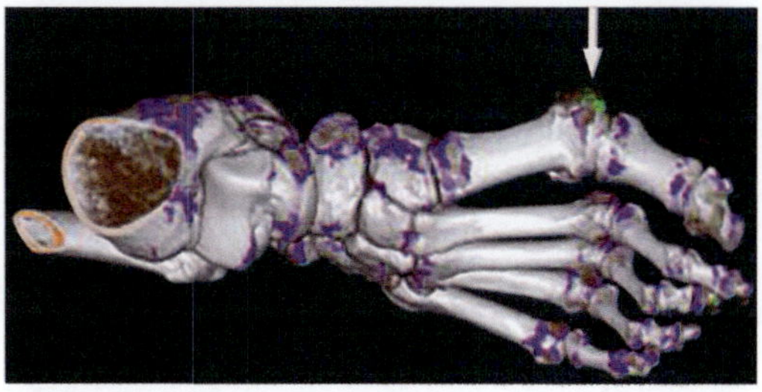

Fig. 3.8 Dual-energy computed tomography of the right foot (gouty arthritis). DECT shows monosodium urate crystals (green color) in the first metatarsophalangeal joint (arrow)

3.5 Magnetic Resonance Imaging

Magnetic resonance imaging (MRI) has the advantages of high soft tissue resolution and no radiation. MRI can show the location, size, border, depth involvement of the lesion, and the relationship between the lesion and the surrounding tissues (Fig. 3.9).

Various parameters constitute different types of sequences. Based on it, MRI scan tissues and organs to obtain images with different contrast (Fig. 3.10). Sequences include T1-weighted imaging (T1WI), T2-weighted imaging (T2WI), proton density weighted imaging (PDWI), diffuse weighted imaging (DWI), susceptibility weighted imaging (SWI), arterial spin labeling (ASL), and so on.

MRI also has some limitations, such as relatively time-consuming and inferior display of bone compared to CT. In addition, patients with metal implants cannot undergo MRI. MRI is

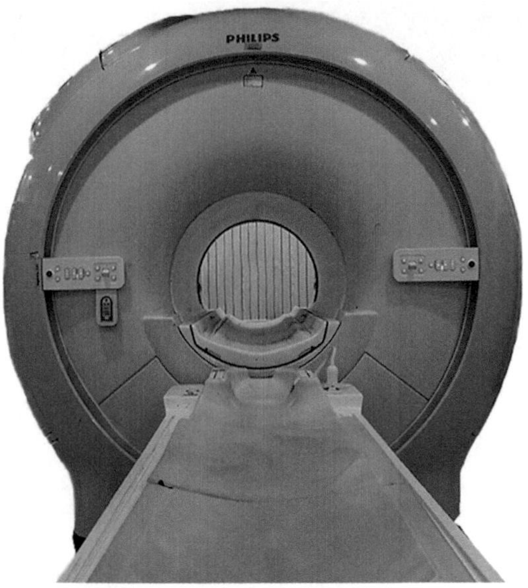

Fig. 3.9 MR (PHILIPS: Ingenia 3.0 T)

rarely used in skin diseases due to the superficial location of most skin diseases.

3.6 Comparison of Various Skin Imaging Techniques

The various skin imaging techniques have their own advantages, but it is often difficult to achieve a balance between resolution and penetration depth. For example, the resolution of CLSM is as high as 1.0 μm, but the imaging depth is less than 1.0 mm. While, the imaging depth of conventional CT or MRI imaging is deeper, but the resolution is low.

Ultrasound can achieve a good balance between imaging depth and resolution. Through the adjustment of transducer frequency, the resolution can span the scale from μm to cm, and the imaging depth can span the scale from mm to cm (Fig. 3.11). Therefore, it has a great potential in the diagnosis of skin diseases (Table 3.1).

Key Points

- Dermoscopy is currently the most widely used imaging modality in dermatology, but it cannot obtain deep information of skin diseases.
- The axial resolution of OCT is as high as 1.0 ~ 15.0 μm, while lesions with a depth of more than 2.0 mm are difficult to be shown.
- CLSM enables imaging at the cell-level, but the depth can only reach the superficial dermis. Simultaneously, CLSM can obtain coronal imaging, while it is difficult to show important demarcation lines in every layer of the skin.
- CT and MRI are rarely used in skin diseases due to the superficial location of most skin diseases.

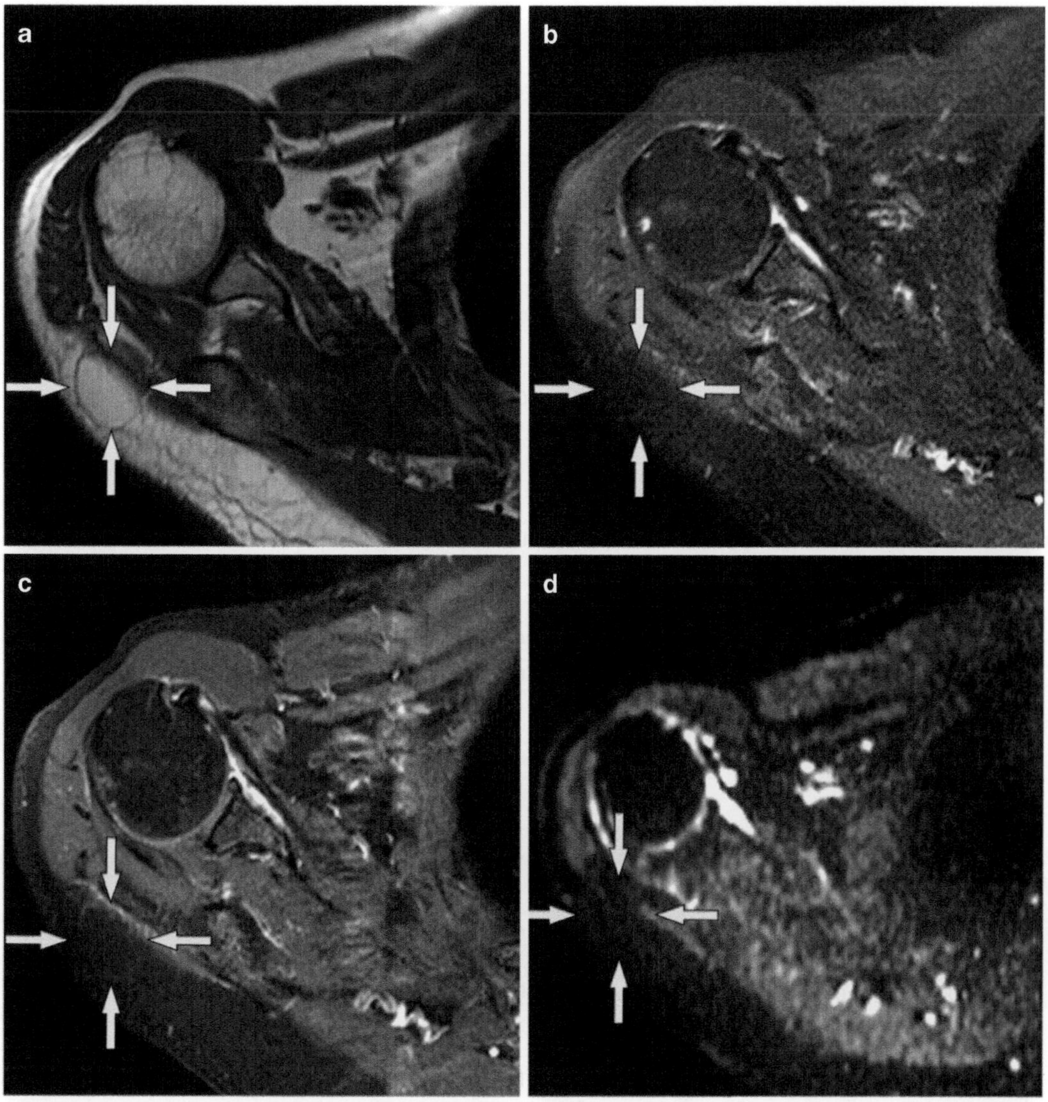

Fig. 3.10 MRI of soft tissue tumor (lipoma). Male, 64 years of age. (**a**) An oval lesion can be seen in the subcutaneous tissue of right shoulder joint (size: 21.5 × 17.2 mm). It is regular and well-defined. The surrounding fat space is clear. And the lesion shows hyperintense signal on T1WI. (**b**) The lesion shows hyperintense signal on T2WI. (**c**) The lesion shows hypointense signal on T2WI-FS. (**d**) Enhanced MR imaging shows no enhancement of the lesion. Lesions are indicated by arrows

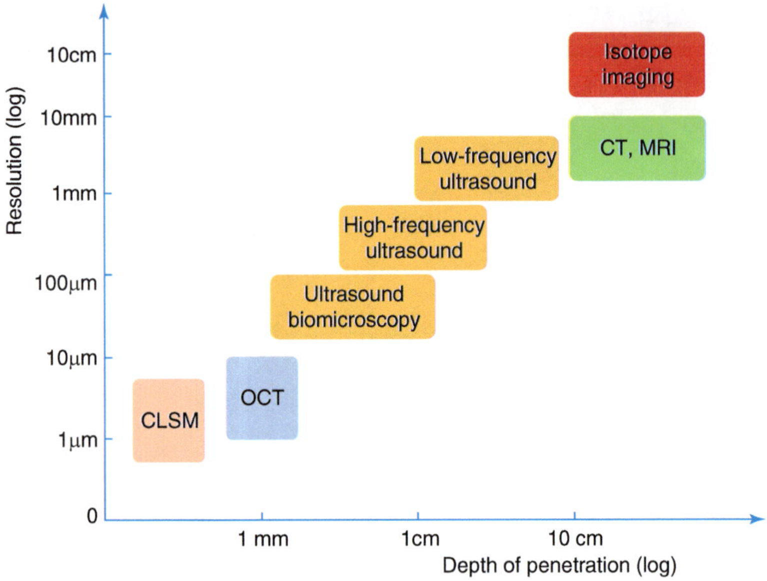

Fig. 3.11 Resolution and imaging depth of various skin imaging technologies

Table 3.1 Principles and characteristics of common skin imaging technologies

	Dermoscopy	CLSM	OCT	Ultrasound
Imaging technologies	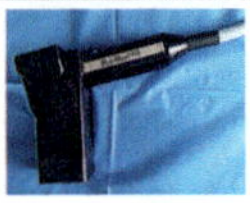	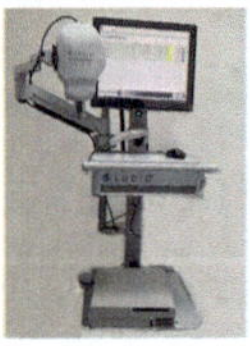	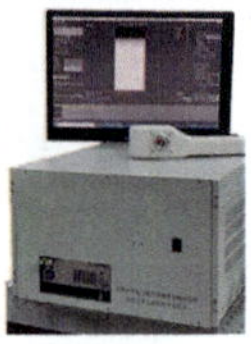	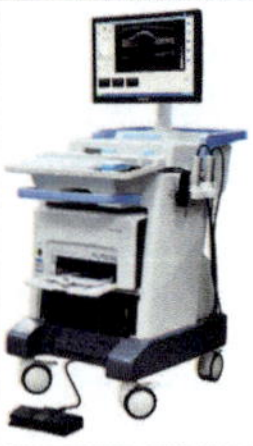
Imaging principles	Optical	Optical	Optical	Acoustic
Imaging depth	0 mm	0 ~ 350 μm	0 ~ 2 mm	1 mm ~ 50 mm
Transverse resolution	< 10 μm	5 μm	5 ~ 15 μm	40 μm ~ 1 mm
Imaging direction	Transversal direction	Transversal direction	Longitudinal direction	Longitudinal direction
Imaging layer	Epidermal surface	Epidermis	Epidermis + superficial dermis	Epidermis + dermis + subcutaneous tissue
Schematic diagram	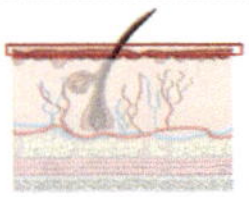	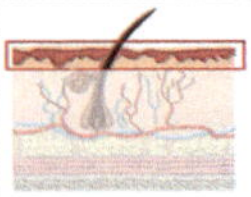	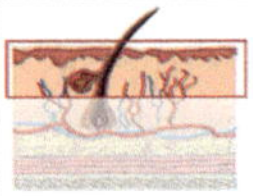	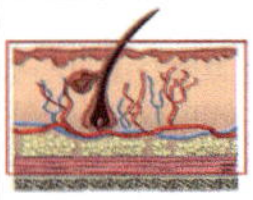

Suggested Reading

1. Yelamos O, Braun RP, Liopyris K, et al. Usefulness of dermoscopy to improve the clinical and histopathologic diagnosis of skin cancers [J]. J Am Acad Dermatol. 2019;80(2):365–77.
2. Reiter O, Mimouni I, Dusza S, et al. Dermoscopic features of basal cell carcinoma and its subtypes: a systematic review [J]. J Am Acad Dermatol. 2021;85(3):653–64.
3. Carducci M, Bozzetti M, De Marco G, et al. Usefulness of margin detection by digital dermoscopy in the traditional surgical excision of basal cell carcinomas of the head and neck including infiltrative/morpheaform type [J]. J Dermatol. 2012;39(4):326–30.
4. Carducci M, Bozzetti M, Foscolo AM, et al. Margin detection using digital dermatoscopy improves the

performance of traditional surgical excision of basal cell carcinomas of the head and neck [J]. Dermatol Surg. 2011;37(2):280–5.
5. MacFarlane D, Shah K, Wysong A, et al. The role of imaging in the management of patients with nonmelanoma skin cancer: diagnostic modalities and applications [J]. J Am Acad Dermatol. 2017;76(4):579–88.
6. Kawaguchi M, Kato H, Matsuo M. CT and MRI features of scalp lesions [J]. Radiol Med. 2019;124(10):1049–61.
7. Koustenis A Jr, Harris A, Gross J, et al. Optical coherence tomography angiography: an overview of the technology and an assessment of applications for clinical research [J]. Br J Ophthalmol. 2017;101(1):16–20.

4 Terminology, Image Interpretation, and Artifacts for Skin Ultrasound

Hui-Xiong Xu, Le-Hang Guo, An-Qi Zhu, Dan-Dan Shan, and Qiao Wang

4.1 Terminology and Image Interpretation

Visual appearance refers to the spatial location and appearance characteristics of the lesion on the body surface under the naked eyes. The above information is significant for skin disease diagnosis.

For example, the perineum is a characteristic site for extramammary Paget's disease. The glans is a predisposed site for diseases such as condyloma acuminatum and squamous cell carcinoma. The face and dorsum of the hands are predisposed sites for diseases such as basal cell carcinoma and solar keratosis. Lesions located in these sites should be considered for associated highly prevalent diseases firstly.

In addition, if there are appearance changes, such as wound surface, ulceration, and erythema, it means that the lesion involves epidermis. The transducer with the higher frequency is preferred to display the surface information during the examination. If there are no appearance changes, it means that the lesion is deeply located and may not involve the dermis and epidermis, then a lower frequency transducer is usually used to observe the lesion.

4.1.1 Gray-Scale Ultrasound

4.1.1.1 Ultrasound Features

Echogenicity

Echogenicity is the basic parameter to be described during ultrasound examination of the lesion and can reflect the property of the lesion to some extent. According to the literatures, during the skin ultrasound examination, echogenicity is divided into anechogenicity, hypoechogenicity, isoechogenicity, hyperechogenicity, and high echogenicity (Fig. 4.1).

Anechogenicity is more common in homogeneous fluid, and typical simple cysts are generally anechogenic, such as hepatic cysts and renal cysts. But the ultrasound findings of epidermoid

H.-X. Xu (✉) · Q. Wang
Department of Medical Ultrasound, Shanghai Skin Disease Hospital, Ultrasound Research and Education Institute, School of Medicine, Tongji University, Shanghai, China

Department of Medical Ultrasound, Shanghai Tenth People's Hospital, Ultrasound Research and Education Institute, School of Medicine, Tongji University, Shanghai, China

L.-H. Guo
Department of Medical Ultrasound, Shanghai Skin Disease Hospital, Ultrasound Research and Education Institute, School of Medicine, Tongji University, Shanghai, China

A.-Q. Zhu · D.-D. Shan
Department of Medical Ultrasound, Shanghai Tenth People's Hospital, Ultrasound Research and Education Institute, School of Medicine, Tongji University, Shanghai, China

H. Xu et al. (eds.), *Diagnostic Ultrasound in Dermatology*,
https://doi.org/10.1007/978-981-16-7345-0_4

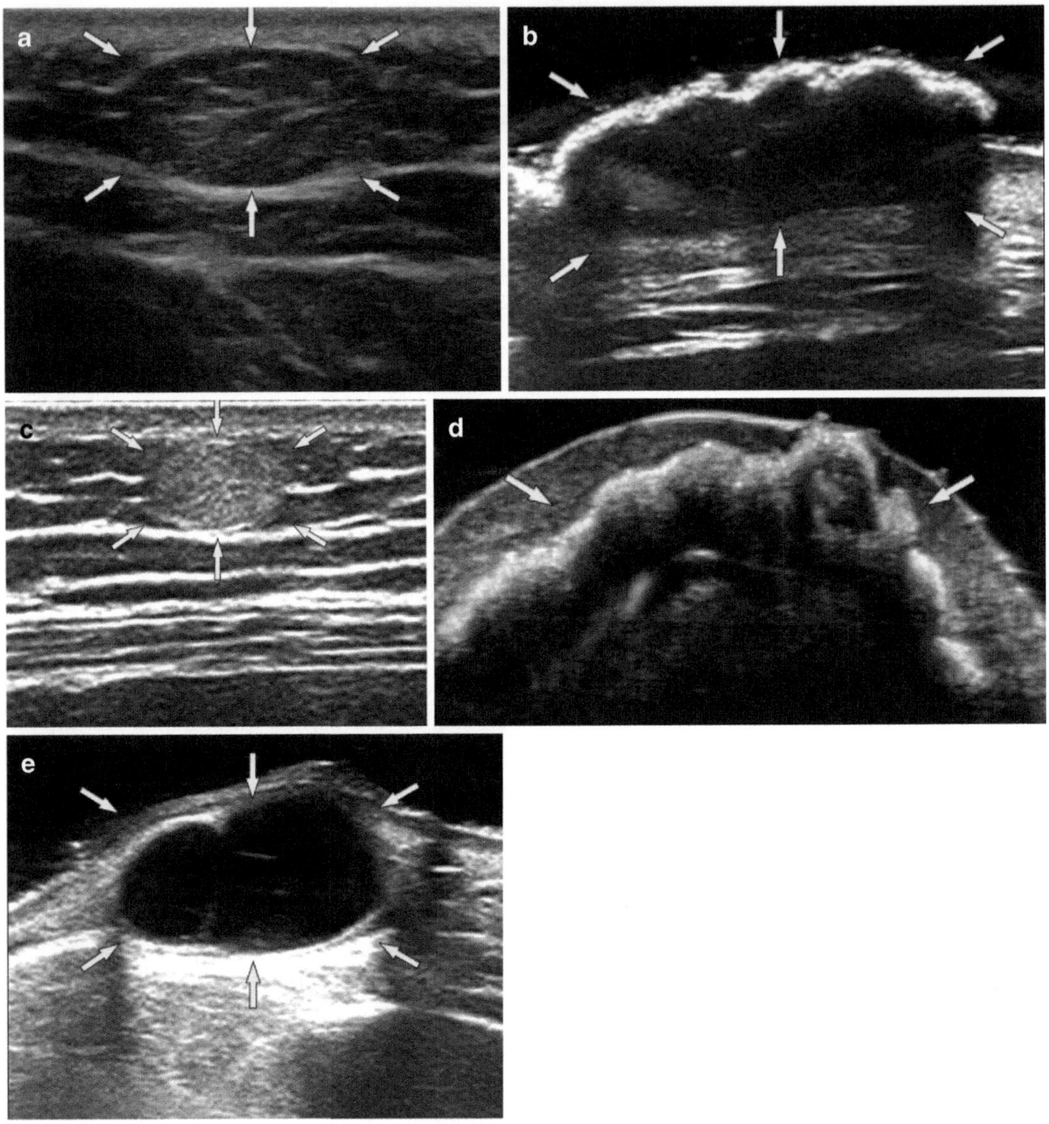

Fig. 4.1 Lesions with different echogenicity. (**a**) Isoechogenic lesion (subcutaneous lipoma). (**b**) Hypoechogenic lesion (cutaneous squamous cell carcinoma). (**c**) Hyperechogenic lesion (subcutaneous lipoma). (**d**) High echogenic lesion (calcinosis cutis). (**e**) Anechogenic lesion (mucous cyst). Lesions are indicated by arrows

cysts are different from those of typical anechogenic cysts, which shows different echogenicity because they are often filled with viscous caseous contents.

Hypoechogenicity can be seen in the adipose tissue. Isoechogenicity is similar to echogenicity of liver and spleen parenchyma. Hyperechogenicity can be seen in subcutaneous lipomas. High echogenicity can be seen in abnormal keratinization on the surface of lesions, often with posterior acoustic shadowing.

Layers of Involvement

The severity of skin disease is highly correlated with the layers of involvement, and breaking through the layer of primary disease means dis-

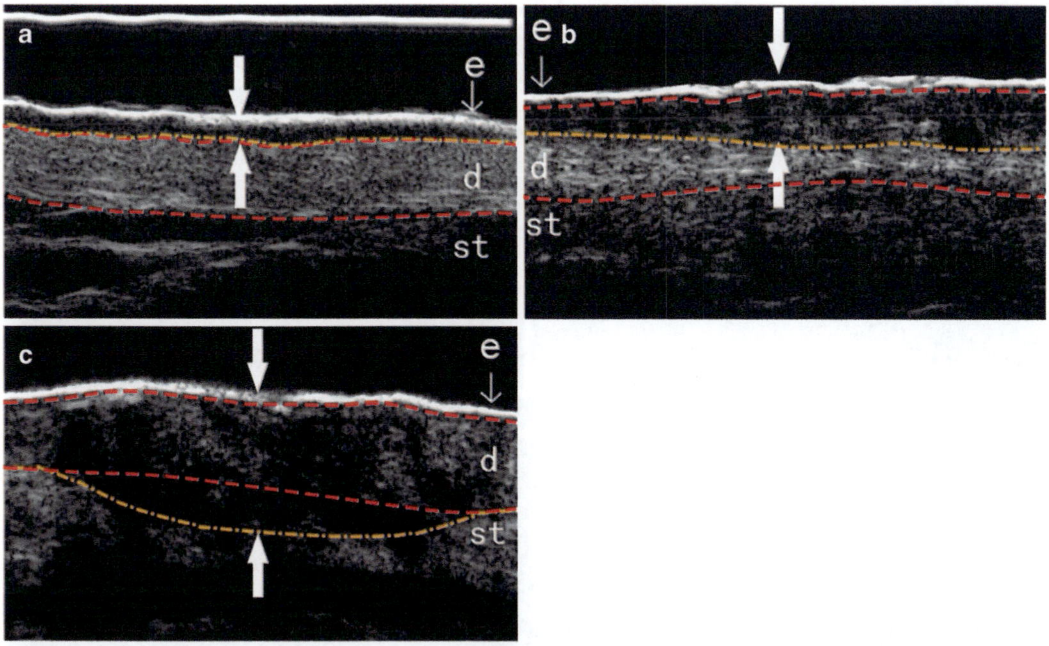

Fig. 4.2 Schematic diagram of lesion involvement layers (Paget's disease). (**a**) Gray-scale ultrasound shows the bottom (yellow dotted line) of the lesion (arrows) reaches the epidermal/dermal junction (upper red dotted line) (Frequency: 50 MHz). (**b**) Gray-scale ultrasound shows the bottom (yellow dotted line) of the lesion (arrows) involves the dermis and is located between the junctions of epidermis/dermis (upper red dotted line) and the dermis/subcutaneous tissue (lower red dotted line) (Frequency: 50 MHz). (**c**) Gray-scale ultrasound shows the bottom (yellow dotted line) of the lesion (arrows) breaks through the junction of dermis/subcutaneous tissue (lower red dotted line) and reaches the subcutaneous tissue layer (Frequency: 50 MHz) [Image cited from Chen ST et al., J Ultrasound Med, 2019, 38(12): 3229–3237]

ease progression. Assessing the layers of involvement of skin disease and the relationship between the lesion and the two key demarcations (i.e., junctions of epidermis/dermis and dermis/subcutaneous tissue) is important (Fig. 4.2).

When describing lesions, it is important to point out the layer where the lesion is located, which layers are involved, and which demarcation lines are broken through. When the boundary of the lesion is ill-defined, it is impossible to determine whether it breaks through a certain demarcation line. The bottom of the lesion to "reach" or "touch" a demarcation line should be described, which will give clinicians sufficient alert.

Surface

The boundary of the lesion is mainly observed through two sides, which are the surface and the bottom.

Surface morphology is usually based on the horizontal plane of the surrounding normal skin as a reference and is divided into four morphologies: elevated, flat, depressed, and wrinkled (Fig. 4.3).

Bottom

The bottom is referenced by the natural morphology and the boundary of the lesion. It may be ill-defined or well-defined, reflecting the degree of involvement of the lesion to deep tissues.

The bottom can be divided into regular and irregular patterns, and the regular bottom appears flat and convex (deep direction) (Fig. 4.4).

Stratum Corneum

The outermost layer of the epidermis is the stratum corneum. Under physiological conditions, the stratum corneum appears as a continuous, smooth, and fine linear hyperechoic band on

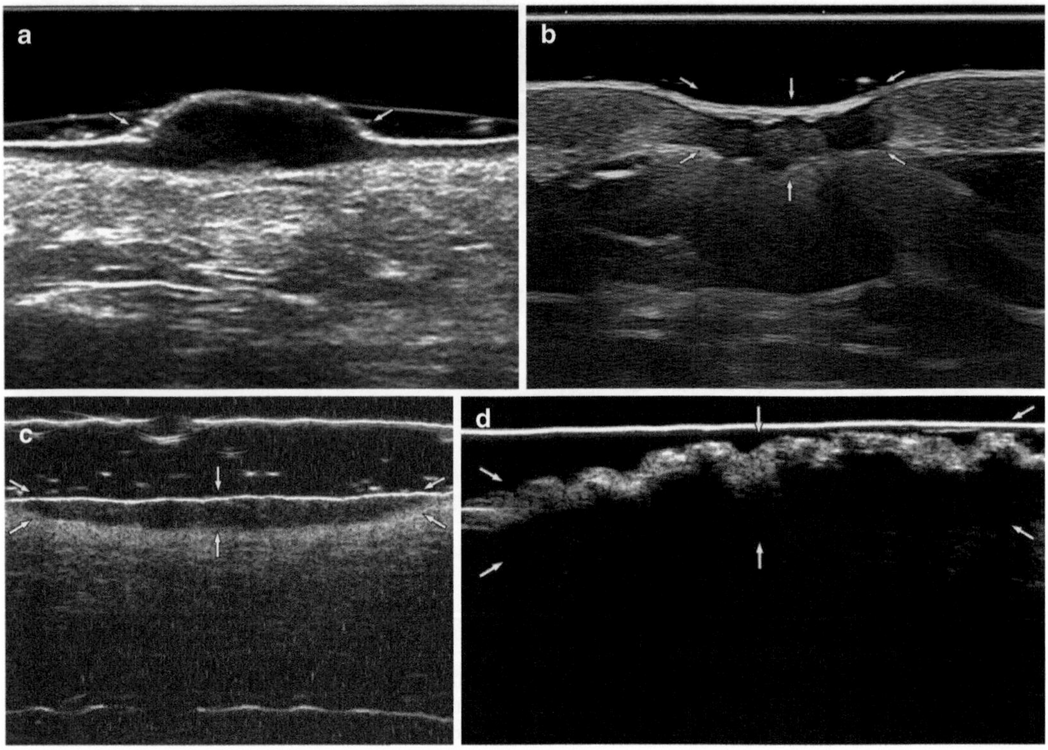

Fig. 4.3 Surface morphology. (**a**) Lesion with elevated surface (basal cell carcinoma). (**b**) Lesion with depressed surface (dermatofibroma). (**c**) Lesion with flat surface (basal cell carcinoma). (**d**) Lesion with wrinkled surface (Bowen's disease). Lesions are indicated by arrows

high-frequency ultrasound without posterior acoustic shadowing.

When abnormal keratinization including hyperkeratosis or parakeratosis occurs, the above hyperechoic band can become thicker, and the surface turns into irregular shape such as roughness or wrinkle. Various degrees of posterior acoustic shadowing induced by hyperechoic band will seriously obstruct the display of deep structure of the lesion and color Doppler flow signals.

Hyperkeratosis or parakeratosis are features of many skin lesions, which can provide important information for disease diagnosis. Therefore, it is not recommended to remove abnormal keratinization in order to rule out posterior acoustic shadowing, otherwise it will lead to changes in the original morphology of the lesion and cause additional damage.

At this point, the internal information of the lesion can be observed from the edge of the lesion or an "ultrasound transmission window" in the stratum corneum space.

On the other hand, the disappearance of linear hyperechoic band is observed on the surface in some lesions, which means the local loss of stratum corneum. It usually appears in uncured wounds or in the postepidermectomy.

It should be pointed out that in some cases, hyperechogenicity thickening with posterior acoustic shadowing does not mean hyperkeratosis or parakeratosis, such as scabs, hair, scars, or air-containing spaces of skin wrinkle. In this condition, the ultrasound findings are similar to pathological keratosis, which needs to be differentiated in combination with visual appearance (Fig. 4.5).

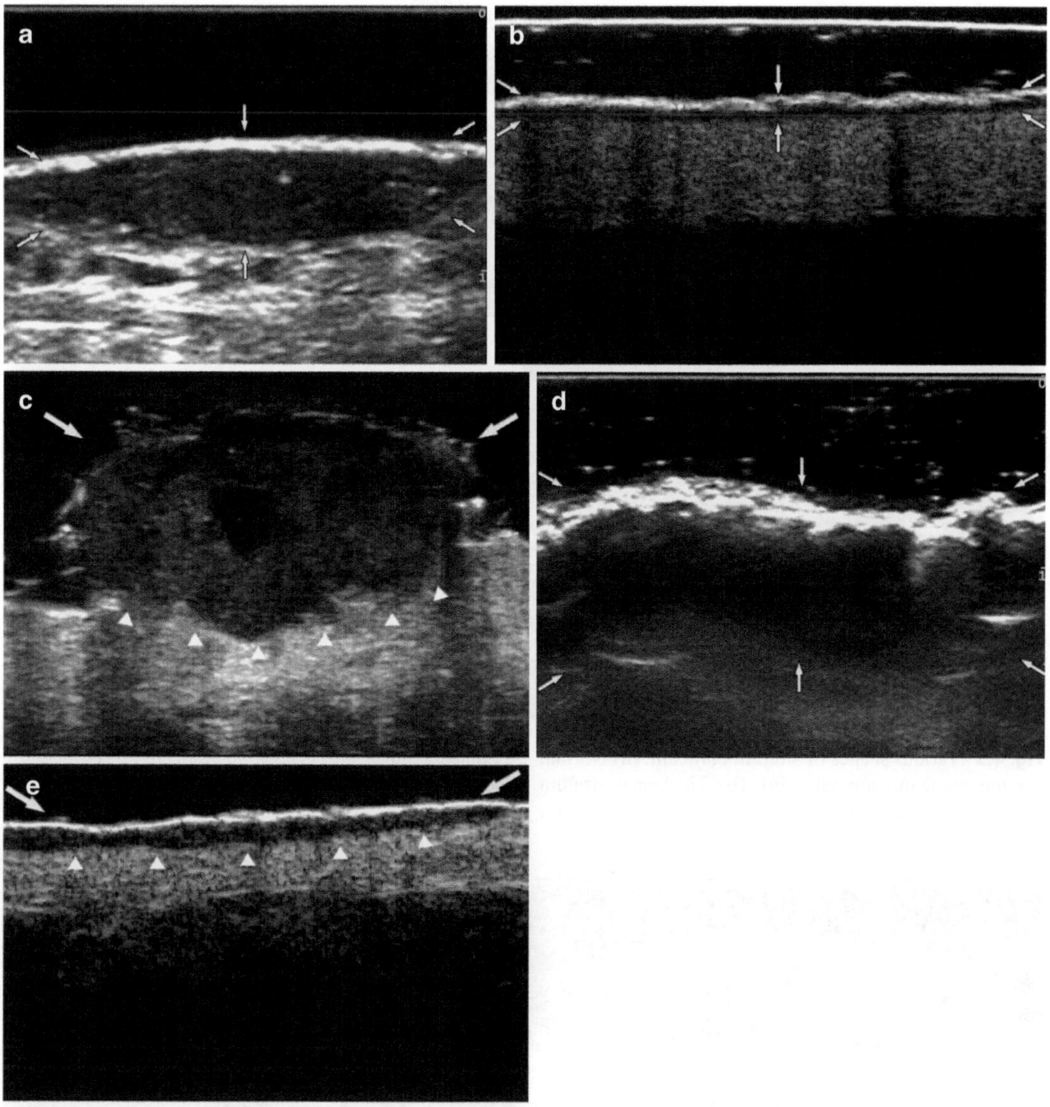

Fig. 4.4 Bottom morphology. (**a**) Lesion with convex bottom (basal cell carcinoma). (**b**) Lesion with flat bottom (Bowen's disease). (**c**) Lesion with irregular bottom (cutaneous squamous cell carcinoma). (**d**) Lesion with ill-defined bottom (cutaneous squamous cell carcinoma). (**e**) Lesion with well-defined bottom (basal cell carcinoma)

Shape

Hemispherical, oval, crawling, and irregular shapes are common.

Hemispherical shape refers specifically to the lesion with a flat bottom and elevated surface, which is common in diseases such as seborrheic keratosis and epidermal nevus (Fig. 4.6a).

Oval shape is common in benign lesions of dermal or subcutaneous tissue (Fig. 4.6b).

Crawling shape is usually confined to the epidermis, manifested as a narrow hypoechogenic band parallel to the body surface. The longitudinal section is significantly smaller than the cross section. The shape is unique for skin diseases, which is common in psoriasis, Bowen's disease, and extramammary Paget's disease (Fig. 4.6c).

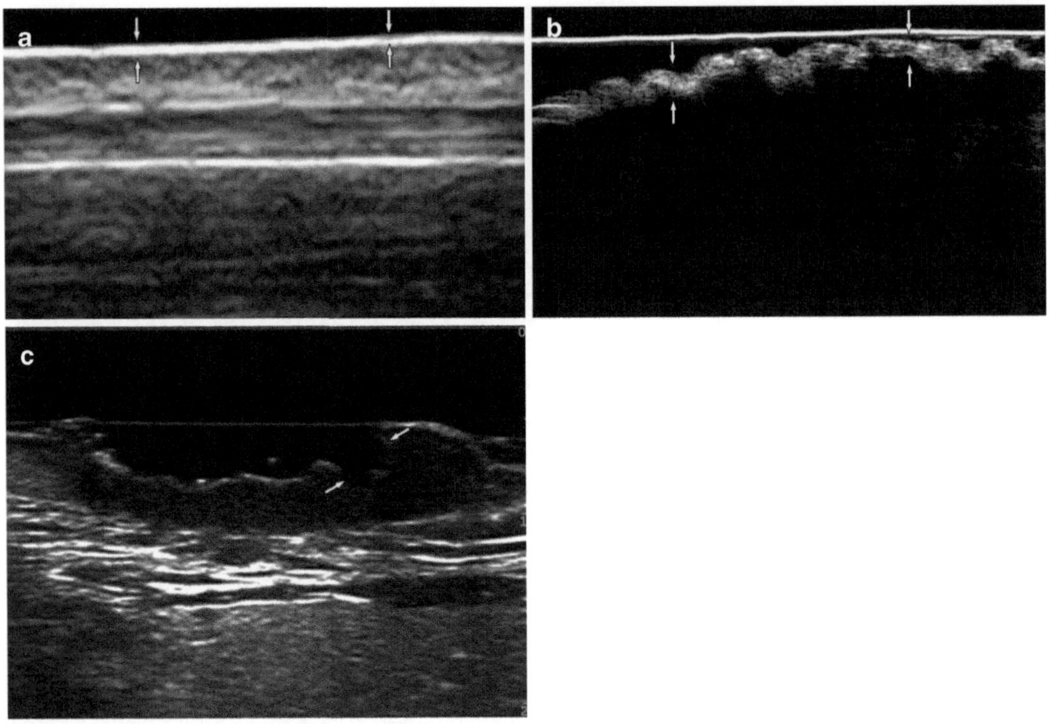

Fig. 4.5 Various shapes of stratum corneum. (**a**) Normal stratum corneum (normal skin). (**b**) Thickened stratum corneum (Bowen's disease). (**c**) Absent stratum corneum (cutaneous squamous cell carcinoma). Arrows point to the location of stratum corneum

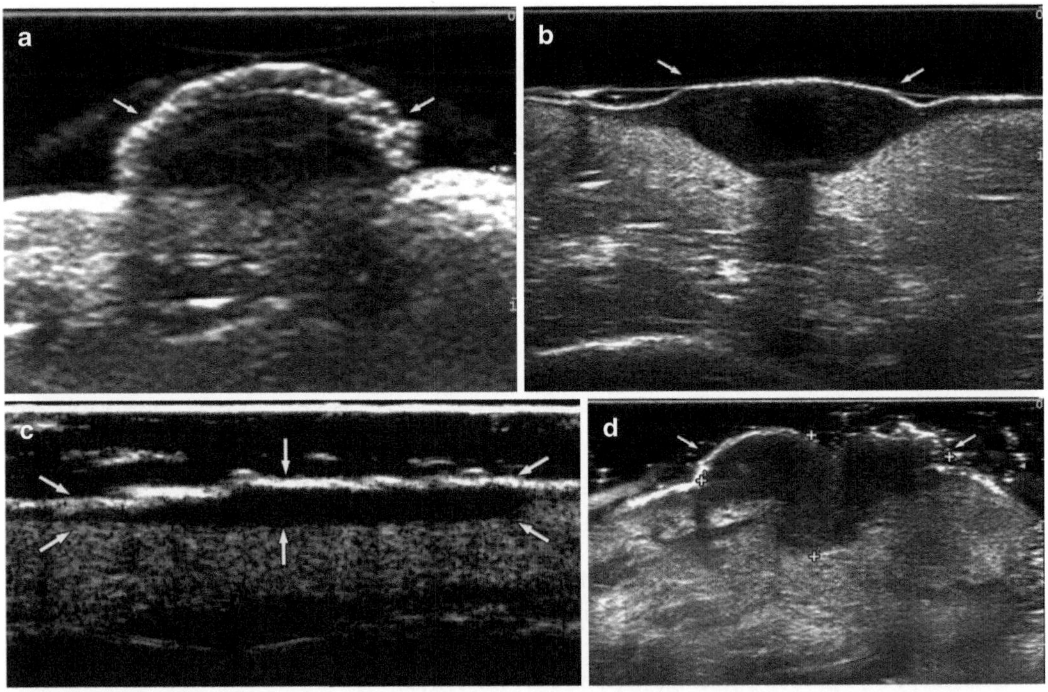

Fig. 4.6 Shapes of lesions. (**a**) Lesion with hemispherical shape (intradermal nevus). (**b**) Lesion with oval shape (cutaneous squamous cell carcinoma). (**c**) Lesion with crawling shape (seborrheic keratosis). (**d**) Lesion with irregular shape (cutaneous squamous cell carcinoma). The lesions are indicated by arrows

Irregular shape is characterized by lobulated or angular bulges with irregular boundary, such as squamous cell carcinoma (Fig. 4.6d).

Internal Composition

The internal composition refers to the composition of the lesion, which is divided into cystic, solid, and mixed composition (Fig. 4.7).

For solid lesions, it is necessary to describe their internal echogenicity, such as hyperechogenicity, isoechogenicity, or hypoechogenicity, and whether the echogenicity is uniform.

For the cystic part of the cystic lesions or the mixed lesions, the degree of ultrasound transmission of the anechoic part needs to be described. In general, anechogenicity with good ultrasound transmission means that the internal fluid is clear. Conversely, hypoechogenicity or hyperechogenicity with poor ultrasound transmission means that the internal fluid is turbid or even gelatinous.

For the solid part of mixed lesions, the internal shape needs to be described, such as papillary, nodular, or septate. And the nodular solid part should be further described according to the requirements for solid nodules.

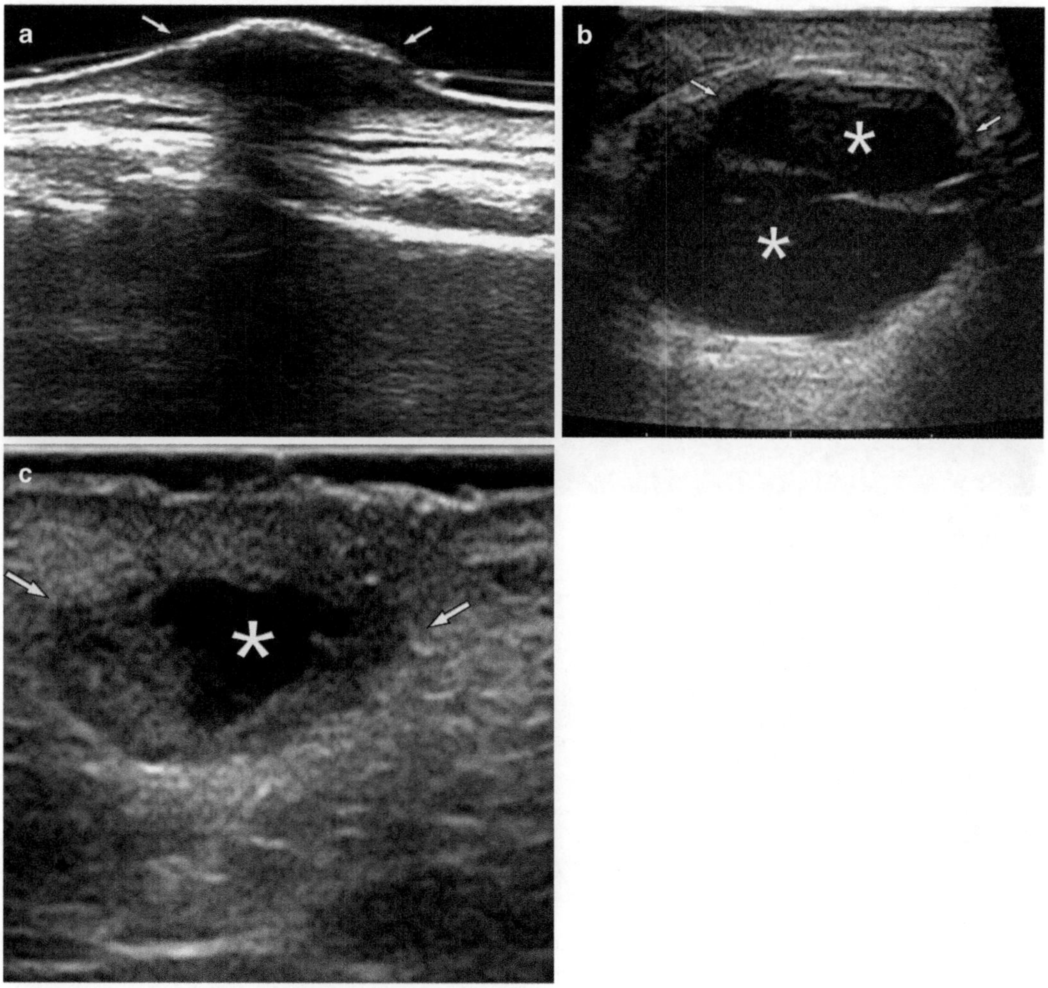

Fig. 4.7 Internal composition. (**a**) Solid lesions (cutaneous squamous cell carcinoma). (**b**) Cystic lesions with banded septa inside (chronic inflammatory lesions). (**c**) Mixed lesions (cutaneous squamous cell carcinoma). Arrows point to lesions, * point to the cystic areas

Special Signs

Some skin diseases have special ultrasound findings:

The characteristic feature of a "cap-like" hypoechogenicity is visible on the top of pilomatricoma (Fig. 4.8a).

A characteristic "wave sign," a hyperechogenic wrinkle, can be seen in Bowen's disease (Fig. 4.8b).

The multiple hyperechoic spots and cystic degeneration zones are characteristic features of basal cell carcinoma (Fig. 4.8c).

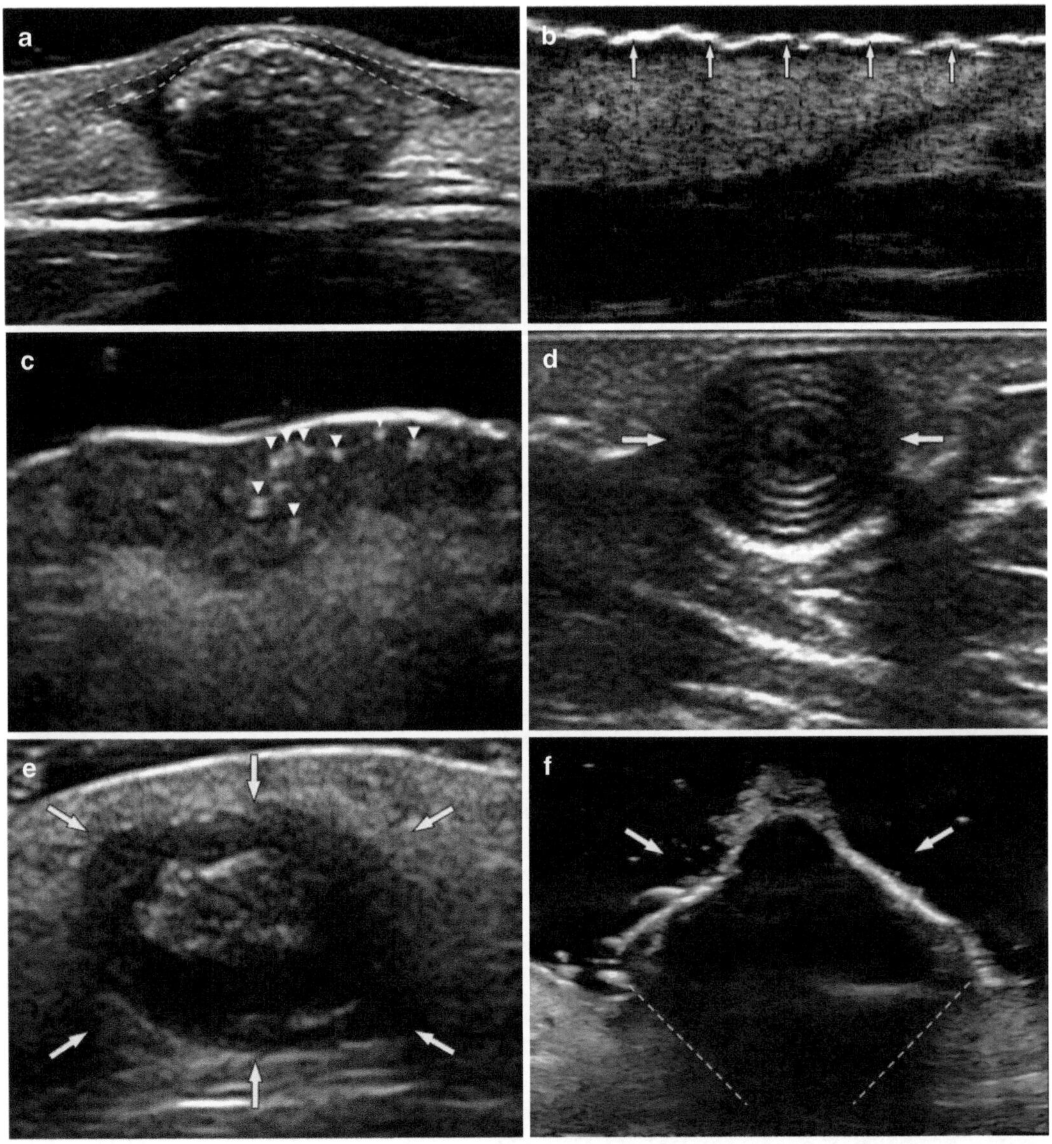

Fig. 4.8 Special signs of lesions. (**a**) A "cap-like" hypoechogenicity (yellow dotted line) of pilomatricoma. (**b**) The "wave sign" (arrows) of Bowen's disease. (**c**) Multiple hyperechoic spots (▽) of basal cell carcinoma. (**d**) The feature of "onion-like" (arrows) in epidermoid cyst. (**e**) The "target sign" (arrows) of trichilemmal cyst. (**f**) "Inverted triangular" posterior acoustic shadowing (dotted line) of keratoacanthoma (arrows). (**g**) The double-contour sign (arrows and ▽) is seen in gouty arthritis. (**h**) Thick (arrows) and fine (△) pseudopodia of dermatofibrosarcoma protuberans (*). (**i**) The "rat tail sign" (△) of neurilemmoma (*)

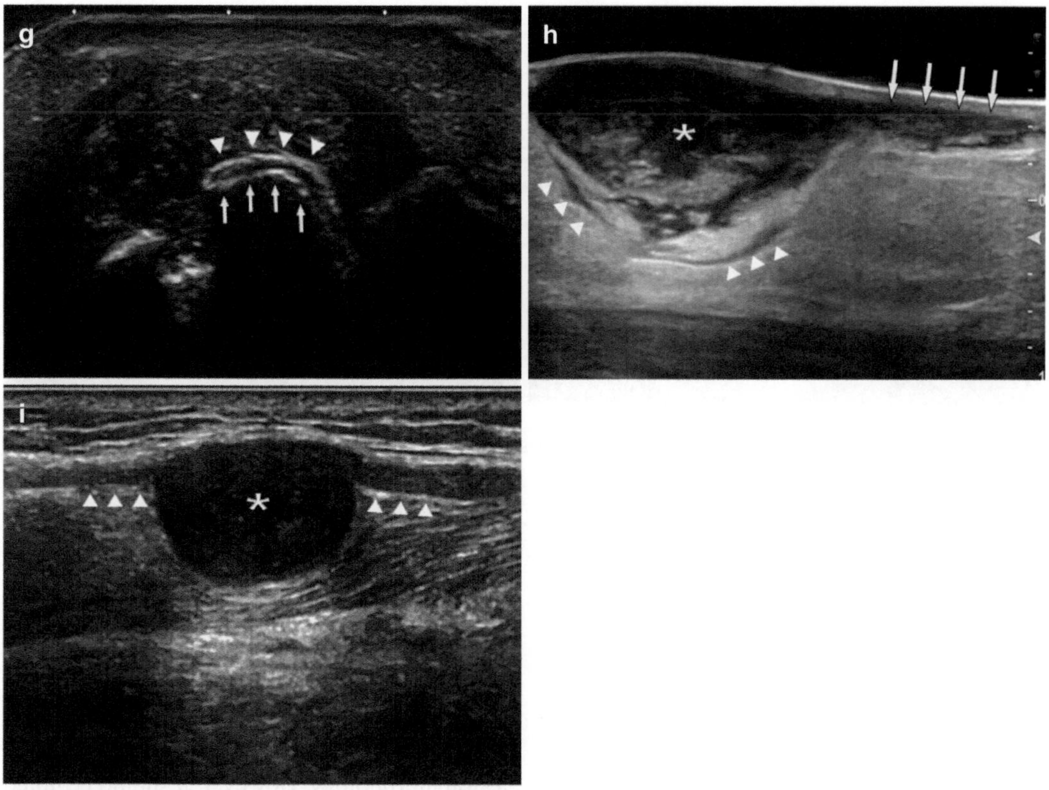

Fig. 4.8 (continued)

"Onion-like" change is a characteristic feature of epidermoid cyst (Fig. 4.8d).

A characteristic "target sign," the center of the lesion is hyperechogenic, surrounded by a ring-like hypoechogenic area that can be visible in trichilemmal cyst (Fig. 4.8e).

"Inverted triangular" posterior acoustic shadowing is a characteristic feature of keratoacanthoma (Fig. 4.8f).

Double-contour sign which consists of a hyperechoic irregular line formed by monosodium urate crystals in hyaline cartilage and a parallel hyperechoic line formed by the cortical bone (independent of the scanning angle of the US transducer) is a characteristic feature of gouty arthritis (Fig. 4.8g).

Pseudopodium means one or more prominences of different lengths, extending from the lesion to the deep tissue (Fig. 4.8h).

"Rat tail sign" is formed by the two ends of the lesion connecting to the hypoechoic nerve, which can be seen in neurilemmoma (Fig. 4.8i).

The above special signs are helpful to provide more diagnostic information in clinical practice.

4.1.1.2 Measurement

Size

Lesion size refers specifically to the two largest diameters of the lesion measured in perpendicular sections on the cross-sectional image (Fig. 4.9). With the improvement of resolution of ultrasound device, especially the application of ultrasound transducer with a frequency ≥ 50 MHz, the spatial resolution reaches sub-millimeter level, and subtle lesions at epidermis, skin appendages can be found.

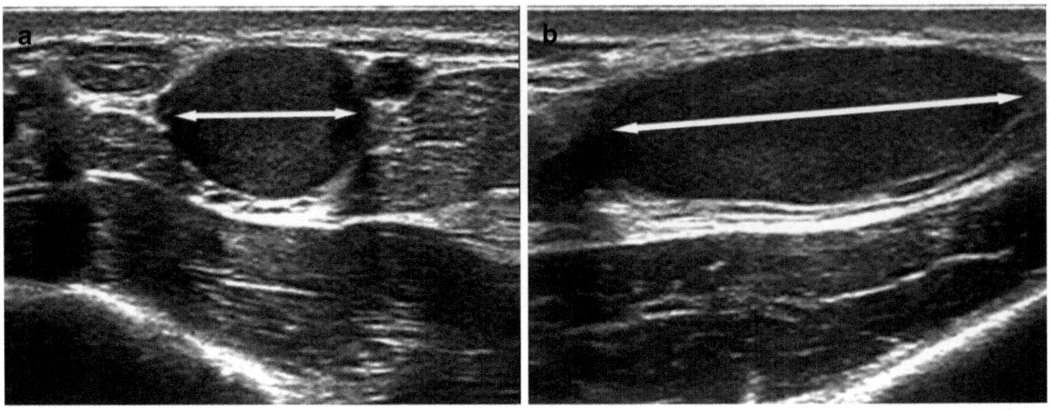

Fig. 4.9 Measurement of size. (**a**) Size measurement of lesion's minimum diameter. (**b**) Size measurement of lesion's maximum diameter

Thickness

Lesion thickness refers to the distance from the shallowest to the deepest part of the lesion on a vertical direction, which is an important indicator of ultrasound examination. This indicator can be obtained by direct measurement on ultrasound images. Before measurement, we should first look for the deepest of the lesion, and keep the transducer stable and perpendicular to the body surface, and then measure when the lesion is clearly displayed as much as possible. Due to the various lesion shapes in different skin diseases, the following four conditions may occur during measurement. The corresponding measurement method is as follows.

Regular Shape

The shallowest and deepest points of a lesion are generally located on a vertical line, and the length of the line between the two points is directly measured as the lesion thickness (Fig. 4.10a).

Crawling

The lesions are not uniform in thickness and need to be measured at multiple points to give a range of thickness. And the location of the thickest point needs to be indicated (Fig. 4.10b).

Irregular Shape

The vertical distance between the shallowest and the deepest points of the lesion is measured (Fig. 4.10c).

Ill-Defined Boundary

Some lesions show ill-defined boundaries and are difficult to be measured accurately. At this point, the approximate contour of the lesion is used as the starting point for measurement. Then, the measurement is performed with reference to the above method according to the lesion morphology. However, it should be noted that the values are not absolutely accurate (Fig. 4.10d).

When the lesion with abnormal keratinization, the distance should be measured from the point beneath the hyperechoic band to the deepest border of the tumor invasion. The presence of pseudopodia at the bottom needs to be described separately and is not considered to be within the overall range of the lesion.

4.1.2 Color Doppler Ultrasound

Blood flow signals can be divided into no blood flow, rare blood flow, and rich blood flow. No blood flow shows no color Doppler blood flow signal inside the lesion. Rare blood flow shows short linear, punctate, and discontinuous blood flow signals distributed in the lesion. Rich blood flow shows dense and abundant color flow signals distributed in the lesion, and even thick nourishing vessels around the lesion are observed (Fig. 4.11).

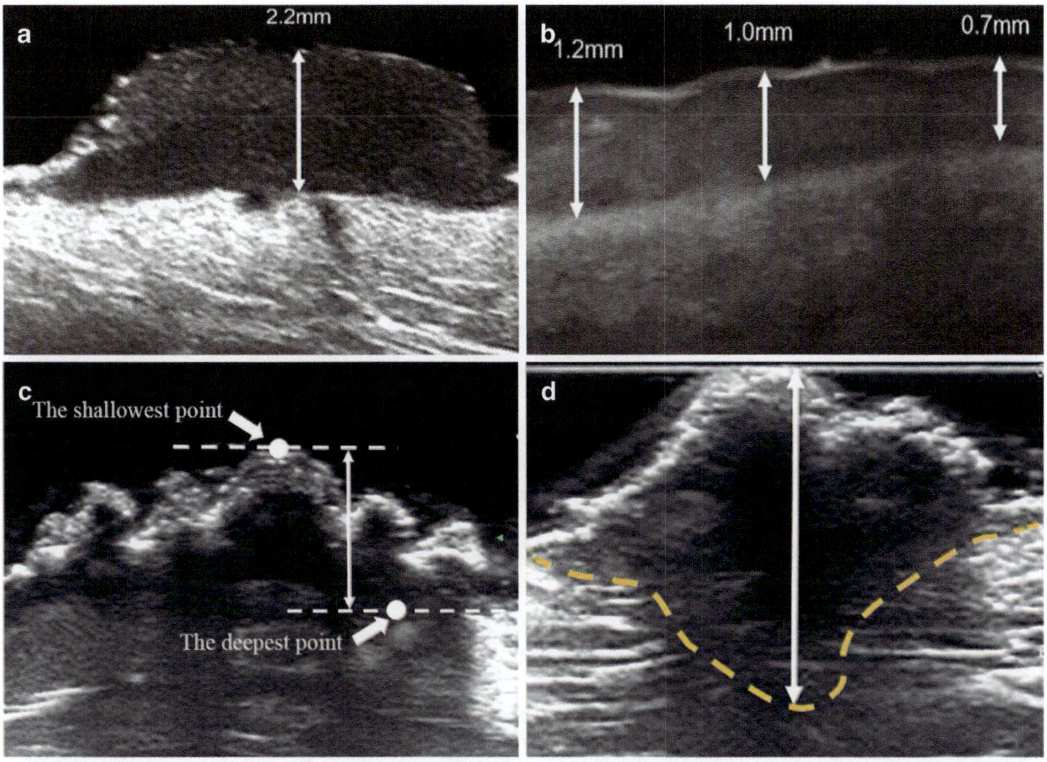

Fig. 4.10 Thickness measurement. (**a**) Thickness measurement of regular lesions. (**b**) Thickness measurement of crawling lesions. (**c**) Thickness measurement of irregular lesions. (**d**) Thickness measurement of ill-defined lesions

4.1.3 Pulsed Doppler Ultrasound

When the blood flow velocity is quantitatively measured in the spectrogram, the blood flow parameters commonly used in clinical practice include peak systolic velocity (V_s), end diastolic velocity (V_d), time-averaged peak velocity, resistance index (RI), pulsatility index (PI), and systolic/diastolic ratio (S/D) (Fig. 4.12).

V_s and V_d can be directly measured in the spectrogram. The time-average peak velocity refers to the time average of the spatial maximum blood flow velocity of the tested vessel sampling volume in a complete cardiac cycle, which can be directly calculated by the ultrasound device. RI and PI reflect the resistance encountered when the blood flows in the blood vessel (Fig. 4.12). S/D is mostly used to evaluate placental function in obstetric ultrasound and is currently less used in skin ultrasound.

RI, PI, and S/D can be calculated from V_s, V_d, and V_{mean} (i.e., mean blood flow velocity over one cardiac cycle), and formulas (4.1) (4.2) (4.3) are as follows:

$$RI = \frac{V_s - V_d}{V_s} \tag{4.1}$$

$$PI = \frac{V_s - V_d}{V_{mean}} \tag{4.2}$$

$$S/D = \left|V_s / V_d\right| \tag{4.3}$$

Key Points

The interpretation of skin ultrasound images describes the general characteristics of the lesion, such as lesion size, boundary, internal composition, and internal blood flow signals.

The interpretation of skin ultrasound images should also describe the special characteristics of

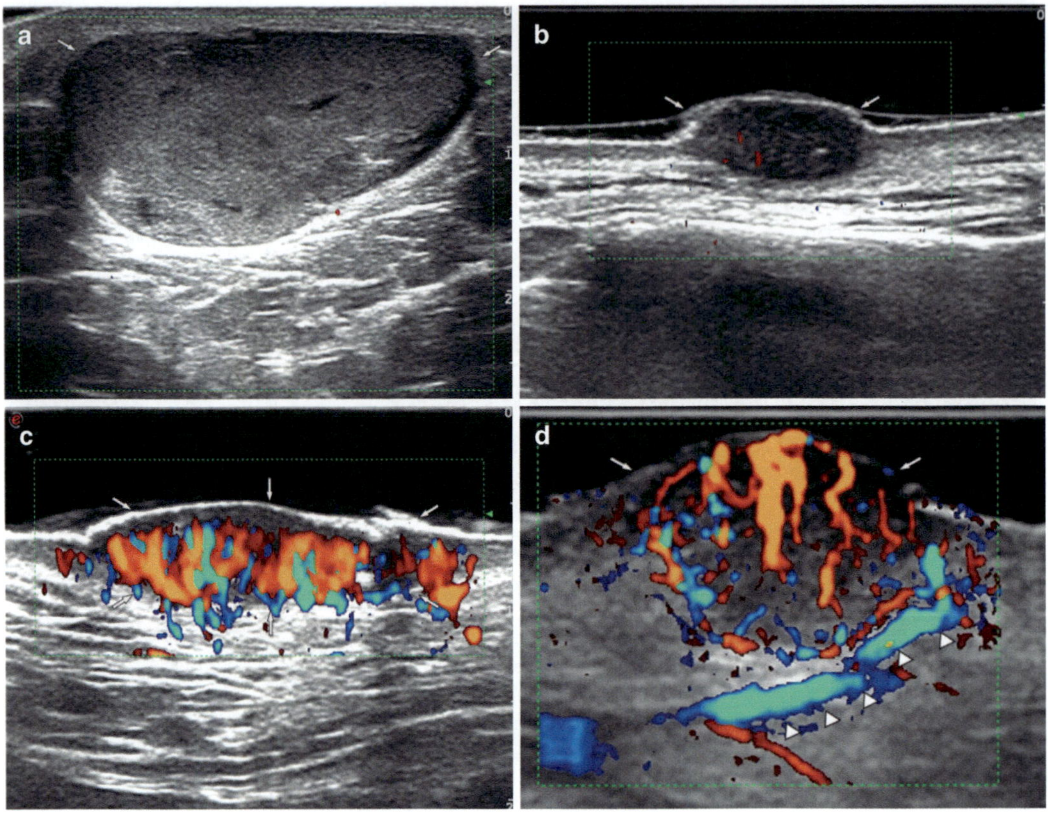

Fig. 4.11 Blood flow signals inside the lesion on color Doppler ultrasound. (**a**) No blood flow signals inside the lesion (epidermoid cyst). (**b**) Rare blood flow signals inside the lesion (compound nevus). (**c**) Rich blood flow signals inside the lesion, and the blood flow signals are radially distributed from the bottom of the lesion to the inside (actinic keratosis combined with cutaneous squamous cell carcinoma). (**d**) Rich blood flow signals inside the lesion, and the blood flow signals are mainly located in the lesion, and large nourishing vessels (basal cell carcinoma) are observed. Arrows point to lesions, △ points to large nourishing vessels

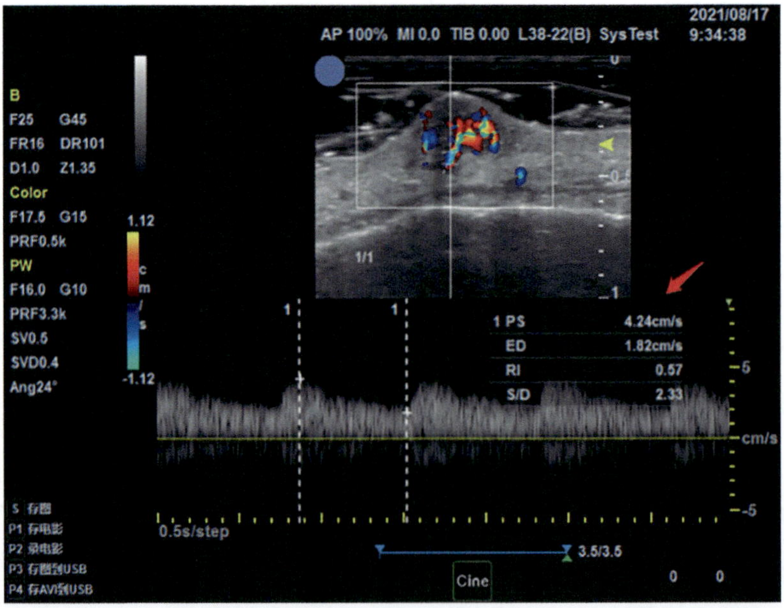

Fig. 4.12 Doppler ultrasound. Quantitative measurement of pulse Doppler blood flow velocity: Vs, V_d, RI, and S/D (Frequency: 34 MHz; red arrow: the hemodynamic values)

skin lesion such as the layer, surface condition, growth morphology, keratinization, and bottom condition of the lesion.

4.2 Artifacts

Ultrasound artifact refers to any unrealistic difference between the ultrasound image and its corresponding anatomical sectional image. In clinical practice, artifacts are common in ultrasound examinations, so as in skin ultrasound. The common skin ultrasound artifacts in clinic mainly include gray-scale ultrasound artifacts and Doppler ultrasound artifacts.

4.2.1 Gray-Scale Ultrasound Artifacts

4.2.1.1 Acoustic Shadowing

In the process of ultrasound transmission, when encountering the medium with greater density, such as stone, bone, or scar, the ultrasound wave is partially or completely reflected due to the large acoustic impedance, and the posterior echogenicity is low or even disappears. Acoustic shadowing suggests that the lesion is characterized by high attenuation or strong reflection. The abnormal keratinization can cause posterior acoustic shadowing of the lesion (Fig. 4.13a).

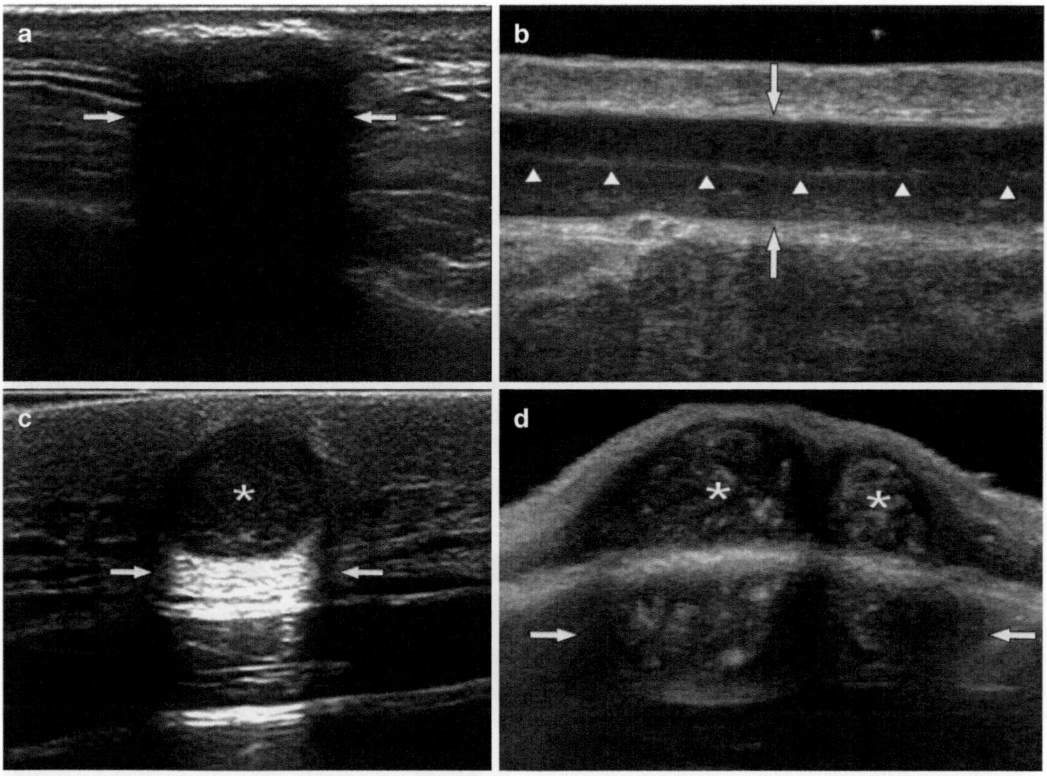

Fig. 4.13 Ultrasound artifacts of skin lesions. (**a**) Artifact of acoustic shadowing (arrows) (calcinosis cutis). (**b**) Reverberation artifact (△) formed in superficial vein (arrows). (**c**) Posterior acoustic enhancement (arrows) of epidermoid cyst (*). (**d**) Mirror effect (arrows) formed in trichilemmal cyst (*)

4.2.1.2 Reverberation Artifact

When the ultrasound wave irradiates vertically on the smooth large interface, the acoustic wave is repeatedly reflected between the transducer and the interface, also known as multiple reflection artifact. It can be seen in the anterior wall of larger cysts (Fig. 4.13b).

4.2.1.3 Side Lobe Artifact

The ultrasound beam is divided into the main lobe and side lobe. Usually, the main lobe is located at the center of the acoustic field, and the axis is perpendicular to the surface of the ultrasound transducer, which is used for ultrasound scanning and imaging. Side lobes are pairs of small lobes symmetrically distributed around the main lobe, followed by the first side lobe, the second side lobe, the third side lobe, and so on, from inside to outside.

Side lobe artifact is produced by the overlap of the first side lobe imaging on the main lobe, and it often appears in liquid areas, such as the gauze-shaped, curved band presented on both sides of the high echogenicity of stones.

4.2.1.4 Partial Volume Effect

Partial volume effect occurs when the size of lesion is smaller than the width of ultrasound beam, or although it is larger than the width of ultrasound beam, only part of it is in the ultrasound beam. In this condition, the echogenicity of normal tissue and the lesion in the ultrasound beam is overlapped and displayed in the same image. Partial volume effect can disturb imaging of the lesion, especially in small cystic lesions.

4.2.1.5 Posterior Acoustic Enhancement

The phenomenon of posterior acoustic enhancement occurs when ultrasound waves pass through a medium with an acoustic attenuation value lower than the assumed acoustic attenuation value, which is more common in the posterior of cysts (Fig. 4.13c).

4.2.1.6 Mirror Effect

Mirror effect is also known as mirror reentrant virtual image. When ultrasound wave encounters a large and relatively smooth surface, the interface reflects ultrasound wave much as a mirror reflects light. This phenomenon is called mirror effect. The mirror effect is usually generated on a large and smooth interface (Fig. 4.13d).

4.2.2 Doppler Ultrasound Artifacts

4.2.2.1 Color Doppler Signal Overflow

Color flow signals may spill from the vessel lumen due to low PRF setting or improper color gain regulation. Color flow signal spillage can be reduced by properly adjusting the PRF and appropriately reducing the color gain (Fig. 1.33).

4.2.2.2 Color Doppler Twinkling Artifact

Color Doppler twinkling artifact is more common in the interference of stones, calcifications, and intestinal gases. The twinkling artifact can be reduced by holding the breath or pressurizing the transducer (Fig. 4.14).

4.2.2.3 Flash Artifact

The flash artifact is pulsatile color signal interference caused by strong mechanical pulsation and respiratory movement of heart and large vessels. Flash artifact can be eliminated using contrast harmonic imaging.

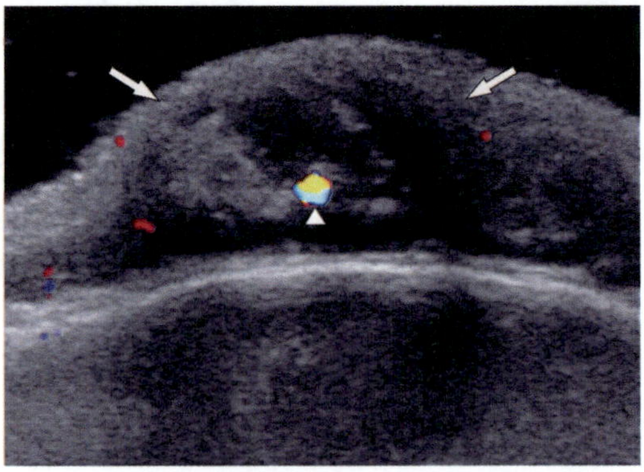

Fig. 4.14 Color Doppler twinkling artifact of skin lesions. Color Doppler twinkling artifact (△) caused by calcification in the lesion (arrows)

4.2.2.4 Aliasing Artifact

If the Doppler shift exceeds 1/2 PRF (Nyquist limit), the portion that exceeds the threshold will be reversed. Proper adjustment of PRF may avoid aliasing artifact.

The above ultrasound artifacts are common in skin ultrasound examination. Understanding various ultrasound artifacts is beneficial to accurately identify the characteristics of the lesion and avoid misdiagnosis.

Suggested Reading

1. Guo WX. Ultrasound medicine [M] (in Chinese). 6th ed. Beijing: People's Military Medical Press; 2011.
2. Harald L, Elisabetta B. WHO manual of diagnostic ultrasound [M]. 2nd. ed. Malta: Gutenberg Press Ltd; 2011.
3. Kremkau FW. Sonography principles and instruments [M]. 8th ed. W.B. Saunders company: St. Louis; 2010.
4. Rukavina B, Mohar N. An approach of ultrasound diagnostic techniques of the skin and subcutaneous tissue [J]. Dermatologica. 1979;158(2):81–92.

Skin Tumors

5

Le-Hang Guo, Hui-Xiong Xu, Qiao Wang, An-Qi Zhu, Li-Fan Wang, Wei-Wei Ren, Xiao-Long Li, Dan-Dan Shan, Ye-Qiang Liu, Jian-Na Yan, Liang Li, Jia Chen, and Pei-Ru Wang

5.1 Benign Skin Tumors

5.1.1 Epidermoid Cyst

5.1.1.1 Clinical Manifestation and Pathology

Epidermoid cyst, also known as keratinous cyst, inclusion cyst, and implantable cyst, is a keratinous tumor in the dermis, the wall of which is composed of epidermis. It is one of the most common subcutaneous masses. The disease is caused by the implantation of epidermal cell fragments into the subcutaneous tissue during trauma or surgery or by epithelial residues and proliferation gradually during embryonic period.

The disease is common and occurs in place where the sebaceous glands distributed densely, such as the head, face, and back. Most of the lesions are hemispherical bumps or have no obvious appearance changes. The lesions are soft and grow slowly (Fig. 5.1). Patients are asymptomatic generally and mostly present with palpable soft or fluctuating masses. If the cyst ruptures, the lesion appears red and swollen. At this time, the

L.-H. Guo (✉)
Department of Medical Ultrasound, Shanghai Skin Disease Hospital, Ultrasound Research and Education Institute, School of Medicine, Tongji University, Shanghai, China

H.-X. Xu
Department of Medical Ultrasound, Shanghai Skin Disease Hospital, Ultrasound Research and Education Institute, School of Medicine, Tongji University, Shanghai, China

A.-Q. Zhu · L.-F. Wang · W.-W. Ren · X.-L. Li
D.-D. Shan
Department of Medical Ultrasound, Shanghai Tenth People's Hospital, Ultrasound Research and Education Institute, School of Medicine, Tongji University, Shanghai, China

Q. Wang
Department of Medical Ultrasound, Shanghai Skin Disease Hospital, Ultrasound Research and Education Institute, School of Medicine, Tongji University, Shanghai, China

Department of Medical Ultrasound, Shanghai Tenth People's Hospital, Ultrasound Research and Education Institute, School of Medicine, Tongji University, Shanghai, China

Y.-Q. Liu · J. Chen
Department of Pathology, Shanghai Skin Disease Hospital, School of Medicine, Tongji University, Shanghai, China

J.-N. Yan · L. Li
Department of Dermatologic Surgery, Shanghai Skin Disease Hospital, School of Medicine, Tongji University, Shanghai, China

P.-R. Wang
Shanghai Skin Disease Hospital, Institute of Photomedicine, School of Medicine, Tongji University, Shanghai, China

H. Xu et al. (eds.), *Diagnostic Ultrasound in Dermatology*,
https://doi.org/10.1007/978-981-16-7345-0_5

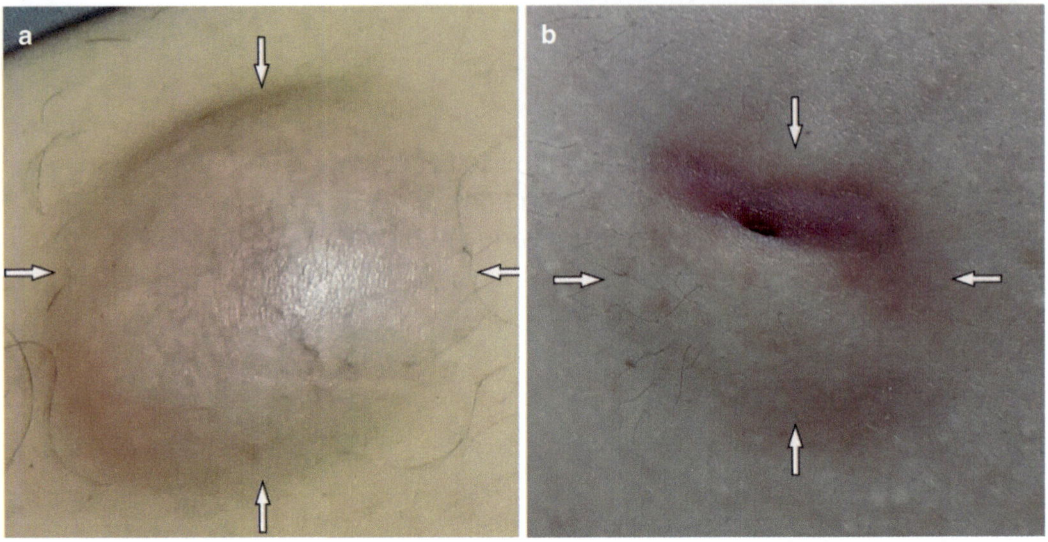

Fig. 5.1 Visual appearance of epidermoid cyst. (**a**) A well-defined hemispherical bump, the size of which is about 38.0 mm in diameter, in the right shoulder, with smooth surface (arrows). (**b**) A skin-colored mass on the right shoulder, which is slightly elevated. A red scar, the size of which is about 20.0 mm in diameter, is observed at the edge of the lesion (the patient underwent incision and drainage half a month ago) (arrows)

diagnosis should be combined with the patient's clinical history, such as a palpable mass and the discharge of bean dregs.

Pathological examination shows that epidermoid cyst is generally a cyst cavity with wall which is composed of lamellar squamous epithelial cells containing keratohyalin granules. The cyst is full of keratoses or white granular oil-like materials, occasionally with calcification.

5.1.1.2 Ultrasound Manifestation

Gray-Scale Ultrasound

Gray-scale ultrasound often shows a nodular mixed echogenic lesion with regular shape located in the subcutaneous tissue. The surface is elevated. Ultrasound shows that the lesion is well-defined owing to the cyst wall. Posterior acoustic shadowing artifact is observed on both sides of the lesion, that is the phenomenon of "acoustic shadows of lateral boundaries". The lesion is usually heterogeneous, showing characteristic anechoic or hypoechoic "fissures" with posterior acoustic enhancement. The lesion is often connected to the surface of skin through the sinus tract, which is usually keeping closed (Figs. 5.2 and 5.3).

Epidermoid cysts rupture due to external forces, which causes leakage of contents, so the cyst wall collapses owing to the tension disappearance. Therefore, epidermoid cyst may appear as an ill-defined, irregular hypoechoic lesion. It is also accompanied by inflammatory findings such as thick peripheral soft tissue, disordered distribution, and increased echogenicity (Fig. 5.4).

Color Doppler Ultrasound

There is often no blood flow signal in the lesion. If the cyst wall ruptures with granulomatous inflammation, blood flow signals are detected in and around the lesion.

5.1.1.3 Differential Diagnosis

Trichilemmal Cyst

The trichilemmal cysts often occur on the scalp, but epidermoid cysts often occur on the head, neck, and trunk. On gray-scale ultrasound epidermoid cysts show specific signs such as dot-like hyperechoic and/or irregular slit-like anechoic areas. However, trichilemmal cysts mostly show a characteristic of "target sign."

In addition, the majority of epidermoid cysts show sinus tracts connected to the epidermis, but rarely visualized in trichilemmal cysts. Ultrasound features can help in differentiation between them.

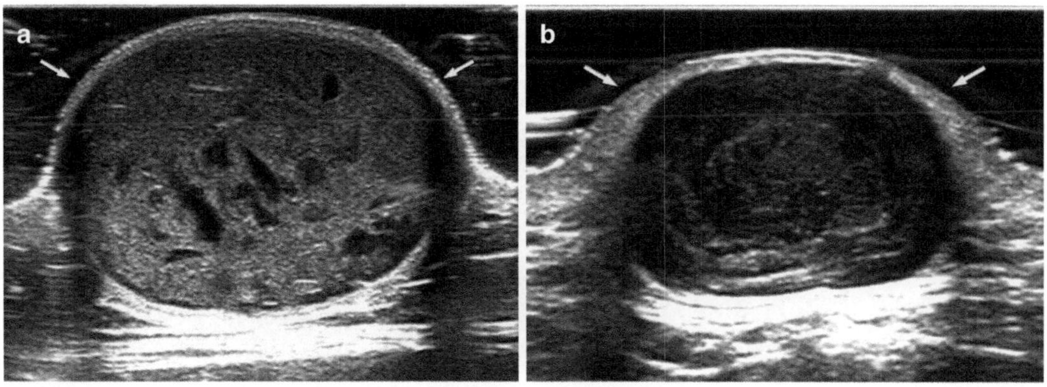

Fig. 5.2 Typical gray-scale ultrasound findings of epidermoid cyst. (**a**) Gray-scale ultrasound shows an oval, well-defined mixed echogenic lesion (arrows) in the subcutaneous tissue (size: 31.0 mm × 30.0 mm; thickness: 28.2 mm). The surface is elevated and smooth. "Slit-like" anechogenic areas are visualized in the lesion, with posterior acoustic enhancement (Frequency: 22 MHz). (**b**) Gray-scale ultrasound shows an oval, well-defined hypoechoic lesion (arrows), which is visualized in the subcutaneous tissue (size: 20.4 mm × 18.5 mm; thickness: 12.2 mm). The surface is elevated and smooth. The lesion is heterogeneous and shows "onion-like" change with posterior acoustic enhancement (Frequency: 22 MHz)

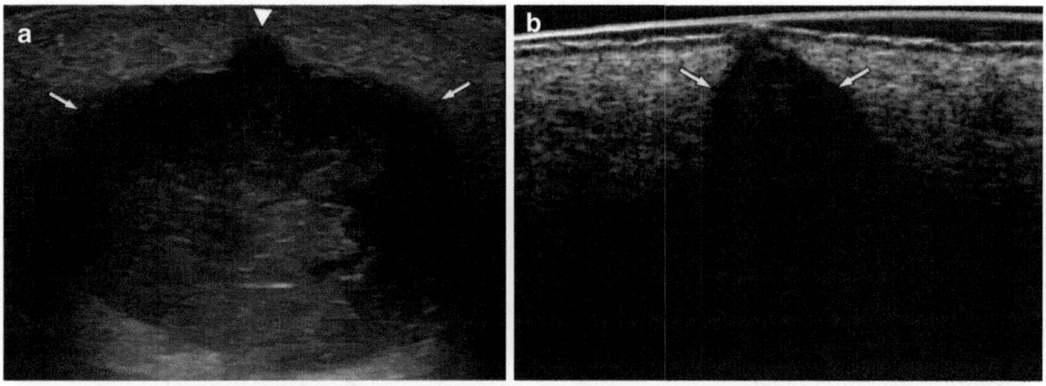

Fig. 5.3 Epidermoid cyst with sinus tract formation. (**a**) Gray-scale ultrasound shows an oval, heterogeneous mixed echogenic lesion (arrows), with posterior acoustic enhancement located in the subcutaneous tissue (size: 20.2 mm × 18.5 mm; thickness: 16.6 mm). The lesion is connected to the surface of skin through a hypoechoic sinus tract (▽) (Frequency: 22 MHz). (**b**) Ultrasound biomicroscopy shows that the lesion is only partially displayed, but it clearly shows the sinus tract (arrows) (Frequency: 50 MHz)

Dermoid Cyst

The location of the lesion is helpful to differentiate them. Dermoid cysts are congenital diseases, and the most common location is the periorbital region, while epidermoid cysts are often located in the sites such as the head, neck, and trunk.

Dermoid cysts show round or oval cystic lesions in the subcutaneous tissue on ultrasound images, with anechogenicity or flocculent echogenicity in some cases. Epidermoid cysts typically show "onion-like" change or irregular "slit-like" anechogenicity. Ultrasound features can help in differentiation between them.

5.1.1.4 Diagnosis Clues

1. Epidermoid cysts can be seen in different locations over the body and are often located in the head, neck, and trunk. Visual appearance shows a well-defined, soft, and hemispherical bump with smooth surface. The patients are usually asymptomatic.

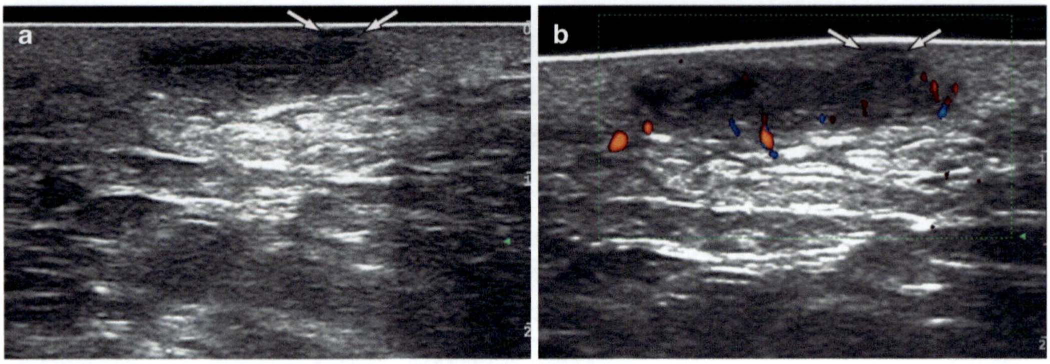

Fig. 5.4 Ruptured epidermoid cyst. (**a**) Gray-scale ultrasound shows a heterogeneous hypoechoic lesion with posterior acoustic enhancement located in the subcutaneous tissue (size: 17.1 mm × 11.5 mm; thickness: 4.1 mm). The shape is still regular. The left edge of the lesion is connected to the epidermis through a sinus tract (arrows) (Frequency: 22 MHz). (**b**) Color Doppler ultrasound shows rare blood flow signals in the lesion (Frequency: 22 MHz)

2. Ultrasound shows a round or oval mixed echogenic lesion in the subcutaneous tissue. "Dot-like" hyperechogenicity and/or "slit-like" anechogenicity are visualized in the lesion. Typically, it may show "onion-like" change. Sinus tracts are common in lesions. The above features are helpful in differentiating them from other tumors.
3. With the leakage of contents due to rupture, the lesion may show ill-defined, irregular features on ultrasound. Sometimes it is also accompanied by inflammatory change of the peripheral soft tissue.
4. There is no blood flow signal in the lesion on color Doppler ultrasound.

Key Points

- Epidermoid cysts are often located in the head, neck, and trunk, and they are well-defined and soft with smooth surface. The lesions usually grow slowly.
- Ultrasound mostly shows a mixed echogenic lesion. They are characterized by irregular "slit-like" anechogenicity, "onion-like" change, and sinus tracts.

5.1.2 Digital Mucous Cyst

5.1.2.1 Clinical Manifestation and Pathology

Digital mucous cyst, also known as myxoid cyst, occurs at the distal interphalangeal joints or in the proximal nail fold and firstly described as synovial lesions in 1883. At present, the mechanism of the disease is still not clear. Most of them are considered to be caused by degeneration of the fibrous capsule and synovial tissue of adjacent joints, or myxoid degeneration of the dermis and subcutaneous tissue.

Digital mucous cyst is divided into two types:

1. Mucous type (superficial type): Dermal fibroblast metaplasia results in excessive hyaluronic acid. This type is not connected to the joint cavity and considered to be local cutaneous mucinosis.
2. Ganglion cyst type (deep type): Hyaluronic acid flows outwards from the degenerated joint through the pedicle-like structure.

The disease is mostly located on the dorsal side of the distal interphalangeal joint of the fingers/toes or at the nail fold. The lesion is a single, soft, and translucent bump growing slowly. It may show fluctuation and mucus flow out after rupture. It is more common in middle-aged and elderly patients.

Patients are asymptomatic usually and mostly present with palpable soft masses at the fingers/toes. Most patients are accompanied by osteophyte on the dorsal surface of the joint, resulting in increased synovial fluid, which may be a factor in the formation of digital mucous cyst. According to the relative literatures, the recurrence rate of this disease is high, with a recurrence rate of 25% to 50% after simple resection.

On pathological examination, there is a pseudocapsule in the fibrous capsule containing myxoid stroma and fibroblasts, and no epithelial cells are found in the inner wall.

5.1.2.2 Ultrasound Manifestation

Gray-Scale Ultrasound

1. Mucous type: It often appears as a round or oval, well-defined, homogeneous, and solitary anechoic lesion with posterior acoustic enhancement, and is located in the subcutaneous tissue without connection to the adjacent joint. The surface of the lesion is elevated and smooth.
2. Ganglion cyst type: It is deeper than mucous type and often appears as a regular or irregular, well-defined and homogeneous anechoic lesion with posterior acoustic enhancement at the joint, connecting to the joint cavity. The surface of the lesion is elevated and smooth.

Color Doppler Ultrasound

There are no blood flow signals in the lesion (Fig. 5.5).

5.1.2.3 Differential Diagnosis

Epidermoid Cyst

Firstly, the age and location are helpful to differentiate the two entities. Epidermoid cysts occur at any age, commonly in the head, neck, and trunk, and it rarely locates in the fingers/toes; while digital mucous cysts often occur in the

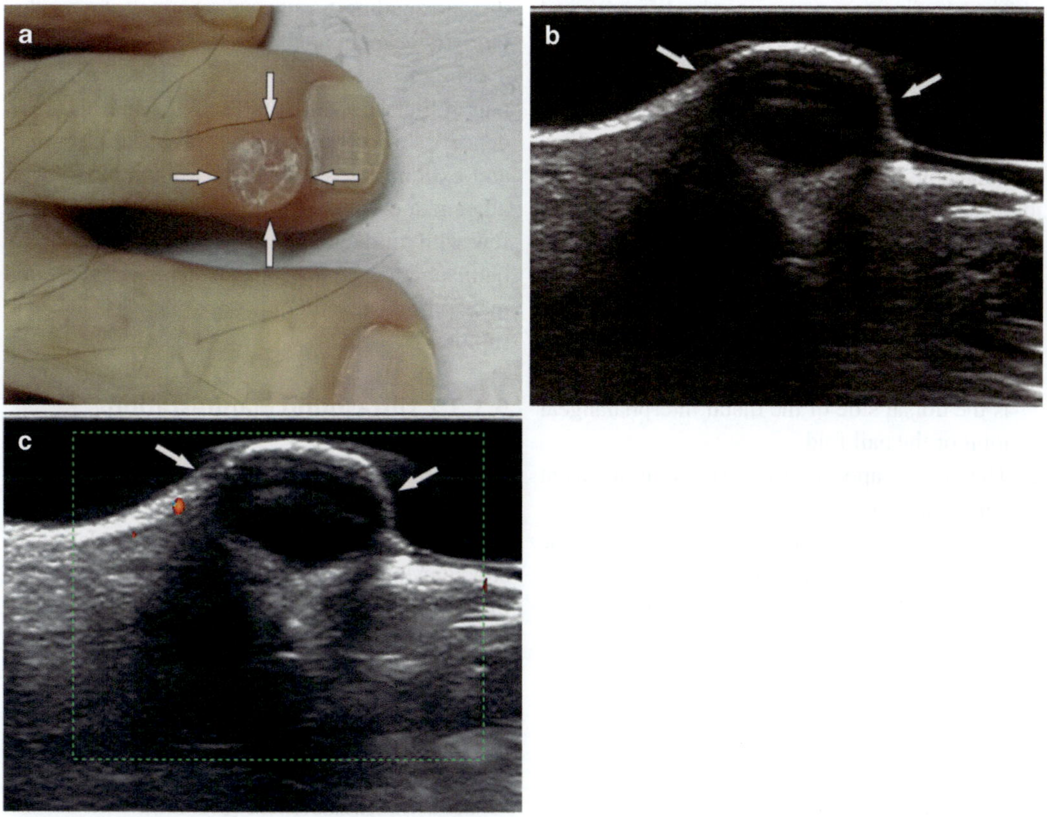

Fig. 5.5 Digital mucous cyst. (**a**) Visual observation shows a well-defined translucent bump in the third toe of the left foot with rough surface (arrows), the size of which is about 6.0 mm × 4.0 mm. (**b**) Gray-scale ultrasound shows a regular, oval, and well-defined anechoic lesion (arrows) in the subcutaneous tissue (size: 5.8 mm × 4.2 mm; thickness: 2.5 mm). The surface is elevated and smooth. The lesion is homogeneous with posterior acoustic enhancement (Frequency: 22 MHz). (**c**) Color Doppler ultrasound shows no blood flow signals inside the lesion (arrows) (Frequency: 22 MHz)

middle-aged and elderly patients, the characteristic location is the dorsal side of the distal interphalangeal joint of the fingers/toes or the nail fold, and most of the lesions are small.

On gray-scale ultrasound, "dot-like" hyperechogenicity, and/or irregular "slit-like" anechogenicity are often visualized in epidermoid cysts. While digital mucous cysts show subcutaneous anechoic lesions with good internal acoustic transmission, which connect to the joint cavity. It is often accompanied by osteoarthritis.

Heberden's Nodes

Heberden's node, appearing as an enlargement located on both sides of the dorsal surface on the distal interphalangeal joint of the finger. It is considered to be a characteristic sign of osteoarthritis and may be accompanied by local tenderness.

The two diseases are easier to be differentiated on gray-scale ultrasound. Heberden's nodes show rough bone cortex, local convexity, and visible osteophyte formation, and are often accompanied by osteoarthritis, while digital mucoceles show subcutaneous anechoic lesions connected to the joint cavity with good internal acoustic transmission and posterior acoustic enhancement.

5.1.2.4 Diagnosis Clues

1. This disease often occurs in middle-aged and elderly patients and the characteristic location is the dorsal side of the distal interphalangeal joint or the nail fold.
2. The lesion appears as a single translucent bump that is usually small.
3. Ultrasound shows an anechoic lesion in the subcutaneous tissue connected to the joint cavity, with posterior acoustic enhancement.
4. It is often accompanied by osteoarthritis.

Key Points

- The characteristic location of digital mucous cyst is the dorsal side of the distal interphalangeal joint of the finger/toe or the nail fold, appearing as a small and translucent nodule.
- Ultrasound shows an anechoic lesion in the subcutaneous soft tissue, with good internal acoustic transmission and posterior acoustic enhancement.
- This disease is often accompanied by osteoarthritis and needs to be differentiated from Heberden's nodes.

5.1.3 Trichilemmal Cyst

5.1.3.1 Clinical Manifestation and Pathology

Trichilemmal cyst is a benign lesion originating from the outer root sheath cells of the hair follicle. It is a tumor of skin appendages. As a relatively rare skin cyst, trichilemmal cyst often occurs in female and the disease progress is slow. It occasionally shows autosomal dominant inheritance. The disease may develop into a benign proliferative tumor, or into a malignant proliferative trichilemmal tumor, which may infiltrate into the surrounding tissues or even metastasize distantly after malignant change.

The disease often occurs in areas with dense hair follicles, 90% in the scalp, while the incidence is low occurring in the face, trunk, groin, and extremities. Patients are asymptomatic usually and mostly present with a palpable mass, and few with mild tenderness. Most of the lesions are hemispherical and pushable bumps. The lesion may present an inflammatory response when it ruptures.

5.1.3.2 Ultrasound Manifestation

Gray-Scale Ultrasound

Trichilemmal cysts appear as regular, oval, and well-defined hypoechoic lesions in the dermis or subcutaneous tissues. According to the internal ultrasound features of the lesions, they are divided into the following three types.

1. "Central target" type: The center of the lesion is hyperechogenic, surrounded by a ring-like hypoechogenic structure, with posterior acoustic enhancement (Fig. 5.6).
2. "Eccentric target" type: The lesion appears as anechogenicity dominantly with an eccentric hyperechoic area in the periphery (Fig. 5.7).
3. Hypoechoic type (rare): The lesion shows heterogeneous hypoechogenicity with punctate

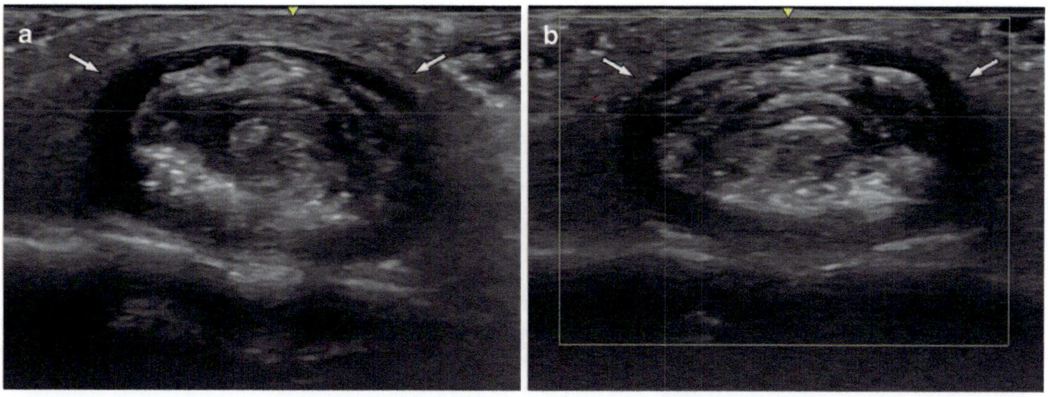

Fig. 5.6 "Central target" type of trichilemmal cyst. (**a**) Gray-scale ultrasound shows that the lesion is a regular, oval, and well-defined mixed echogenic lesion (arrows) located in the subcutaneous tissue (size: 14.2 mm × 15.2 mm; thickness: 8.1 mm). The periphery of the lesion is hypoechoic, the center is hyperechoic, with posterior acoustic enhancement (Frequency: 22 MHz). (**b**) Color Doppler ultrasound shows no blood flow signals in the lesion (arrows) (Frequency: 22 MHz)

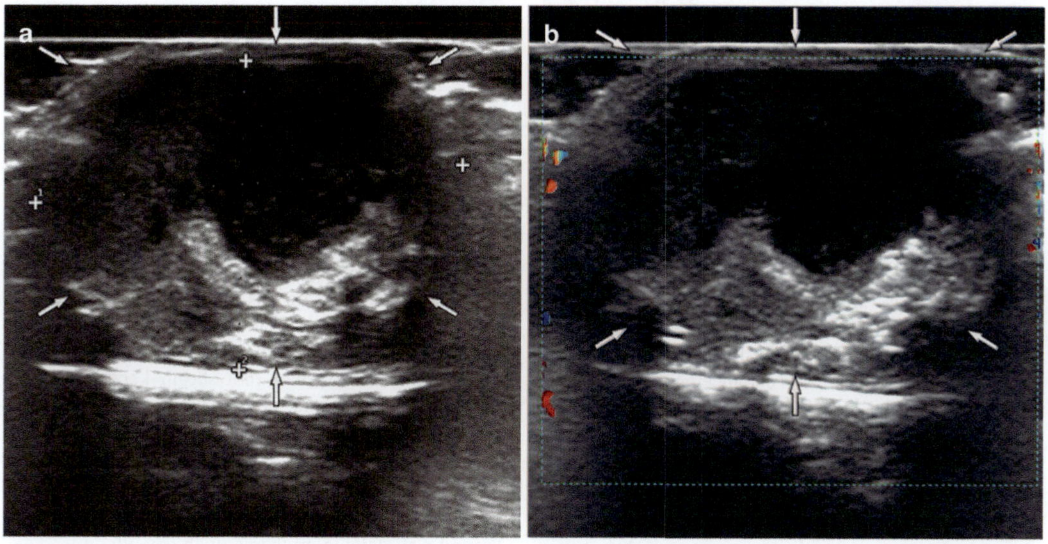

Fig. 5.7 "Eccentric target" type of trichilemmal cyst. (**a**) Gray-scale ultrasound shows a regular and well-defined mixed echogenic lesion (arrows) located in the subcutaneous tissue (size: 17.6 mm × 12.5 mm; thickness: 9.2 mm). The lesion is heterogeneous, appearing as anechoic dominantly with an eccentric hyperechoic area in the periphery, with posterior acoustic enhancement (Frequency: 22 MHz). (**b**) Color Doppler ultrasound shows no blood flow signals in the lesion (arrows) (Frequency: 22 MHz)

calcifications, without "target" sign (Fig. 5.8). When the cyst ruptures with granulomatous reaction, the lesion is irregular and ill-defined.

Color Doppler Ultrasound

There are no blood flow signals in the lesion. When the cyst ruptures with granulomatous reaction, the blood flow signals are increased in the periphery.

5.1.3.3 Differential Diagnosis

Epidermoid Cyst

The diseases often occur in the head, neck, and trunk, while the trichilemmal cysts often occur in

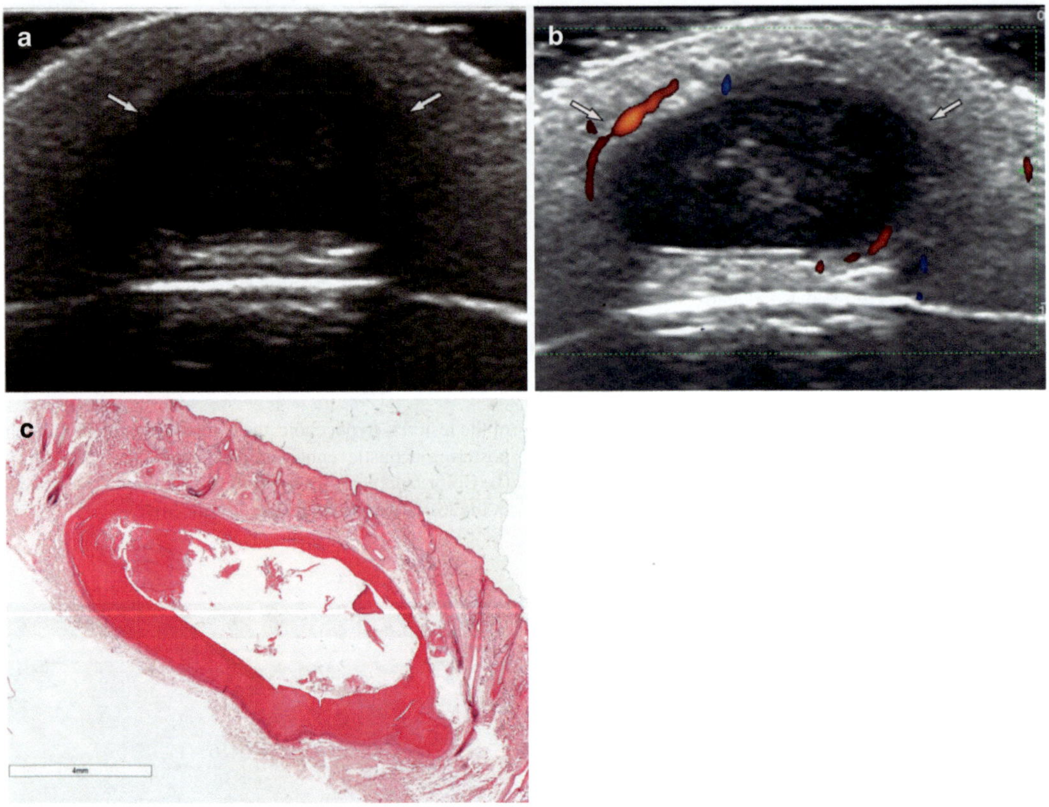

Fig. 5.8 Hypoechoic type of trichilemmal cyst. (**a**) Gray-scale ultrasound shows a regular, oval, and well-defined hypoechoic lesion (arrows) located in the subcutaneous tissue (size: 12.2 mm × 9.8 mm; thickness: 5.7 mm). The lesion is heterogeneous, with dot-like hyperechoic structures and posterior acoustic enhancement (Frequency: 22 MHz). (**b**) Color Doppler ultrasound shows no blood flow signals in the lesion, and rare blood flow signals in the periphery (arrows) (Frequency: 22 MHz). (**c**) Histopathology (HE staining, panoramic scanning): A cyst is observed in the dermis. The cyst wall is composed of squamous epithelium. The granular layer is not visible. The cells near the cyst cavity are large. The cytoplasm is lightly stained. The outer root sheath keratinization is visualized. The contents of the cyst are uniformly red-stained and densely arranged keratin

the scalp. On gray-scale ultrasound, specific features such as dot-like hyperechogenicity and/or irregular slit-like anechogenicity are often visualized in epidermoid cysts. However, trichilemmal cysts mostly show a characteristic "target" sign. In addition, the majority of epidermoid cysts show sinus tracts connected to the epidermis, but sinus tracts are rarely visualized in trichilemmal cysts.

Dermoid Cyst

The location of disease is helpful to differentiate the two entities. Dermoid cysts are congenital diseases. The most common location is the periorbital region, while trichilemmal cysts are often located in the scalp. On ultrasound, dermoid cysts show round or oval lesions in the subcutaneous tissue with anechogenicity and flocculent echo. The ultrasound findings are similar to those of the "eccentric target" type of trichilemmal cysts, thus, ultrasound differentiation is difficult. The clinical history and location of the disease should be considered.

Pilomatricoma

It often occurs in children and adolescents; visual appearance shows skin-colored, erythematous or blue, and firm nodules. Gray-scale ultrasound shows solid nodules with dot-like, patchy, or massive calcifications, without posterior acoustic enhancement. However, visual appearance of the trichilemmal cyst shows skin color. The presence of calcification and posterior acoustic enhancement could be used to differentiate them.

5.1.3.4 Diagnosis Clues

1. The location of the disease is characteristic, which often occurs in the hairy area and 90% of the lesions are located in the scalp. It is often a skin-colored, hemispherical and pushable bump in the subcutaneous tissue.
2. Gray-scale ultrasound shows round or oval heterogeneous hypoechoic or anechoic lesions in the subcutaneous tissue with posterior acoustic enhancement. The "central target" and "eccentric target" are characteristic signs.

Key Points

- Trichilemmal cyst is a benign lesion originating from the cells of the outer root sheath cells of the hair follicle. It is a tumor from the skin appendages. It may develop into a benign proliferative tumor, but also may develop into a malignant proliferative trichilemmal outer hair root sheath tumor.
- It often occurs in the hairy area, and 90% of the lesions are located in the scalp.
- Ultrasound findings of "central target" and "eccentric target" are characteristic signs.

5.1.4 Steatocystoma

5.1.4.1 Clinical Manifestation and Pathology

Steatocystoma, also known as sebaceous cyst adenoma, is a rare skin hamartoma. It is a retention cyst formed by obstruction of the opening of the sebaceous glands.

It is single or multiple. Single steatocystoma is a non-hereditary disease. Steatocystoma multiplex (SM), also known as multiple sebaceous cysts, was first named by Pringle in 1899. It is manifested as multiple sebaceous cysts in the body region with rich sebaceous glands. Steatocystoma multiplex is mostly inherited in an autosomal dominant manner. This disease occurs most frequently in the young people, and is common in the chest, upper extremities, and axillas. It is also seen in the inguinal, buttocks, scrotum, and vulva. The etiology of SM is not yet clear, but it is currently believed to be caused by mutations of KRT17, and may also be related to androgens and environmental factors.

Clinically, the disease is mostly manifested as a local painless mass, which is a hemispherical bulge, with skin-colored, light yellow, or blue surface. Sometimes, a small hole is seen in the center of the lesion, and odorless sebum-like content is extruded. The lesions may be secondary to infection due to trauma or spontaneous rupture, followed by redness and local tenderness.

Histologically, steatocystoma is a cyst in the middle and lower layers of dermis. The cyst wall is composed of a stratified squamous epithelium without a granular layer. The cyst wall connects to the sebaceous glands, and there are lobules of the sebaceous glands in the cyst wall and its surroundings. The oil- and cheese-like content of the cyst is most common with keratin, followed by hair-like structure, and occasionally sebaceous gland fragments are visible.

5.1.4.2 Ultrasound Manifestation

Gray-Scale Ultrasound

Gray-scale ultrasound often shows multiple, oval or round, well-defined lesions distributed in clusters. The lesion is usually located in the dermis and subcutaneous tissues with posterior acoustic enhancement.

Because the content of the lesion is complex, the ultrasound features are diverse. The lesion appears as anechogenicity when the content is oil-like. Flocculent, lumpy, or cord-like hyperechogenicity is visualized when it contains keratin, hair, and sebaceous gland fragments. Steatocystoma appears as an ill-defined, irregular hypoechoic lesion when it is ruptured and is infected.

Color Doppler Ultrasound

Usually, there are no blood flow signals in the lesion. If the lesion presented with granulomatous inflammation, blood flow signals are visualized (Figs. 5.9 and 5.10).

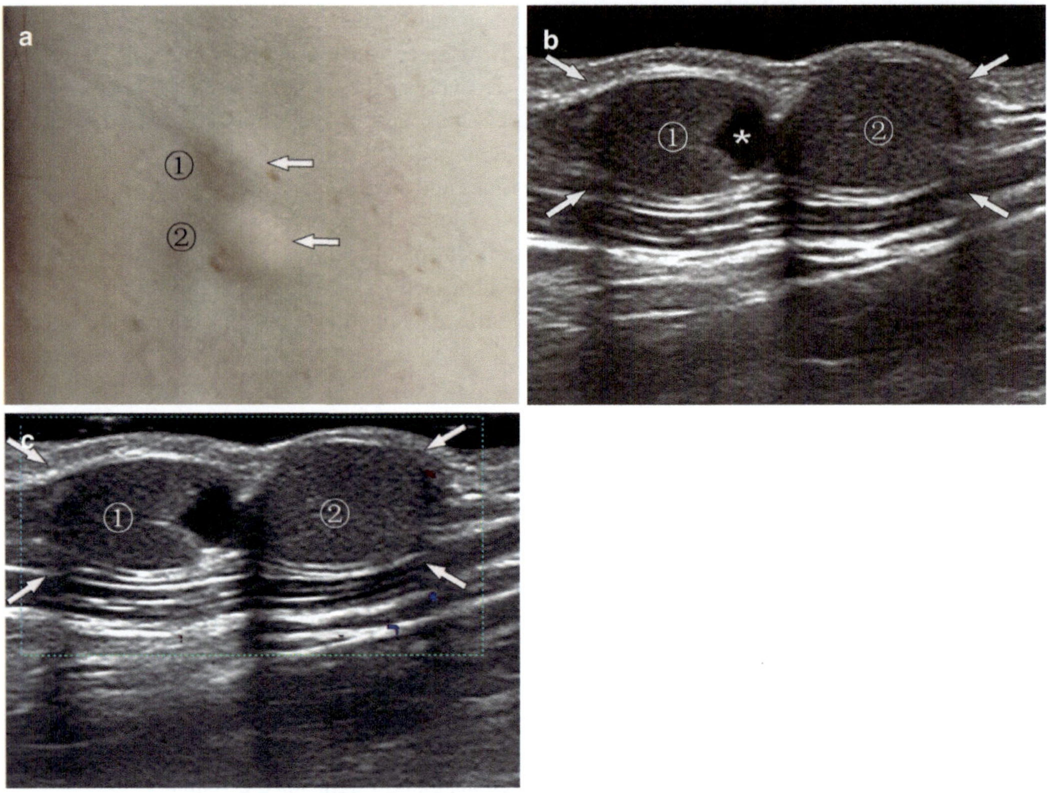

Fig. 5.9 Steatocystoma multiplex. Female, 49 years of age. (**a**) Visual observation shows two soybean-sized hemispherical bumps on the right side of the neck. It is skin-colored and well-defined without ulceration (arrows). (**b**) Gray-scale ultrasound shows two adjacent hypoechoic lesions (arrows) in the subcutaneous tissue (lesion ① size: 9.1 mm × 9.3 mm; thickness: 5.5 mm; lesion ② size: 10.4 mm × 9.7 mm; thickness: 6.0 mm). They are oval and well-defined. An anechoic zone (*) is visible inside the lesion ① (Frequency: 22 MHz). (**c**) Color Doppler ultrasound shows no blood flow signals in the lesion (arrows) (Frequency: 22 MHz)

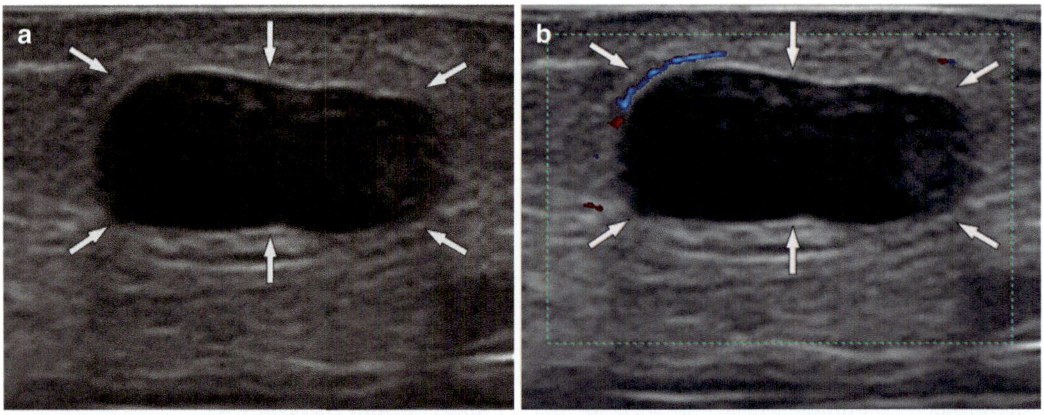

Fig. 5.10 Steatocystoma. Female, 66 years of age. (**a**) Gray-scale ultrasound shows an oval and well-defined anechoic lesion (arrows) in the subcutaneous tissue (size: 8.6 mm × 4.6 mm; thickness: 3.9 mm). The lesion shows good internal acoustic transmission without posterior acoustic enhancement (Frequency: 22 MHz). (**b**) Color Doppler ultrasound shows no blood flow signals inside the lesion (arrows) (Frequency: 22 MHz)

5.1.4.3 Differential Diagnosis

Epidermoid Cyst

The contents of both entities can be squeezed out; the difference is that the contents of epidermoid cysts are odorous, while the contents of steatocystoma are odorless.

On gray-scale ultrasound, "dot-like" hyperechogenicity and/or irregular "slit-like" anechogenicity are often visualized in epidermoid cysts, while the ultrasound features of steatocystoma are diverse. When steatocystoma only contains oil-like materials, it shows homogenous anechogenicity, which is easy to identify; when the content of steatocystoma is complex, it is difficult to distinguish between the two entities. In addition, the majority of epidermoid cysts show sinus tracts connected to the epidermis, but sinus tracts are rarely visualized in steatocystomas. This feature is helpful to distinguish the two entities.

Trichilemmal Cyst

The trichilemmal cyst often occurs in the scalp, but steatocystoma often occurs in the chest, upper extremities, and axillas. The image findings of steatocystomas are diverse on gray-scale ultrasound. However, most of trichilemmal cysts show a characteristic feature of "target sign." Ultrasound features can help in differentiation between the two entities.

Dermoid Cyst

The location of disease helps to differentiate the two entities. Dermoid cyst is a congenital disease. The most common location is the periorbital region. It is usually single. However, steatocystoma is often located in the chest, upper extremities, and axillas. It is usually multiple. Ultrasound features of the two entities are similar.

5.1.4.4 Diagnosis Clues

1. This disease occurs frequently in the young people, and its location is common in the chest, upper extremities, and axillas. It is usually manifested as a painless mass.
2. Gray-scale ultrasound often shows multiple, regular, and well-defined lesions. Flocculent, lumpy, or cord-like hyperechogenicity is visualized inside some lesions. They are usually located in the layers of dermis and subcutaneous tissues with posterior acoustic enhancement. There is often no blood flow signal in the lesion.
3. Steatocystoma may appear as an ill-defined and irregular hypoechoic lesion when ruptured and infected. Blood flow signals are visualized.

Key Points

- Steatocystoma is a retention cyst formed by obstruction of the opening of the sebaceous glands. Steatocystoma multiplex is mostly inherited in an autosomal dominant manner.
- It is common in the chest, upper extremities, and axillas.
- Gray-scale ultrasound often shows a hypoechoic lesion with flocculent, lumpy, or cord-like hyperechogenicity inside. There is often no blood flow signal in the lesion.

5.1.5 Lipoma

5.1.5.1 Clinical Manifestation and Pathology

Lipoma is a common benign soft tissue tumor composed of mature adipocytes. It occurs at all ages and is more common in the middle-aged adults from 40 to 60 years old and rare in children. Lipoma occurs all over the body with fat tissue, mostly in the chest, abdominal wall, scapular, and extremities.

According to the anatomical location of the lesion, lipomas are divided into superficial lipomas and deep lipomas. Superficial lipomas primarily are located on the subcutaneous tissue. Deep lipomas are located on deep tissue or intermuscle in the extremities, mostly growing along the muscles and it can be deep to the periosteum, but rarely invade the bones. Superficial lipomas are well-defined and soft. Some lesions may be elevated (Fig. 5.11).

Patients are asymptomatic usually and some may have local soreness and pain. Patients usually present with palpable mass. Lipomas rarely become malignant and are easily excised by surgery.

5.1.5.2 Ultrasound Manifestation

Gray-Scale Ultrasound

It is characterized by hypoechoic, isoechoic, or hyperechoic solid lesions in the subcutaneous fat layer. The lesions are spindle-shaped, oval, or round, with well-defined boundary. Lipomas showing hypoechogenicity are often single, and most are deeper in location and bulker in size. Short linear and banded hyperechogenicity is visualized inside the lesion, as well as the capsule. However, lipomas showing hyperechogenicity are often multiple, and most are more superficial and smaller. There is no posterior acoustic enhancement (Figs. 5.12, 5.13, and 5.14).

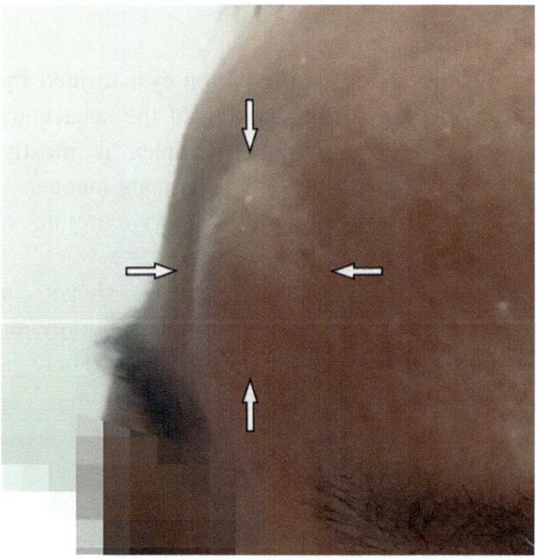

Fig. 5.11 Visual appearance of superficial lipoma. Visual observation shows an oval and skin-colored nodule in the forehead (arrows), the size of which is about 25.0 mm × 20.0 mm

Color Doppler Ultrasound

Color Doppler ultrasound shows no or rare blood flow signals in the periphery and interior of the lesion.

5.1.5.3 Differential Diagnosis

Liposarcoma

Most of the patients present with a palpable and painless mass with similar clinical symptoms to lipoma. Liposarcomas are mostly bulky, irregular, ill-defined, and rapidly growing.

Ultrasound findings are diverse, according to their different degrees of differentiation. Liposarcoma shows hyperechoic, mixed echogenic or hypoechoic lesions, with thin septa inside. Lesions often show rich blood flow signals. While lipomas mostly grow slowly and on ultrasound, the lipomas are regular and well-defined, which are features of benign tumors.

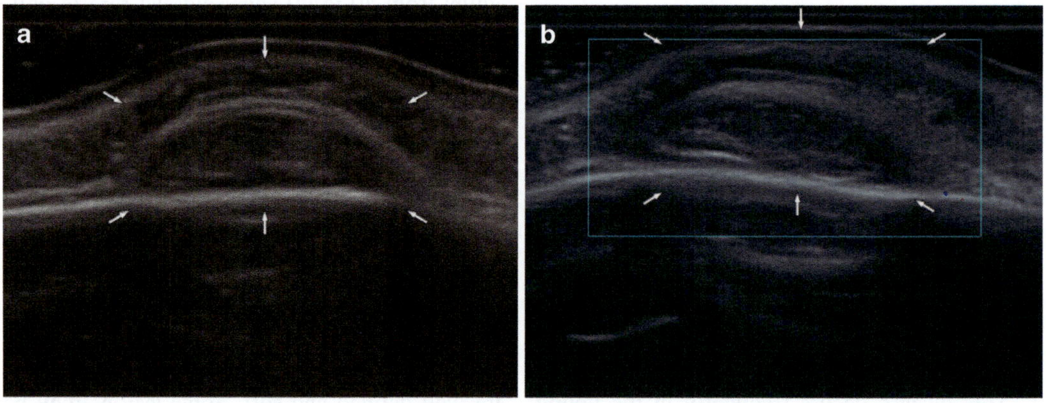

Fig. 5.12 Hypoechoic type lipoma. (**a**) Gray-scale ultrasound shows a regular, well-defined, and oval hypoechoic lesion with capsule (arrows) located in the subcutaneous fat layer (size: 22.5 mm × 19.2 mm; thickness: 10.2 mm). The lesion is heterogeneous, and short linear hyperechogenicity is visualized inside (Frequency: 18 MHz). (**b**) Color Doppler ultrasound shows no blood flow signals in the lesion (arrows) (Frequency: 18 MHz)

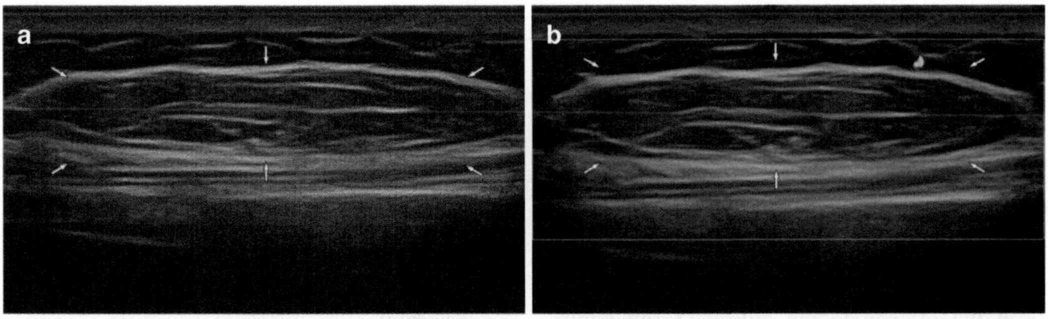

Fig. 5.13 Isoechoic type lipoma. (**a**) Gray-scale ultrasound shows a regular, well-defined, and spindle-shaped isoechoic lesion with capsule (arrows) located in the subcutaneous fat layer (size: 41.6 mm × 39.0 mm; thickness: 16.2 mm). The lesion is heterogeneous, and banded hyperechogenicity is visualized inside (Frequency: 18 MHz). (**b**) Color Doppler ultrasound shows no blood flow signals in the lesion (arrows) (Frequency: 18 MHz)

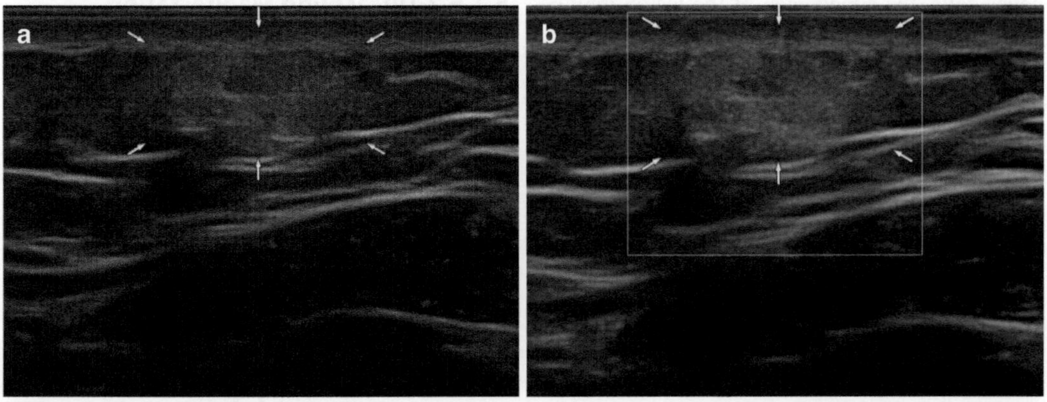

Fig. 5.14 Hyperechoic type lipoma. (**a**) Gray-scale ultrasound shows an oval and well-defined hyperechoic lesion without capsule, located in the subcutaneous fat layer (arrows) (size: 15.4 mm × 13.2 mm; thickness: 11.5 mm). The lesion is homogeneous (Frequency: 18 MHz). (**b**) Color Doppler ultrasound shows no blood flow signals in the lesion (arrows) (Frequency: 18 MHz)

Epidermoid Cyst

The two diseases appear as soft nodules in the subcutaneous tissue. On ultrasound, epidermoid cyst shows a round or oval mixed echogenic lesion in the subcutaneous tissue. "Dot-like" hyperechogenicity and/or "slit-like" anechogenicity are visualized in the lesion. Typically, it shows "onion-like" change. Sinus tracts are common in lesions. However, the superficial lipoma is well-defined and heterogeneous. Banded hyperechogenicity is visualized in the lesion, and there are no sinus tracts.

5.1.5.4 Diagnosis Clues

1. Most lesions appear as skin-colored, palpable, and soft masses. Patients are usually asymptomatic and some present with soreness or pain.
2. On ultrasound, the lesions are located in the subcutaneous tissue and appear as spindle-shaped, oval, or round hyperechoic nodules. Short linear and banded hyperechogenicity is visualized in the lesion.

Key Points

- Lipoma is a common benign soft tissue tumor in clinical practice, which is regular, well-defined, and growing slowly.
- On ultrasound, lipomas show different echogenicity depending on the anatomical location. The lesions located superficially tend to be hyperechoic and multiple, while the lesions located deeply tend to be hypoechoic and single.

5.1.6 Pigmented Nevus

5.1.6.1 Clinical Manifestation and Pathology

Pigmented nevus, also known as melanocytic nevus, cellular nevus, and nevocellular nevus, is a benign tumor composed of nevus cells. It is relatively common in clinical practice and occurs in all parts of the body surface. It occurs at all ages from the infancy to the elderly. From adolescence, the number of lesions gradually increases with age. It is more prevalent in women than in men and in whites than in blacks.

Due to the different content of pigment in nevus cells, the appearance of the lesion may be black, brown, blue-black, and a few are skin-colored or reddish. The surface of the lesion is rough and shows fine granular changes (Fig. 5.15). Pigmented nevus results from the gathering of melanocytes unexpectedly when the melanocytes move from the neural crest to the epidermis. The process of nevus cells nests moving from the basal layer to the dermis is also the process of nevus cells maturation. It is usually believed that the more mature the pigmented nevus is, the lower the probability of malignant transformation is.

According to the location of nevus cells histologically, pigmented nevi are divided into three types:

1. Junctional nevus: Regular and well-defined nevus cell nests are mainly located between the epidermis and dermis.
2. Intradermal nevus: Nevus cell nests are located only in the dermis and the epidermis is normal.
3. Mixed nevus: It contains the dual characteristics of junctional nevus and intradermal nevus.

5.1.6.2 Ultrasound Manifestation

Gray-Scale Ultrasound

Pigmented nevus appears as a regular or irregular and well-defined hypoechoic lesion located in the epidermis and/or dermis, with an elevated surface. It has no obvious keratinization. It may be jagged-like due to small slits and may form irregular acoustic shadowing due to gas between slits. The lesions are heterogeneous with flat bottoms. Sometimes cord-like hyperechogenicity is visualized in the lesion.

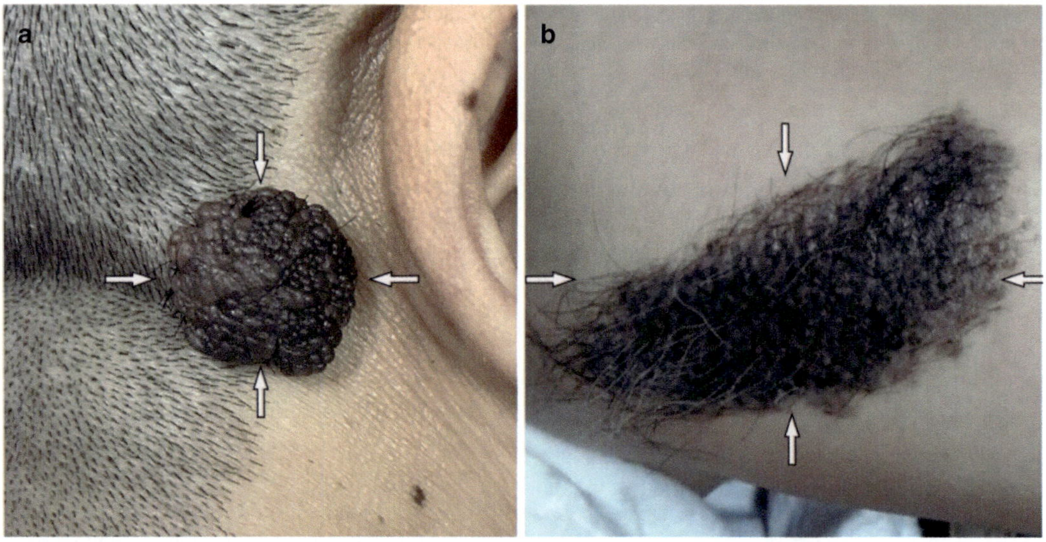

Fig. 5.15 Visual appearance of pigmented nevus. (**a**) A spherical, convex, and brown mass, the size of which is about 25.0 mm × 25.0 mm, is located near the right ear, with a rough and fine granular surface (arrows). (**b**) A black patch, the size of which is about 40.0 mm × 25.0 mm, is located in the right leg, with a rough and fine granular surface and black hairs (arrows)

Color Doppler Ultrasound

There are blood flow signals in the lesion (Figs. 5.16, 5.17 and 5.18).

5.1.6.3 Differential Diagnosis

Seborrheic Keratosis (SK)

Pigmented nevi are mostly black or brown bumps with rough and fine granular surface. In the late stage of SK, the lesions become dark brown with a rough surface, typically with "cerebriform-like" changes. It is difficult to differentiate SK from pigmented nevi when the lesion is atypical.

On gray-scale ultrasound, SK is characterized by regular hypoechogenic lesions in the epidermis. The ultrasound features of hyperkeratosis on the surface and posterior acoustic shadowing are helpful to differentiate the two entities. There are no blood flow signals in the lesion on color Doppler ultrasound. However, there are blood flow signals in the nevi due to that no abnormal keratinization is present on the surface.

Malignant Melanoma (MM)

The visual appearances of cutaneous MM in the early stage and pigmented nevus are similar. MM originates from the malignant transformation of melanocytic nevus. If the original melanocytic nevus grows rapidly, and shows uneven or

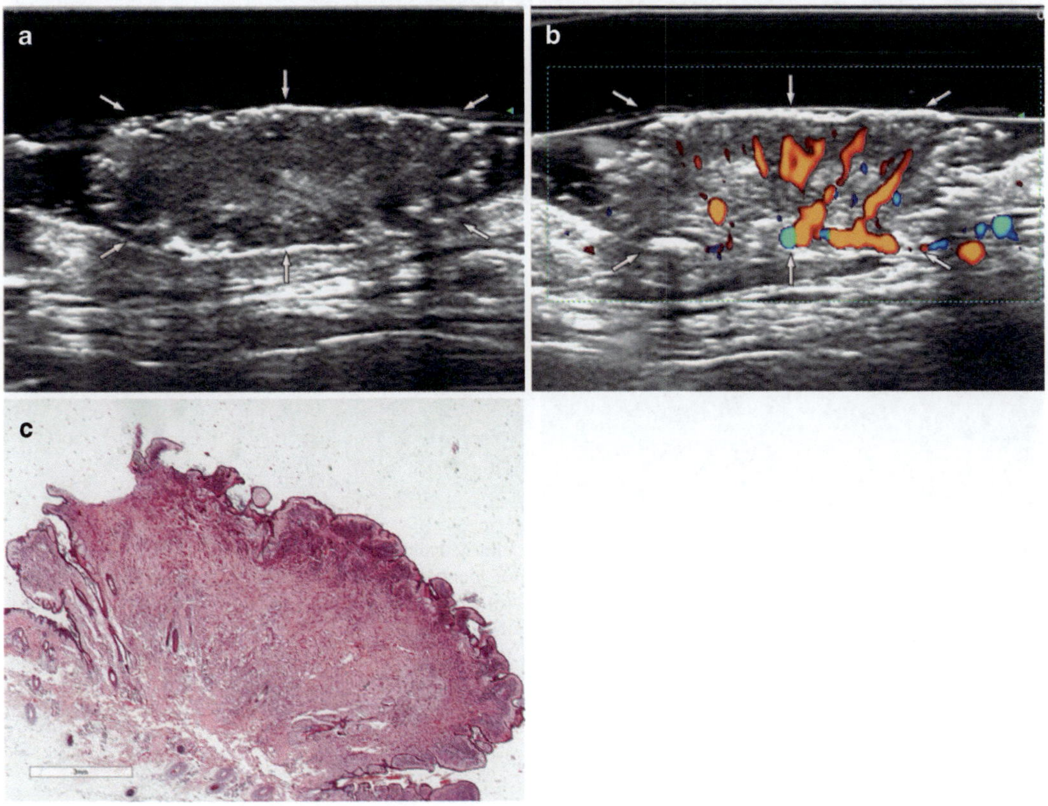

Fig. 5.16 Intradermal nevus. Male, 45 years of age. (**a**) Gray-scale ultrasound shows a regular and well-defined hypoechoic lesion (arrows) located in the dermis (size: 23.2 mm × 20.5 mm; thickness: 8.2 mm). The whole lesion protrudes outward. The lesion is heterogeneous, meanwhile dot and linear hyperechogenicity with posterior acoustic shadowing are visualized in the periphery, which are the ultrasound findings of air in the slits of the lesion (Frequency: 22 MHz). (**b**) Color Doppler ultrasound shows rich blood flow signals in the lesion (arrows) (Frequency: 22 MHz). (**c**) Histopathology (HE staining, panoramic scanning) shows that the epidermis is nearly normal and a large number of proliferated nevus cells are seen in the dermis. Nevus cells show nested and scattered distribution with maturation phenomenon. Nevus cells in the superficial layer contain pigment granules

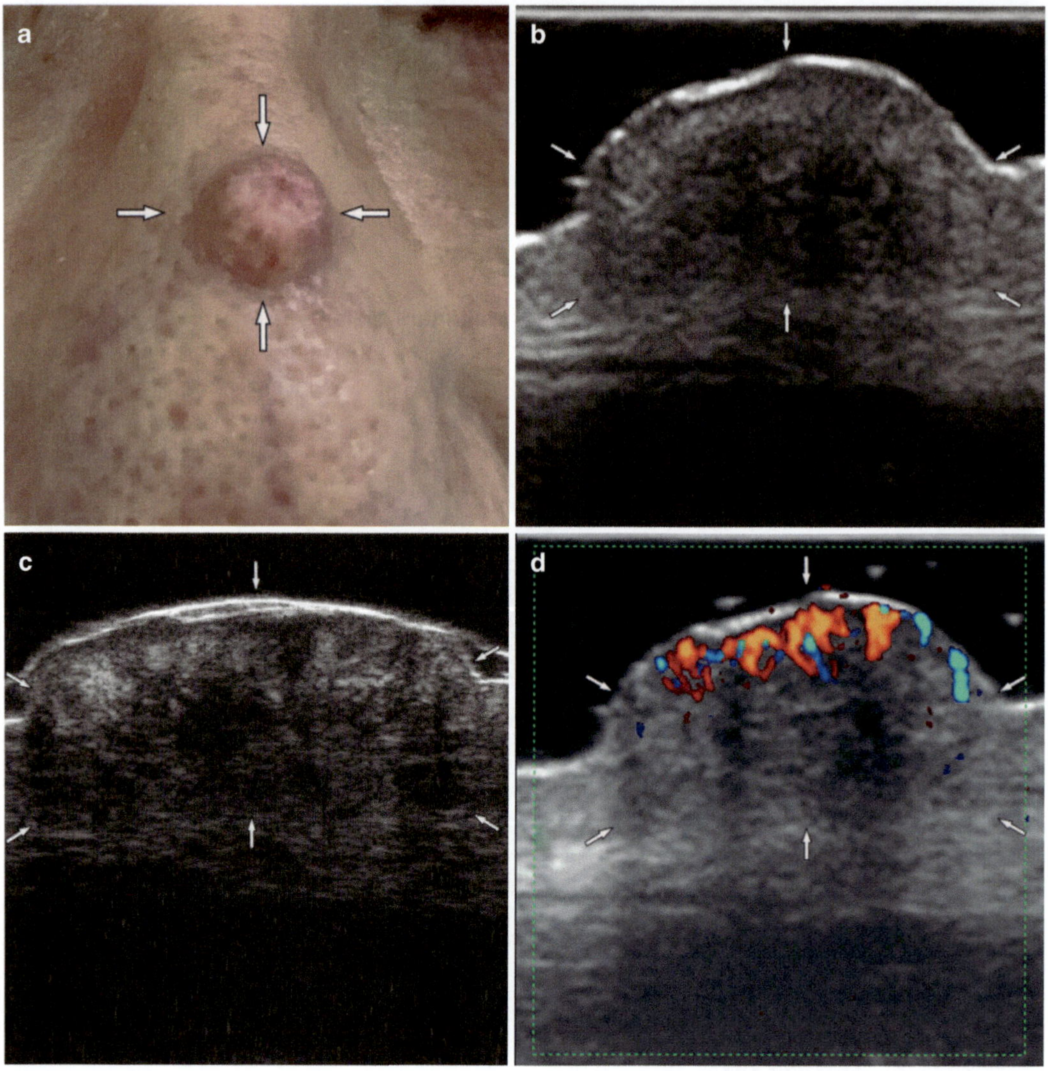

Fig. 5.17 Intradermal nevus. Male, 56 years of age. (**a**) Visual observation shows a skin-colored, well-defined, and soybean-sized hemispherical bump in the middle of the nose, without rupture (arrows). (**b**) Gray-scale ultrasound shows a regular, well-defined, and heterogeneous hypoechoic lesion (arrows) located in the dermis (size: 9.6 mm × 8.2 mm; thickness: 5.2 mm). The surface is elevated and smooth. The bottom is located in the junction of dermis/subcutaneous tissue (Frequency: 22 MHz). (**c**) Ultrasound biomicroscopy shows clearly the bottom of the lesion (arrows) (Frequency: 50 MHz). (**d**) Color Doppler ultrasound shows rich blood flow signals in the lesion (arrows) (Frequency: 22 MHz)

increased pigmentation, and irregular margin, the malignant transformation of melanocytic nevus should be highly suspected. Also, if pigmented nevus appears as an irregular, ill-defined, and heterogeneous lesion with rich blood flow signals on ultrasound, the diagnosis of MM is highly suspicious.

5.1.6.4 Diagnosis Clues

1. Visual appearance of nevus shows a black or brown patch or papule, and a few are skin-colored or reddish. On ultrasound, the lesions are regular, well-defined, and homogeneous. The slit-like structures are visualized on the surface.

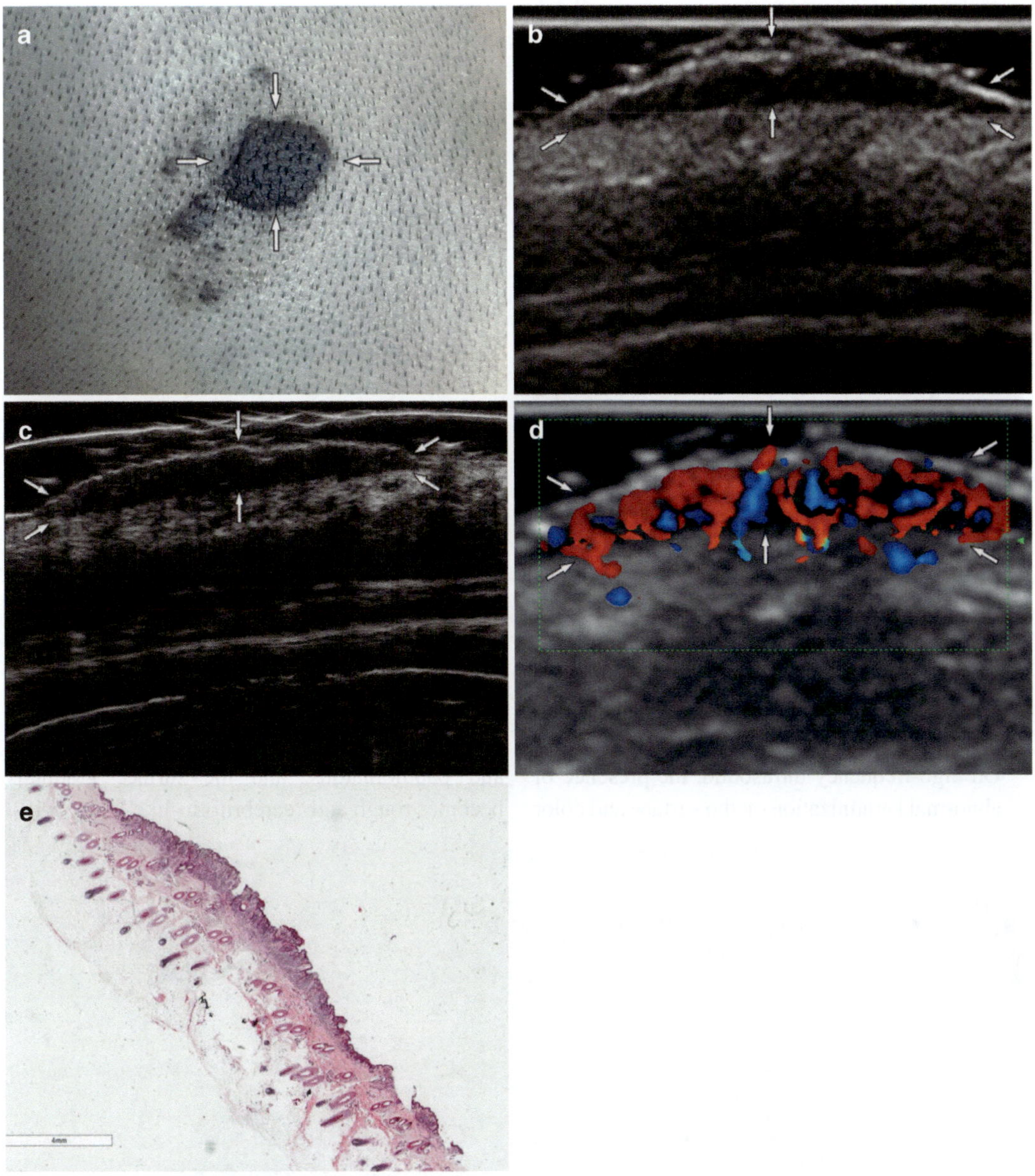

Fig. 5.18 Mixed nevus. Female, 7 years of age. (**a**) Visual observation shows an elevated, well-defined, and bean-sized black papule on the right scalp (arrows). Several rice-sized black patches are scattered at its margin. (**b**) Gray-scale ultrasound shows a regular, well-defined, and homogeneous hypoechoic lesion (arrows) located in the epidermis (size: 15.2 mm × 13.2 mm; thickness: 5.4 mm). The surface is elevated and rough without abnormal keratinization. The bottom is located in the dermo-epidermal junction (Frequency: 22 MHz). (**c**) Ultrasound biomicroscopy shows the bottom of the lesion clearly (arrows) (Frequency: 50 MHz). (**d**) Color Doppler ultrasound shows rich blood flow signals in the lesion (arrows) (Frequency: 22 MHz). (**e**) Histopathology (HE staining, panoramic scanning): The epidermis is nearly normal. Scattered or nested nevus cells distribute in the basal layer and dermis. The maturation phenomenon is visible and superficial nevus cells contain pigment granules

2. On ultrasound, it is mainly characterized by nodular or crawling and well-defined hypoechogenic lesion in the epidermis and/or dermis with an elevated and rough surface.
3. Color Doppler ultrasound shows blood flow signals in the lesion.

5.1.6.5 Clinical Significance

Histologically, pigmented nevi are divided into junctional nevi, intradermal nevi, and mixed nevi according to the location of nevus cells, but they cannot be differentiated by high-frequency ultrasound at present.

Sometimes, high-frequency ultrasound findings identify the involvement layer of the lesion bottom. The ultrasound feature of abnormal keratinization on the surface helps to differentiate pigmented nevus from SK. For pigmented nevi, it is important to identify its malignant change. Changes in visual appearances of the lesion (rapid growth, uneven or darker pigment, irregular shape) and changes in ultrasound features (irregular shape, ill-defined boundary) are helpful for the assessment of malignant change.

Key Points

- Pigmented nevi are classified as junctional, intradermal, and mixed nevi. The ultrasound findings are diverse and lack of characteristic features.
- On high-frequency ultrasound, the presence of abnormal keratinization on the surface and color Doppler ultrasound blood flow signals are helpful in differentiating pigmented nevus from SK.
- Changes in the visual appearances of the lesion (rapid growth, uneven or darker pigment, irregular shape) and changes in ultrasound features (irregular shape, ill-defined boundary) are helpful for the assessment of malignant change.

5.1.7 Seborrheic Keratosis

5.1.7.1 Clinical Manifestation and Pathology

Seborrheic keratosis (SK), also known as senile warts, is a benign skin tumor due to retarded maturation of keratinocytes. It has been reported that SK may have a potential tendency to occur malignant change. Most of the lesions are single, small, flat, well-defined, and yellowish or appear as brown patches with smooth or finely verrucous surface in the early stage. As the disease progressing, the lesions gradually enlarge. Most of them are regular and papillomatous, and the surface gradually becomes rough and "cerebriform-like" (Fig. 5.19).

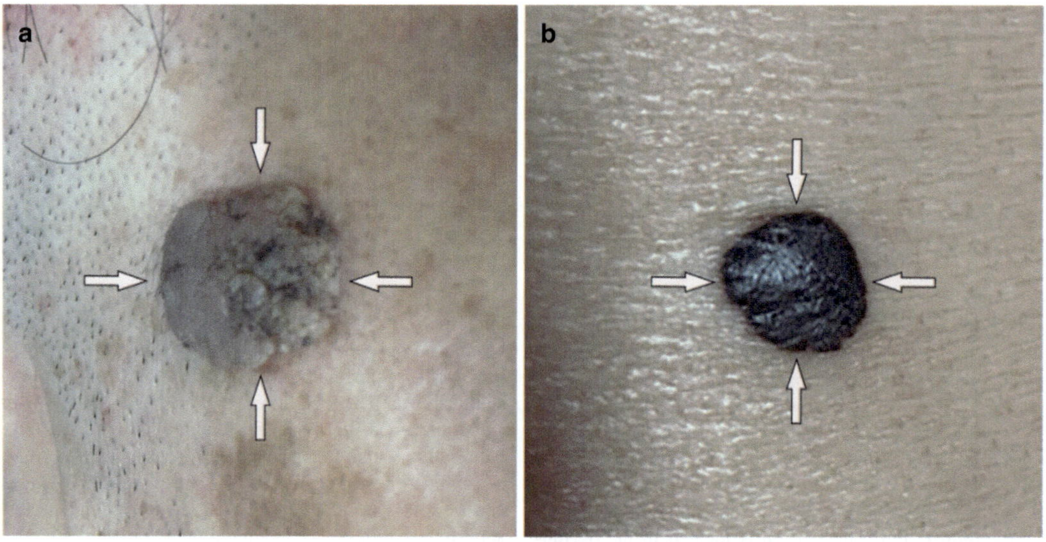

Fig. 5.19 Visual appearance of seborrheic keratosis. (**a**) A well-defined, brown, and patchy papule is in the right tempus with rough surface (arrows), the size of which is about 10.0 mm in diameter. (**b**) A verrucous and dark brown papule, the size of which is about 8.0 mm in diameter, is in the left shoulder, with rough surface showing the "cerebriform-like" change (arrows)

SK occurs all over the body. The majority of patients are usually asymptomatic and some present with pruritus or pain. Histopathologically, they are classified into the following subtypes: acanthotic, hyperkeratotic, adenoid, clonal, bowenoid, irritative, and so on. There are many histologic subtypes of SK, but their high-frequency ultrasound findings are similar.

5.1.7.2 Ultrasound Manifestation

Gray-Scale Ultrasound

SK appears as a hypoechoic lesion confined to the epidermis, showing a typical morphology of arcuate elevation with hyperechogenicity on the surface and various degrees of posterior acoustic shadowing. However, due to the presence of "cerebriform-like" crumple on the surface, it shows "serrated" changes locally based on the morphology of arcuate elevation.

The bottom of SK is well-defined and flat, and does not break through the dermo-epidermal junction. But sometimes the bottom is not clearly visualized due to acoustic shadowing caused by abnormal keratinization.

Color Doppler Ultrasound

There are blood flow signals in the lesion, but sometimes abnormal keratinization disturbs the visualization of blood flow signals (Figs. 5.20 and 5.21).

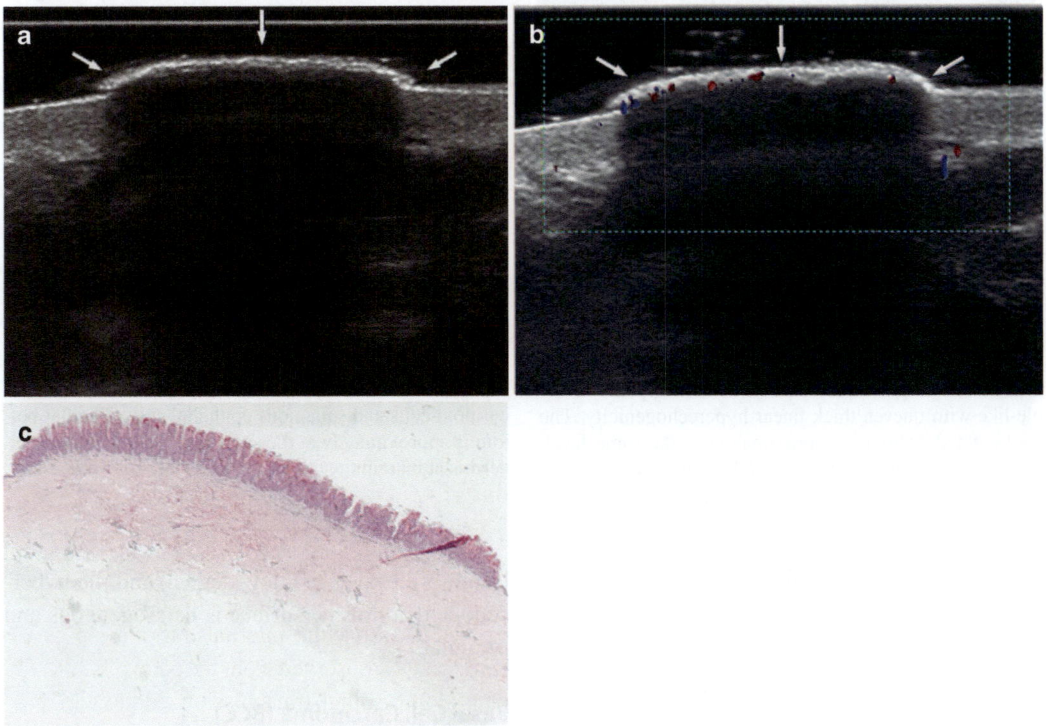

Fig. 5.20 Seborrheic keratosis. (**a**) Gray-scale ultrasound shows the lesion is arcuately elevated (arrows) (size: 18.2 mm × 15.2 mm; thickness: 3.1 mm). The surface shows a thick linear hyperechoic structure with posterior acoustic shadowing, which disturbs the visualization of the bottom (Frequency: 22 MHz). (**b**) Color Doppler ultrasound shows no blood flow signals in the lesion (arrows) (Frequency: 22 MHz). (**c**) Histopathology (HE staining, panoramic scanning) shows exophytic growth of the lesion with acanthosis and marked hyperkeratosis. Horn pseudocysts, pigmented granules, and lymphocytic infiltration in the superficial dermis are visualized. The proliferate cells are basaloid cells and squamous epithelial cells. The flat bottom is approximately at the same level as the normal epidermis at margins

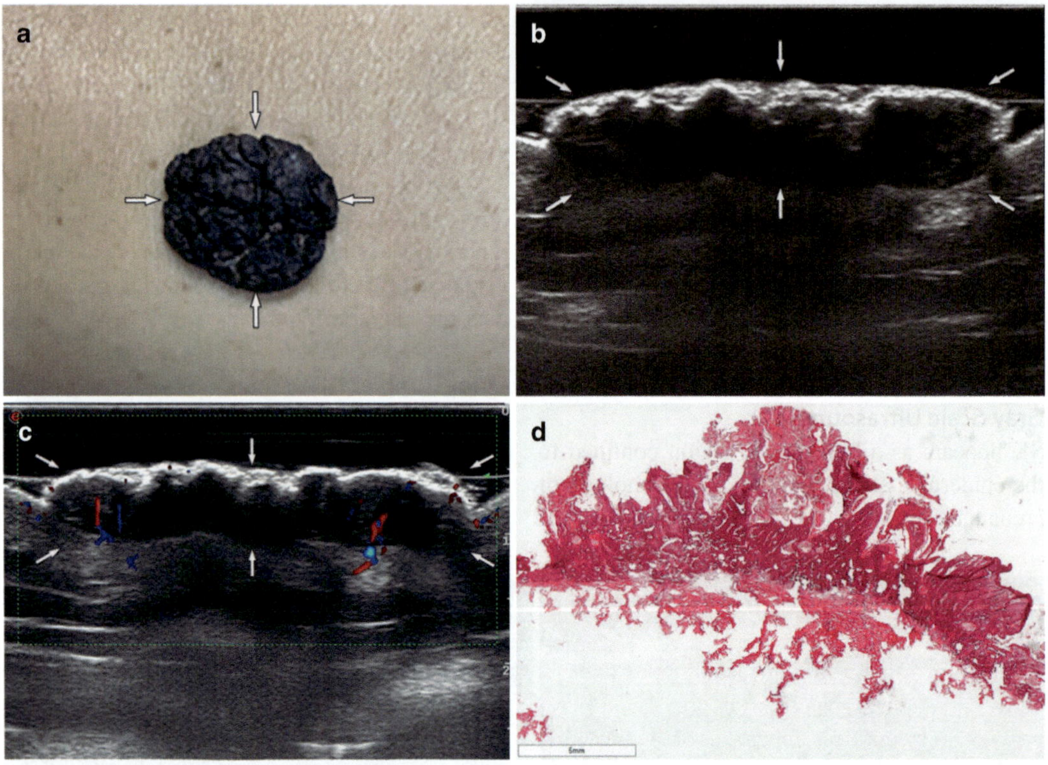

Fig. 5.21 Seborrheic keratosis. Male, 67 years of age. (**a**) Visual observation shows a black papule in the left buttock with a rough and "cerebriform-like" surface (arrows), the size of which is about 40.0 mm in diameter. (**b**) Gray-scale ultrasound shows an irregular hypoechoic lesion (arrows) in the epidermis (size: 40.2 mm × 39.4 mm; thickness: 7.5 mm). The elevated surface appears crumple-like with uneven thick linear hyperechogenicity. The well-defined bottom is approximately at the same level, and the echogenicity of dermis beneath the lesion is decreased. The lesion is homogeneous (Frequency: 22 MHz). (**c**) Color Doppler ultrasound shows rare blood flow signals in the lesion (arrows) (Frequency: 22 MHz). (**d**) Histopathology (HE staining, panoramic scanning) shows exophytic growth of the lesion with pronounced acanthosis and marked hyperkeratosis. Horn pseudocysts, pigmented granules, and lymphocytic infiltration in the superficial dermis are visualized. The proliferate cells are basaloid cells and squamous epithelial cells. The flat bottom is approximately at the same level as the normal epidermis at margins

5.1.7.3 Differential Diagnosis

Actinic Keratosis (AK)

In the early stage, both entities appear as a small and black patch, which is difficult to distinguish by the naked eyes. As the disease progressing, SK may show "cerebriform-like" appearance, which is helpful to differentiate them.

On gray-scale ultrasound, most of the two diseases appear as hypoechoic lesions within the epidermis with abnormal keratinization. SK is obviously elevated, the hyperechogenicity of the surface is serrated or lobulated, and the bottom is flat. However, the bottom of AK is ambiguous, and it seems to reach the superficial dermis. The lesion is elevated in a low degree, and the hyperechogenicity of the surface is heterogeneous and irregular.

Basal Cell Carcinoma (BCC)

BCC is located in the epidermis and/or dermis. On ultrasound, the surface is flat or elevated, and smooth. Most of them have no abnormal keratinization. Hyperechoic spots and anechoic areas are frequently observed in the lesion.

SK is hypoechoic and confined to the epidermis and has a rough surface with various degrees of hyperkeratosis on ultrasound. The internal blood flow signals of BCC are richer than that of SK.

Bowen's Disease (BD)

On ultrasound, the two entities are confined to the epidermis and the bottoms are clearly demarcated from the dermis. Different degrees of keratinization are visualized on the surface, with posterior acoustic shadowing. SK is elevated. However, BD is mostly crawling. Color Doppler ultrasound can help to differentiate them, and the internal blood flow signals of BD are richer than SK.

In addition, visual appearance of the lesions also helps to differentiate them. BD appears as a reddish or dark red papule or patch and may have scales on the surface; SK appears as a small, flat, and yellowish or brown patch in the early stage, and a characteristic "cerebriform-like" appearance in the late stage.

5.1.7.4 Diagnosis Clues

1. The lesion appears as a small, flat, well-defined, and yellowish or brown patch in the early stage. The surface is smooth or verrucous. In the late stage, the lesions gradually enlarge, and the surface gradually becomes dry and rough, showing "cerebriform-like" appearance.
2. On ultrasound, SK confines to the epidermis. The lesion is elevated, with lobulated or serrated hyperechogenicity on the surface and posterior acoustic shadowing.
3. On color Doppler ultrasound, there are no or rare blood flow signals in lesions.

Key Points

- SK is a benign tumor of the skin with a potential tendency to be malignancy. The "cerebriform-like" appearance on the surface is characteristic.
- Typically, ultrasound shows a hypoechoic lesion confined to the epidermis, demonstrating a typical morphology of arcuate elevation with hyperechogenicity on the surface and various degrees of posterior acoustic shadowing. The bottoms are clearly demarcated from the dermis and do not break through the dermo-epidermal junction.
- It should be differentiated from AK, BCC, and BD.

5.1.8 Pilomatricoma

5.1.8.1 Clinical Manifestation and Pathology

Pilomatricoma, also known as calcified epithelioma, originates from the hair matrix cells in the hair follicle and is a benign tumor located in the dermis or subcutaneous tissue. The disease often occurs in children and adolescents, and is commonly located in the head, neck, and extremities.

Clinically, it is usually single, occasionally multiple. It appears as a skin-colored, erythematous or bluish, and firm nodule. The lesion is slightly elevated and grows slowly. Most patients are asymptomatic. Histologically, the tumor is composed of cellular components and calcium. Sometimes, the tumor has a capsule. Malignant change is rare.

5.1.8.2 Ultrasound Manifestation

Gray-Scale Ultrasound

Gray-scale ultrasound shows an oval, well-defined, and solid lesion in the dermis or subcutaneous tissue. Patchy or scattered punctate hyperechogenicity is visualized in the interior caused by calcium deposition, surrounded by a ring-like hypoechogenic structure, with varying degrees of posterior acoustic shadowing. Studies showed that punctate calcifications are visible in 68% to 80% of cases (Figs. 5.22 and 5.23).

There are anechoic areas in some lesions, which are caused by intralesional hemorrhage or accumulation of anucleated cells without calcium deposition (Fig. 5.24).

Color Doppler Ultrasound

There are rich blood flow signals in the lesion. But sometimes calcification disturbs the display of blood flow signals.

5.1.8.3 Differential Diagnosis

Superficial Lymph Node

Superficial lymph nodes are the most commonly palpable superficial masses, and gray-scale ultrasound shows a subcutaneous hypoechoic lesion

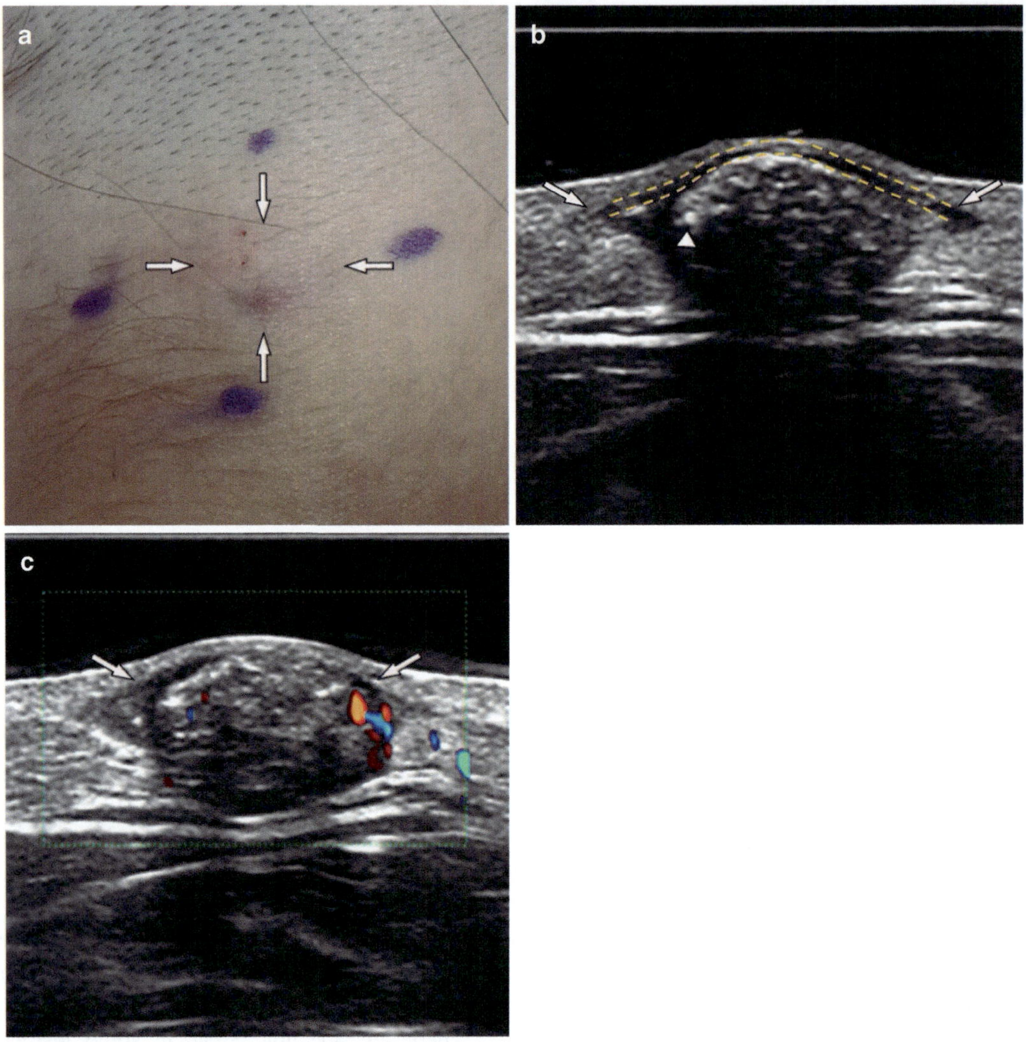

Fig. 5.22 Typical ultrasound findings of pilomatricoma. Female, 7 years of age. (**a**) Visual observation shows a slightly elevated lesion in the left neck, without redness and swelling (arrows), the size of which is about 15.0 mm in diameter. (**b**) Gray-scale ultrasound shows a regular, oval, and well-defined hypoechoic lesion (arrows) in the subcutaneous tissue (size: 16.2 mm × 14.5 mm; thickness: 7.5 mm). The lesion is heterogeneous and multiple punctate hyperechogenicity (▽) is visualized, with posterior acoustic shadowing. Ring-like hypoechogenicity is visible in the periphery of the lesion, and "cap-like" hypoechogenicity is visible on the top of the lesion (virtual line) (Frequency: 22 MHz). (**c**) Color Doppler ultrasound shows rare blood flow signals in the lesion (arrows) (Frequency: 22 MHz)

with a lymphatic hilum. Color Doppler ultrasound shows "portal type" blood flow signals.

However, typical pilomatrixoma does not have the above ultrasound features. Multiple punctate hyperechogenicity is visualized, with posterior acoustic shadowing. Ring-like hypoechogenicity is visible in the periphery of the lesion, and "cap-like" hypoechogenicity is visible on the top of the lesion. If a single lymph node is accompanied by calcification, it is difficult to differentiate the two entities and clinical history is fundamental.

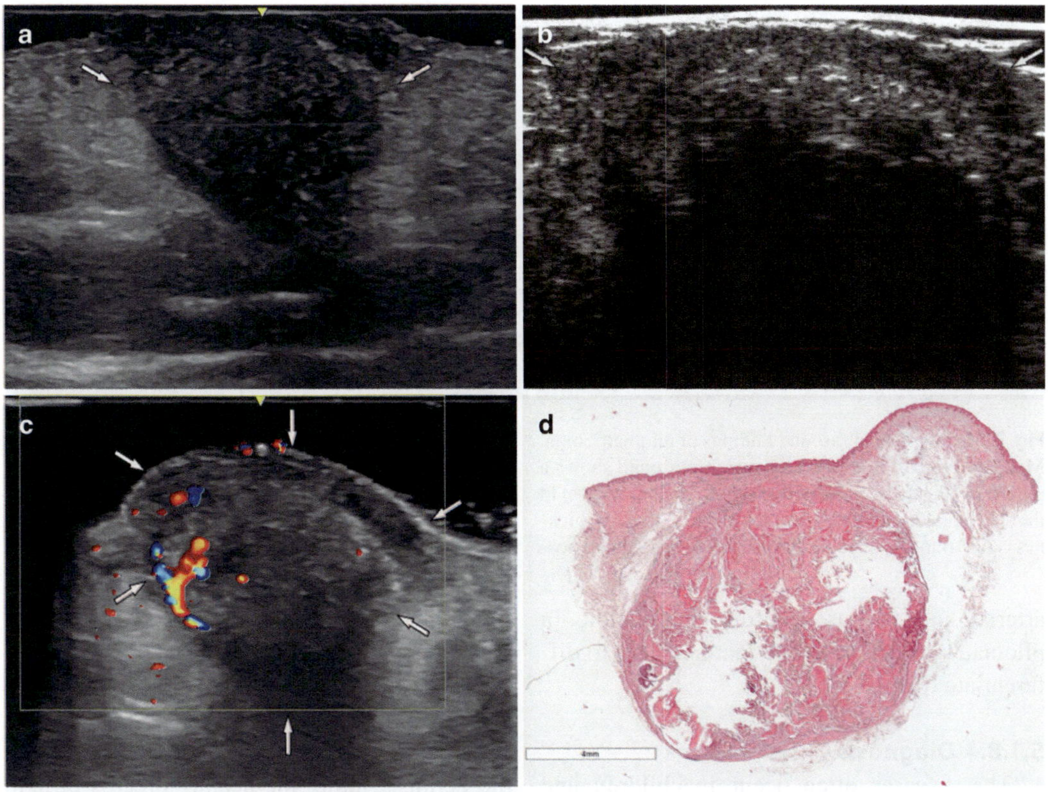

Fig. 5.23 Typical ultrasound findings of pilomatricoma. Male, 32 years of age. (**a**) Gray-scale ultrasound shows a regular, oval, and well-defined hypoechoic lesion (arrows) in the subcutaneous tissue (size: 11.5 mm × 9.2 mm; thickness: 9.6 mm). The lesion is heterogeneous and multiple punctate hyperechogenicity is visualized, with posterior acoustic shadowing. Ring-like hypoechogenicity is visible in the periphery of the lesion, and "cap-like" hypoechogenicity is visible on the top of the lesion (Frequency: 22 MHz). (**b**) Ultrasound biomicroscopy shows that part of the lesion and the punctate hyperechogenicity are visualized inside with posterior acoustic shadowing (arrows) (Frequency: 50 MHz). (**c**) Color Doppler ultrasound shows blood flow signals in the lesion (arrows) (Frequency: 22 MHz). (**d**) Histopathology (HE staining, panoramic scanning) shows that the well-defined lesion is located in the dermis. It is composed of a lot of eosinophilic ghost cells and a little of basaloid cells, as well as transitional cells, shadow cells, keratinization, and calcifications

Epidermoid Cyst

Epidermoid cysts need to be differentiated from atypical pilomatrixomas. Epidermoid cysts show heterogeneous mixed echogenic lesions in the subcutaneous tissue, with posterior acoustic enhancement. Dot-like hyperechogenicity and/or irregular slit-like anechogenicity are often visualized in epidermoid cysts specifically. Usually, there are no blood flow signals in the lesion.

However, ring-like hypoechogenicity is visible in the periphery of atypical pilomatrixoma. Sometimes, blood flow signals are detected in the periphery and interior of the lesion.

Hemangioma with Calcification

It needs to be differentiated from hemangioma when rich blood flow signals are shown in pilomatrixoma on color Doppler ultrasound. At this time, the gray-scale ultrasound of the two entities shows hypoechoic lesions in the subcutaneous tissue with internal hyperechogenicity.

Hemangioma is irregular and soft, without space-occupying effect. It can deform under the compression. While, pilomatrixoma is regular and firm with space-occupying effect. Spectral Doppler ultrasound of hemangiomas mostly shows a venous spectrum, while the

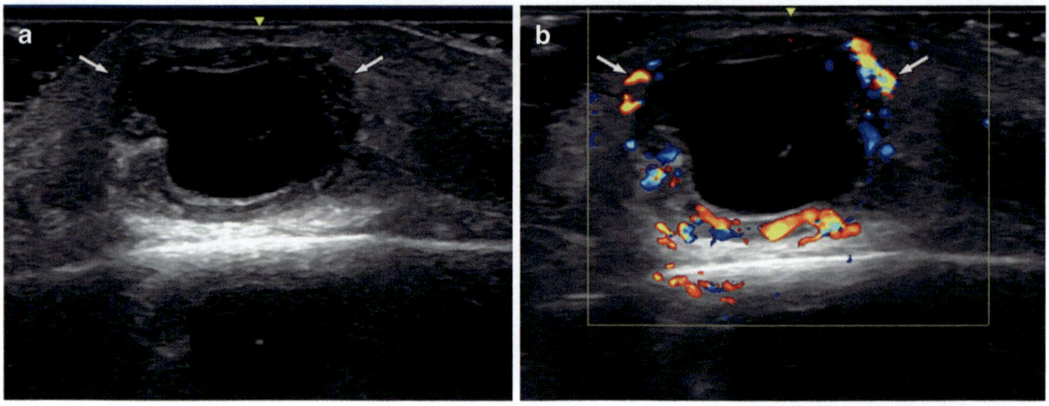

Fig. 5.24 Atypical ultrasound findings of pilomatricoma. Male, 24 years of age. (**a**) Gray-scale ultrasound shows a regular, oval, and well-defined anechoic lesion (arrows) in the subcutaneous tissue (size: 14.5 mm × 13.5 mm; thickness: 10.7 mm), with good acoustic transmission and posterior acoustic enhancement. Ring-like hypoechogenicity is visible in the periphery of the lesion (Frequency: 22 MHz). (**b**) Color Doppler ultrasound shows circular blood flow signals in the periphery of the lesion, but no blood flow signals inside (arrows) (Frequency: 22 MHz)

arterial and venous spectrum are visible in pilomatrixoma. The above features help to differentiate them.

5.1.8.4 Diagnosis Clues

1. The diseases often occur in children and adolescents, and lesions appear as skin-colored, erythematous or bluish, and firm nodules.
2. On gray-scale ultrasound, patchy or scattered dot-like hyperechogenicity is visualized in the interior. The peripheral "ring-like" or "cap-like" hypoechogenicity is its characteristic feature. When the lesion appears as anechoic change, it is difficult to diagnose.

Key Points

- Pilomatrixoma is a benign tumor located in the dermis or subcutaneous tissues, usually found in children and adolescents. It is often located in the head, neck, and extremities. It is firm.
- Typically, ultrasound shows a hypoechoic lesion in the subcutaneous tissue, and patchy or scattered dot-like hyperechogenicity is visualized in the interior. The peripheral "ring-like" or "cap-like" hypoechogenicity is its characteristic feature.

5.1.9 Scar

5.1.9.1 Clinical Manifestation and Pathology

Skin scar is a unique fibrometabolic disease in the dermis. During the healing process of skin injury, collagen synthesis and metabolism are disturbed and remain in an exuberant state resulting in excessive fiber proliferation. It is also known as desmoplasia.

The pathological changes of skin scar are massive proliferation of fibroblasts and excessive deposition of collagen in the dermis. Histologically, it is divided into:

1. Superficial scars: It occurs in the epidermis or dermis and is usually flat without dysfunction.
2. Hypertrophic scar: It occurs in the deep dermis and protrudes outward, but limited to the original extent of injury.
3. Atrophic scar: It occurs in the soft tissue and may involve the whole layers of skin. It has great contractility and can cause severe dysfunction by dragging the adjacent tissues and organs.
4. Keloids: Most keloids occur after the local injury 1 year later. It usually appears as a red

and firm bump, protruding outwards. Lesions are diverse in shape, usually do not regress spontaneously, and sometimes accompanied with pruritus or pain.

5.1.9.2 Ultrasound Manifestation

Gray-Scale Ultrasound

The lesion is nodular or irregularly elevated. Depending on the depth of injury, blurring or disappearance of the two demarcations (between the epidermis and dermis, or between the dermis and subcutaneous tissue) may occur in turn.

If it is confined to the epidermis, there are no characteristic findings on ultrasound. If the dermis is involved, the lesion appears as significantly thickened dermis with plaque-like hypoechogenicity. The lesion has no space-occupying effect. The skin appendages often disappear. When it involves into subcutaneous tissue, the above findings extend to the depth.

Color Doppler Ultrasound

There are no or rare blood flow signals in the lesion (Figs. 5.25 and 5.26).

5.1.9.3 Differential Diagnosis

The disease can be diagnosed based on clinical history. However, it still needs to be differentiated from dermatofibrosarcoma protuberans on visual appearance. Most of the two entities appear as red, firm, and elevated bumps.

Gray-scale ultrasound findings help to differentiate them. Dermatofibrosarcoma protuberans is mainly located in the subcutaneous tissue. Hyperechogenic and hypoechogenic bands are

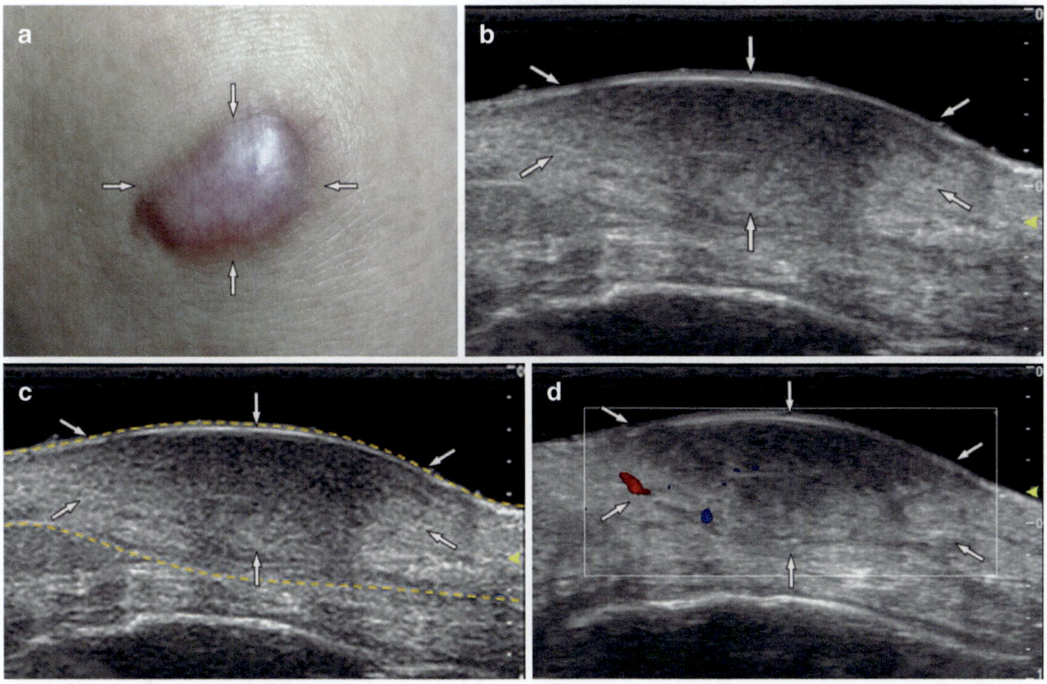

Fig. 5.25 Keloid. Female, 35 years of age. (**a**) Visual observation shows a reddish and slightly elevated lesion in the left knee, with a smooth surface (arrows), the size of which is about 15.2 mm in diameter. (**b**) Gray-scale ultrasound shows that the dermis thickens obviously where this lesion is located (thickness of the lesion: 7.3 mm; thickness of adjacent normal dermis: 3.0 mm). The lesion is heterogeneous with an irregular hypoechoic area (arrows) visualized in the center (size: 6.2 mm × 5.2 mm; thickness: 3.4 mm). The epidermis, where the lesion is located, is smooth and continuous, without abnormal keratinization (Frequency: 34 MHz). (**c**) The ill-defined lesion is located in the dermis, without obvious space-occupying effect (arrows). Its top and bottom naturally continue with the junctions of dermis/epidermis and dermis/subcutaneous tissue, respectively (yellow dotted line) (Frequency: 34 MHz). (**d**) Color Doppler ultrasound shows rare blood flow signals in and around the lesion (arrows) (Frequency: 34 MHz)

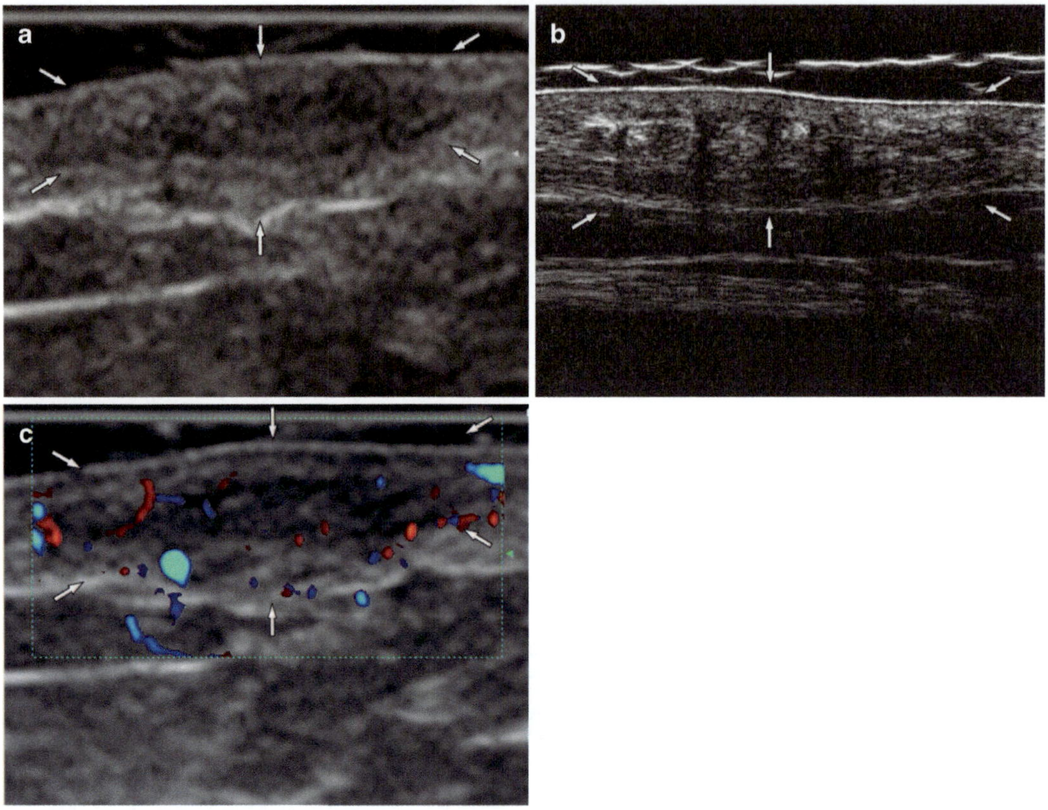

Fig. 5.26 Superficial scar. Female, 20 years of age. (**a**) Gray-scale ultrasound shows that the thickened dermis appears as an irregular and ill-defined hypoechoic lesion (arrows) (size: 20.5 mm × 16.4 mm; thickness: 4.2 mm). The lesion has no space-occupying effect. The lesion is heterogeneous (Frequency: 22 MHz). (**b**) Ultrasound biomicroscopy shows that the dermis is thickened and the lesion is irregular and ill-defined without space-occupying effect. The lesion is heterogeneous, showing hyperechogenicity and plaque-like hypoechogenicity, with banded posterior acoustic shadowing (arrows) (Frequency: 50 MHz). (**c**) Color Doppler ultrasound shows rare blood flow signals in the lesion (arrows) (Frequency: 22 MHz)

visualized in the lesion, and the pseudopodia-like protrusions extending to adipose tissue in the periphery, forming a typical characteristic of "whirlpool sign." However, the scar shows significantly thickened dermis with plaque-like hypoechogenicity. The lesion has no space-occupying effect.

5.1.9.4 Diagnosis Clues

1. With a definite clinical history, most of scars appear as elevated, irregular, skin-colored, and firm nodules, and some of lesions appear as flat and reddish patches.
2. On ultrasound, the stratum corneum of the lesion is continuous but irregularly elevated. The dermis is thickened, with local echogenicity decreased. The lesion has no space-occupying effect.
3. On color Doppler ultrasound, most of the lesions have no blood flow signals inside, and some show rare blood flow signals. Most keloids show rare blood flow signals.

5.1.9.5 Clinical Significance

Clinical history and the visual appearance of the lesions are helpful for the diagnosis of scars. High-frequency ultrasound provides information such as the size, thickness, and blood flow signals of the scar, and facilitates evaluation of the therapeutic effect. SWE might be an ideal method for assessing the stiffness of keloids and their therapeutic effects.

Key Points

- Most of the scars have a definite clinical history and are firm.
- Typical ultrasound findings are thickened dermis with local echogenicity decreased. The lesion is well-defined without obvious space-occupying effect.
- It should be differentiated from dermatofibrosarcoma protuberans.

5.1.10 Keratoacanthoma

5.1.10.1 Clinical Manifestation and Pathology

Keratoacanthoma (KA) is a common skin tumor that remains controversial regarding classification. It is thought to originate from the infundibulum of hair follicles. The disease grows rapidly and tends to regress spontaneously. KA mostly occurs in the middle-aged and elderly patients, and it commonly occurs in the naked areas of the body. It is currently considered to be possibly related to viral infection and ultraviolet exposure.

Clinically, KA is usually divided into three types: solitary, multiple, and special, of which the solitary type is more common. The lesion often appears as a firm, well-defined, reddish, elevated, and hemispherical nodule. The center of the lesion is filled with keratin plug, and appears "volcano-like" when the keratin is stripped, with dilation of the capillaries in the periphery.

There are three steps of KA development: proliferation, maturation, and regression. Most lesions regress spontaneously within 6 months then leaving scars. Histopathologically, KA has been considered as a variant of cutaneous squamous cell carcinoma (cSCC) and is often reported as KA-type cSCC. However, due to the penchant for regression, KA also has been considered as biologically benign tumor with distinct pathophysiological mechanism from malignant cSCC.

5.1.10.2 Ultrasound Manifestation

Gray-Scale Ultrasound

Gray-scale ultrasound shows a nodular and well-defined hypoechoic lesion in the epidermis and dermis. The surface of the lesion is elevated, with a characteristic central hyperkeratotic area, forming an "inverted triangle" posterior acoustic shadowing, which disturbs the visualization of the interior and bottom of the lesion.

After changing the scanning direction to avoiding acoustic shadowing, the bottom of the lesion is visualized, which bulges to the deep tissue.

Color Doppler Ultrasound

Rich blood flow signals are detected in the periphery and interior of the lesion, but sometimes the hyperkeratosis disturb the visualization of blood flow signals in the area of acoustic shadowing (Figs. 5.27 and 5.28).

5.1.10.3 Differential Diagnosis

Squamous Cell Carcinoma (SCC)

KA is easily confused with SCC both clinically and histopathologically. The central ulcer of KA is relatively regular, and it tends to regress spontaneously. However, the margin of ulceration in SCC may be cauliflower-like. But actually, differentiation is still difficult in real clinical practice.

On gray-scale ultrasound, SCC appears as a heterogeneous and ill-defined hypoechoic lesion, that often involves the whole layer of the skin, even deep tissues. While KA forms a characteristic "inverted triangular" posterior acoustic shadowing, and is clearly demarcated from the surrounding tissue. KA usually does not involve the subcutaneous tissue.

Nodular Basal Cell Carcinoma (BCC)

The lesions of nodular BCC show light brown, pearl-like, or patchy papules. KA often shows reddish, elevated, and hemispherical nodules with keratin plug in the center, which is "volcano-like" after stripping the keratin.

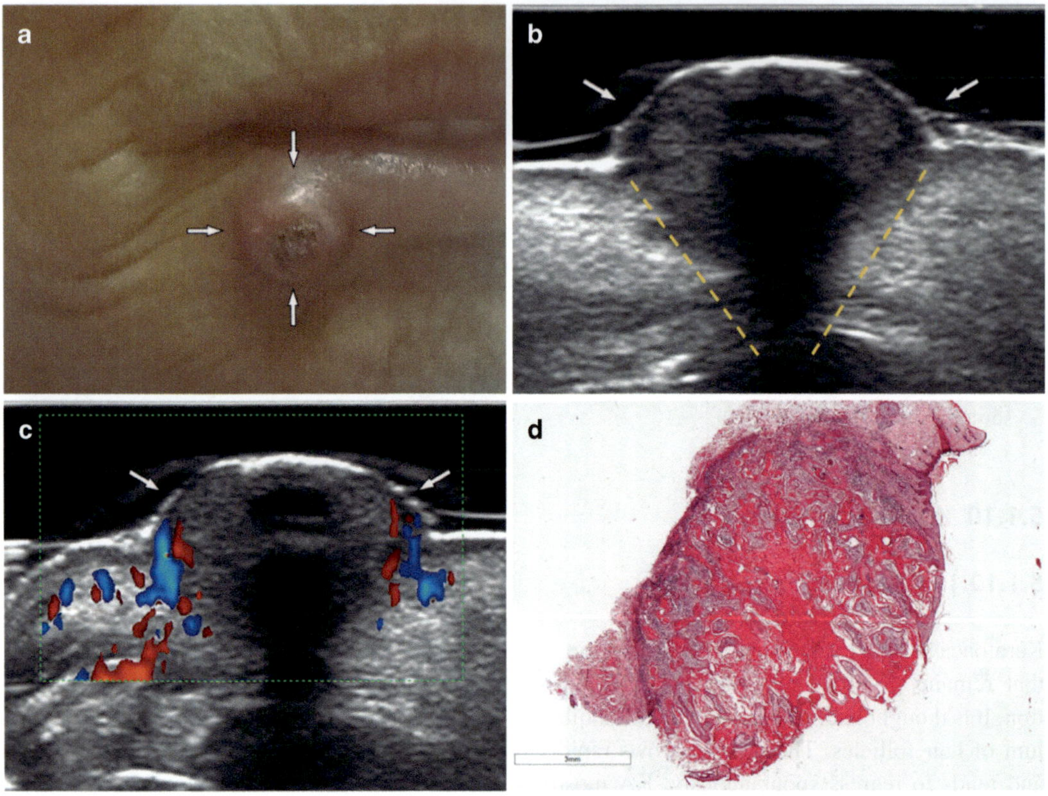

Fig. 5.27 Keratoacanthoma. Female, 63 years of age. (**a**) Visual observation shows a hemispherical and reddish lesion located in the lower jaw, with a scab in the center of the surface (arrows), the size of which is about 13.0 mm in diameter. (**b**) Gray-scale ultrasound shows a nodular, elevated, homogeneous, and well-defined hypoechoic lesion (arrows) located in the epidermis and dermis (size: 13.2 mm × 12.6 mm; thickness: 8.5 mm). Fine linear hyperechogenicity is visualized in the center, with "inverted triangle" posterior acoustic shadowing (dotted line) (Frequency: 22 MHz). (**c**) Color Doppler ultrasound shows that local hyperkeratosis disturbs the visualization of blood flow signals at the bottom of the lesion. Rich blood flow signals are only showed in the periphery of the lesion (arrows) (Frequency: 22 MHz). (**d**) Histopathology (HE staining, panoramic scanning) shows that the lesion has no obvious boundary and is composed of proliferation of squamous cells in lobules. Hyperkeratosis is visible, with lymphocytes and Langhans cells infiltration in the interstitium. The cells have obvious atypia, with infiltrative growth in some areas

On gray-scale ultrasound, sometimes both nodular BCC and KA show regular and well-defined hypoechoic lesions located in the epidermis and dermis. KA forms a characteristic "inverted triangular" posterior acoustic shadowing due to the keratin plugs in the center of the lesion. Most of the nodular BCC show hyperechoic spots and/or anechoic areas inside, without abnormal keratinization on the surface. The gray-scale ultrasound findings of the two diseases are characteristic and easily differentiated from each other.

5.1.10.4 Diagnosis Clues

1. Visual appearance shows a reddish, elevated, and hemispherical nodule with keratin plug and scab in the center of the rough surface. After stripping the keratin, the center of the lesion is "volcano-like" and well-defined. Some lesions regress spontaneously, only leaving scar.

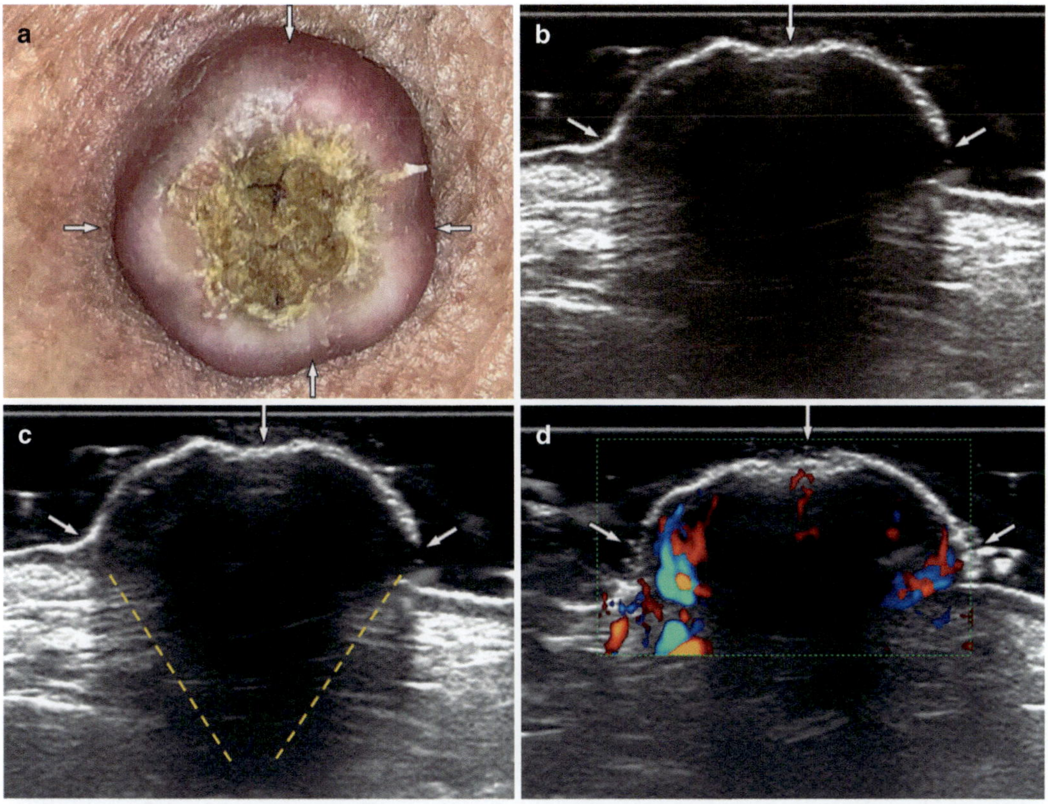

Fig. 5.28 Keratoacanthoma. Female, 63 years of age. (**a**) Visual observation shows a lesion in the middle of the right cheek (arrows), the size of which is about 12.0 mm in diameter. A "volcano-like" surface is visible in the center of the lesion, which is filled with keratin plugs. The edge of the lesion shows a dike-like elevation. (**b**) Gray-scale ultrasound shows a nodular and heterogeneous hypoechoic lesion (arrows) located in the epidermis and dermis (size: 12.2 mm × 10.5 mm; thickness: 7.6 mm). The lesion is elevated, with a slight hollow in the center of the surface and linear hyperechogenicity. (**c**) The linear hyperechogenicity is accompanied by "inverted triangle" posterior acoustic shadowing (dotted line) (Frequency: 22 MHz). (**d**) Color Doppler ultrasound shows rich blood flow signals in the periphery of the lesion (arrows) (Frequency: 22 MHz)

2. On gray-scale ultrasound, KA shows a hypoechoic lesion in the epidermis and dermis, with an elevated surface and a characteristic central hyperkeratotic area, forming a characteristic "inverted triangle" posterior acoustic shadowing.

Key Points

- KA is a common skin tumor that remains controversial regarding classification and has a tendency to regress spontaneously.
- Visual observation shows a reddish, elevated, and hemispherical nodule with keratin plug and scab in the center. After stripping the keratin, the center of the lesion is "volcano-like."
- Typical ultrasound features are hypoechoic lesions in the epidermis and dermis, with characteristic central hyperkeratotic areas on the surface and characteristic "inverted triangular" posterior acoustic shadowing.
- It should be differentiated from SCC and nodular BCC.

5.1.11 Dermatofibroma

5.1.11.1 Clinical Manifestation and Pathology

Dermatofibroma is a benign skin tumor characterized by the proliferation of collagen fibers and fibroblasts in the dermis. Its etiology is uncertain, but it can result from an inflammatory change of reactive proliferation of fibroblasts caused by trauma. It often has no tendency of spontaneous regression, so it is still considered as a tumor.

It occurs in both men and women, commonly in the young and middle-aged patients. It is often located in the extremities. The lesions are often single or multiple. Visual appearance shows skin-colored, yellowish-brown or dark brown, oblate or button-shaped, small and firm nodule, which protrudes outward. The lesion is pushable and grows slowly. Patients are usually asymptomatic and some present with pruritus and mild pain.

5.1.11.2 Ultrasound Manifestation

Gray-Scale Ultrasound

Gray-scale ultrasound shows a regular, ill-defined, and homogeneous hypoechoic lesion located in the dermis with a slightly elevated surface. The epidermis is continuous without abnormal keratinization.

Color Doppler Ultrasound

There is no or rare blood flow signals in the lesion (Figs. 5.29 and 5.30).

5.1.11.3 Differential Diagnosis

Dermatofibrosarcoma Protuberans (DFSP)

DFSP appear as brownish-red and reddish subcutaneous painless nodules. The lesion grows rapidly. On high-frequency ultrasound, banded hyperechogenicity and hypoechogenicity are visualized in the lesion, and characteristic hypoechoic "pseudopodia" extends to adipose tissue in the periphery to form a "whirlpool sign."

However, most dermatofibromas appear as small, brown, firm, and protrusive nodules. On high-frequency ultrasound, although the demarcation between the lesion and the surrounding tissue is not clear, there is no "pseudopodia" extending to the adipose tissue.

Cavernous Hemangioma

It often occurs after birth, and it is always found on the scalp, face, and oral mucosa. The lesion appears as round or irregular, skin-colored or red-blue, soft and elevated patch on the skin. The lesion invades deeply and widely. Most dermatofibromas appear as yellow-brown or dark brown, small, firm, and protrusive nodules.

Color Doppler ultrasound is helpful to differentiate them. Cavernous hemangioma has characteristic high-frequency ultrasound features: the compression by transducer can cause deformation of the lesion; when the transducer rapidly squeezes the lesion, the blood flow signals increased transiently on color Doppler ultrasound, followed by decrease or even disappearance of blood flow signals in the lesion. However, there is usually no or rare blood flow signals in the dermatofibroma.

Verrucous Epidermal Nevus

Verrucous epidermal nevus is known as linear verrucous epidermal nevus. It is composed of keratinocytes that arise from pluripotential germ cells in the basal layer of the embryonic ectoderm and results from mosaic postzygotic mutations. It is usually present at birth or within the first year of life.

Visual appearance shows pale to dark brown papules with rough and verrucous keratinization on the surface. Most dermatofibromas appear as yellow-brown or dark brown, small and firm nodules. On high-frequency ultrasound, verrucous nevi appear as hypoechoic lesions located in the epidermis. The surface is irregular and elevated with hyperkeratosis and posterior acoustic shadowing. But dermatofibromas are located in the dermis with a curved elevation of the surface without hyperkeratosis.

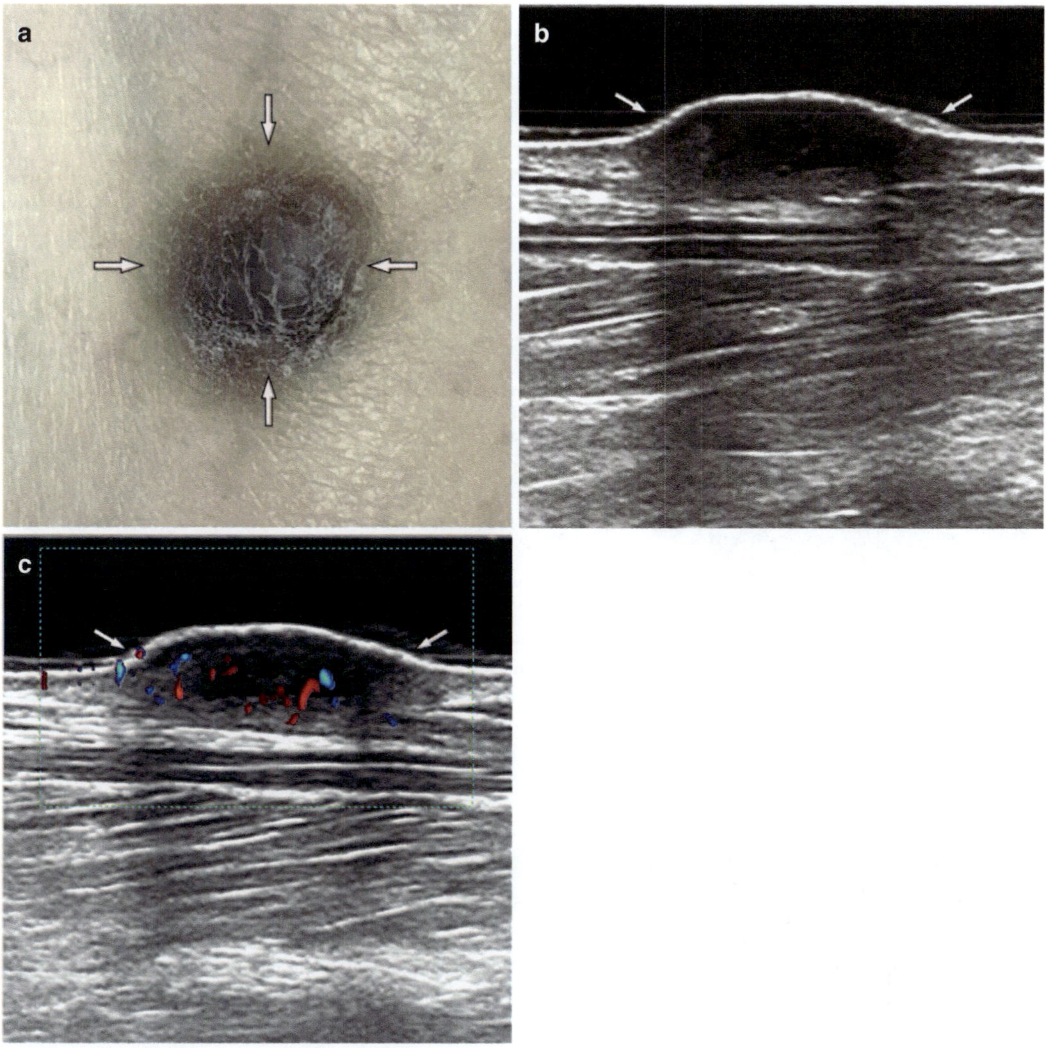

Fig. 5.29 Dermatofibroma. Female, 64 years of age. (**a**) Visual observation shows a dark brown and well-defined patch in the left pretibial, protruding outward (arrows), the size of which is about 15.0 mm × 14.0 mm. (**b**) Gray-scale ultrasound shows a regular, nodular, ill-defined, and heterogeneous hypoechoic lesion (arrows) located in the dermis (size: 13.2 mm × 12.5 mm; thickness: 7.8 mm). The surface of the lesion is elevated and the stratum corneum is continuous without abnormal keratinization (Frequency: 22 MHz). (**c**) Color Doppler ultrasound shows rare blood flow signals in the lesion (arrows) (Frequency: 22 MHz)

5.1.11.4 Diagnosis Clues

1. Visual appearance shows an oblate or button-shaped, protrusive, small, firm, and brown nodule. Patients may present with pruritus, mild pain, or other discomfort.
2. High-frequency ultrasound shows an oval hypoechoic lesion in the dermis with continuous stratum corneum and an unclear demarcation between the bottom and the surrounding tissue. There is no or rare blood flow signals in the lesion.

Key Points

- Dermatofibroma is a benign skin tumor characterized by proliferation of collagen fibers and fibroblasts in the dermis.
- Ultrasound shows an oval hypoechoic lesion in the dermis with continuous stratum cor-

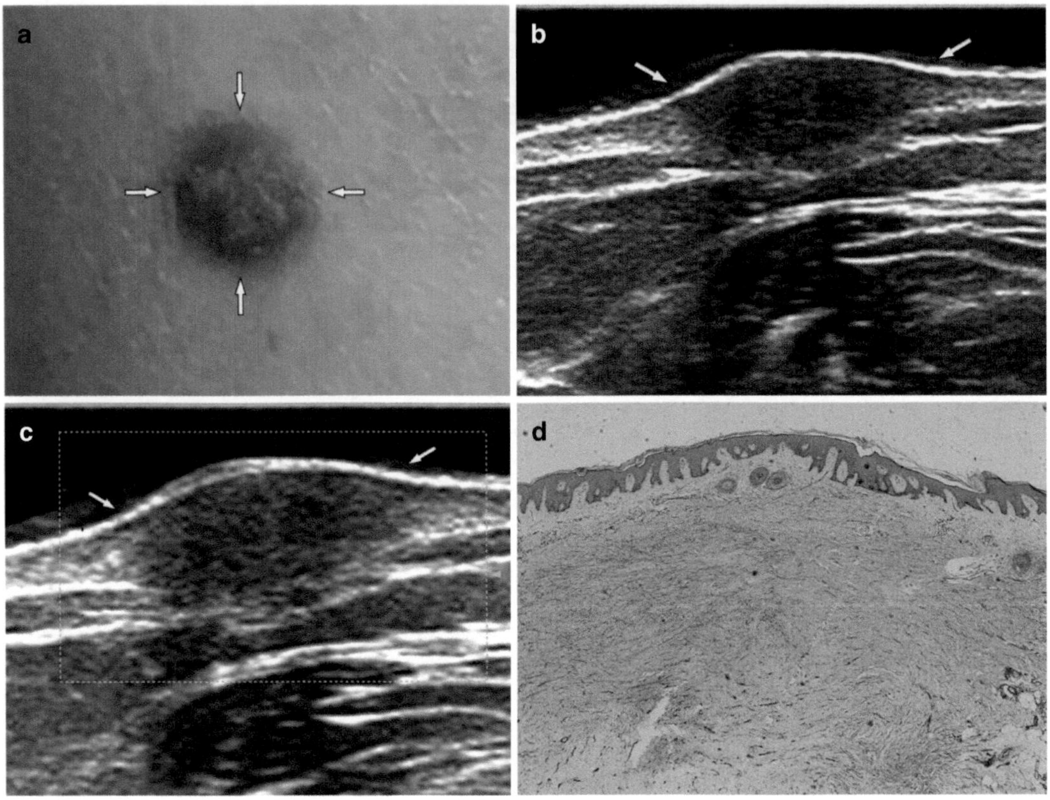

Fig. 5.30 Dermatofibroma. Female, 44 years of age. (**a**) Visual observation shows an oblate, coin-sized, and brown papule in the right leg. The surface is smooth without bleeding and exudates (arrows). (**b**) Gray-scale ultrasound shows a regular, nodular, homogeneous, and ill-defined hypoechoic lesion (arrows) located in the dermis (size: 11.2 mm × 9.5 mm; thickness: 4.5 mm). The surface is elevated and the stratum corneum is continuous without abnormal keratinization. The bottom reaches the dermis/subcutaneous tissue junction (Frequency: 22 MHz). (**c**) Color Doppler ultrasound shows no blood flow signal in the lesion (arrows) (Frequency: 22 MHz). (**d**) Histopathology (HE staining, panoramic scanning) shows proliferative epidermis, prolonged dermatome, and increased pigment in the basal layer. There are proliferation of a large number of fibroblasts and collagen fibers in the dermis. Collagen fenestration is visible

neum and an unclear demarcation between the bottom and the surrounding tissue. There is no or rare blood flow signals in the lesion.

- It should be differentiated from DFSP, cavernous hemangioma, and verrucous nevus.

5.1.12 Neurofibroma (Neurofibromatosis)

5.1.12.1 Clinical Manifestation and Pathology

Neurofibroma originates from peripheral nerve sheath cells and is a common benign tumor. It may be located in the dermis, subcutaneous tissue, or muscular layer. The lesion is often single and is called solitary neurofibroma. If multiple, it is called neurofibromatosis type I, or von Recklinghausen's disease, which is an autosomal dominant pattern of inheritance. Besides multiple peripheral neurofibromas, type I neurofibromatosis is accompanied by changes of skin pigmentation with café-au-lait spots (Fig. 5.31).

Neurofibromatoses are often located in the neck and extremities. The lesions are significantly elevated and most grow slowly. Most patients present with painless masses. When the lesion enlarges and compresses the nerve, patients may have symptoms such as local soreness and limb numbness.

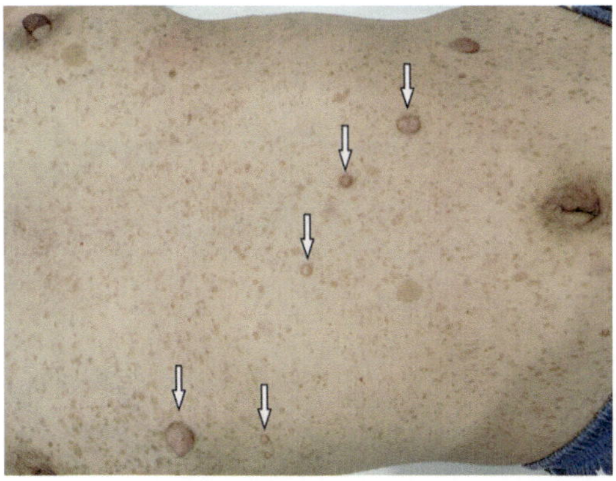

Fig. 5.31 Visual appearance of neurofibromatosis. Visual observation shows skin pigmentation with café-au-lait spots and many nodules (arrows) in the skin of chest wall and abdominal wall

5.1.12.2 Ultrasound Manifestation

Gray-Scale Ultrasound

According to the morphology of the lesion, neurofibroma is divided into the following types.

1. Elevated type: It shows an oval and well-defined hypoechoic lesion located in the dermis, with elevated and smooth surface. The lesion usually is more homogeneous than other cutaneous tumors (Figs. 5.32, 5.33, and 5.34).
2. Fungoides type: The lesion is significantly elevated. The whole fungoides lesion is divided into an extradermal elevated part and an intradermal basal part, which are con-

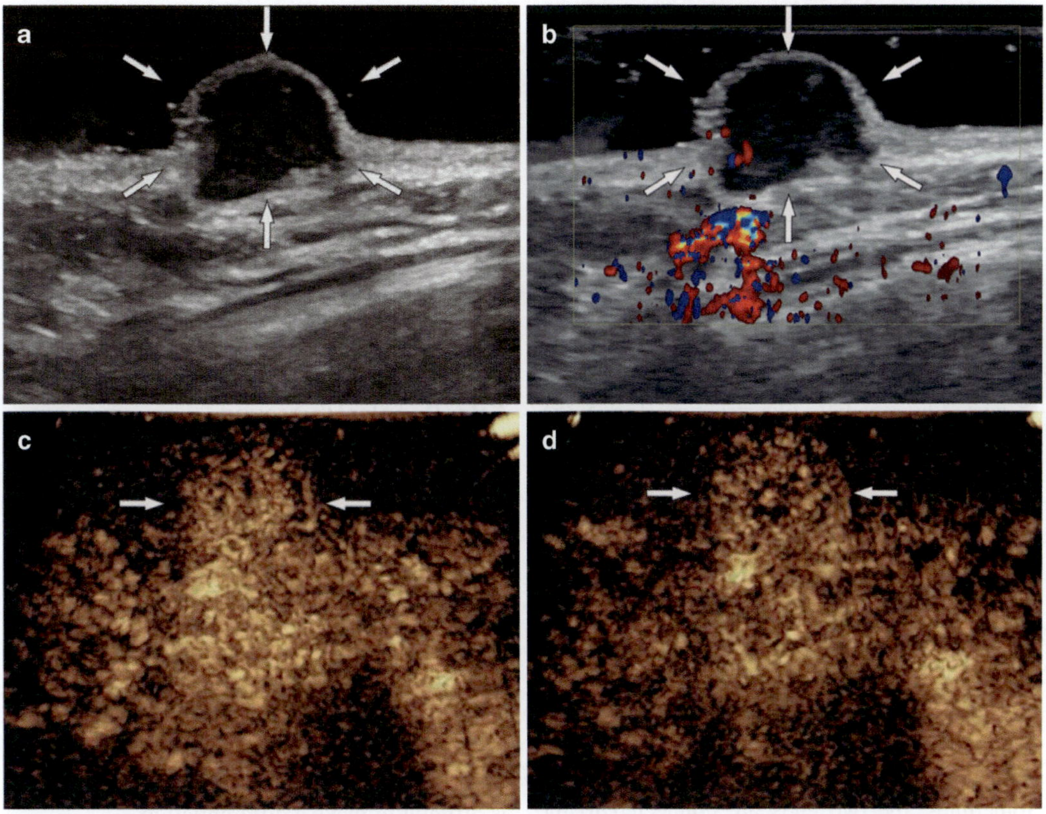

Fig. 5.32 Type I neurofibromatosis. Female, 67 years of age. (**a**) Gray-scale ultrasound shows a regular, semicircular, elevated, well-defined, and homogeneous hypoechoic lesion (arrows) in the dermis (size: 10.1 mm × 9.8 mm; thickness: 4.2 mm) (Frequency: 18 MHz). (**b**) Color Doppler ultrasound shows rare blood flow signals in the lesion (arrows) (Frequency: 18 MHz). (**c**) Contrast-enhanced ultrasound (the early phase of enhancement, 20th second after contrast agent administration) shows that the lesion (arrows) is homogeneously slightly hyperenhanced in comparison with the surrounding dermis (Frequency: 9 MHz). (**d**) In the late phase of enhancement (56th second), the lesion is also homogeneously and slightly hyperenhanced (arrows) (Frequency: 9 MHz)

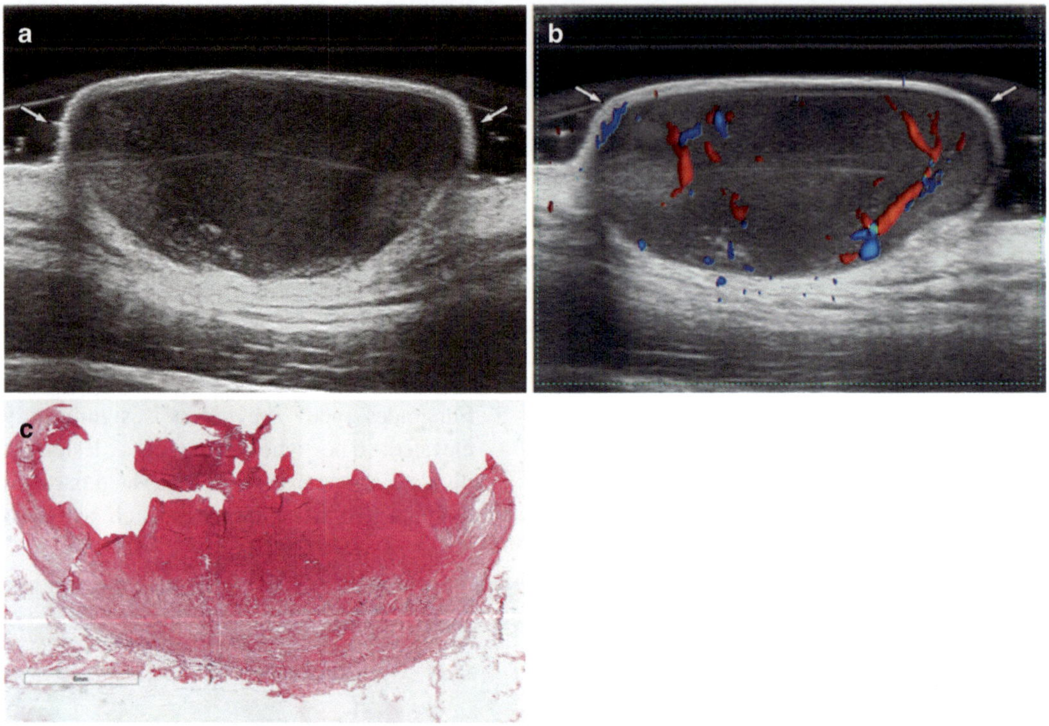

Fig. 5.33 Elevated neurofibroma. (**a**) Gray-scale ultrasound shows an oval, elevated, well-defined, and homogeneous hypoechoic lesion (arrows) located in the dermis (size: 38.6 mm × 35.2 mm; thickness: 5.4 mm) (Frequency: 22 MHz). (**b**) Color Doppler ultrasound shows rich blood flow signals in the lesion (arrows) (Frequency: 22 MHz). (**c**) Histopathology (HE staining, panoramic scanning): The well-defined lesion is located in the dermis without capsule. The tumor is composed of a large number of cells with short fusiform nuclei and lightly stained cytoplasm, as well as a few mast cells

nected by a pedicle-like structure (Fig. 5.35). The extradermal elevated part shows similar ultrasound findings to solitary neurofibroma; the intradermal part located in the dermis is ill-defined without space-occupying effect. Due to the extremely fine nerve branches in the dermis, the lesion usually does not show a rat tail sign.

When the lesion is deeper and located in the subcutaneous tissue or muscular layer, there is usually no change in the appearance of the skin. Sometimes, the two ends are connected to the hypoechoic nerve, forming the rat tail sign. The ultrasound findings of a single lesion of neurofibromatosis are similar to that of a solitary neurofibroma.

Color Doppler Ultrasound

There are various degrees of blood flow signals in the lesion. When the lesion is protruding outward, nourishing vessel is visible in the pedicle-like structure.

5.1.12.3 Differential Diagnosis

Schwannoma

The deeply located neurofibromas need to be differentiated from schwannomas. On gray-scale ultrasound, both of them show rat tail sign, which is difficult to make a differentiation.

However, schwannoma mainly grows eccentrically along the nerve. Cystic change, necrosis, and hemorrhage are common in the lesion. Neurofibroma grows surrounded the nerve,

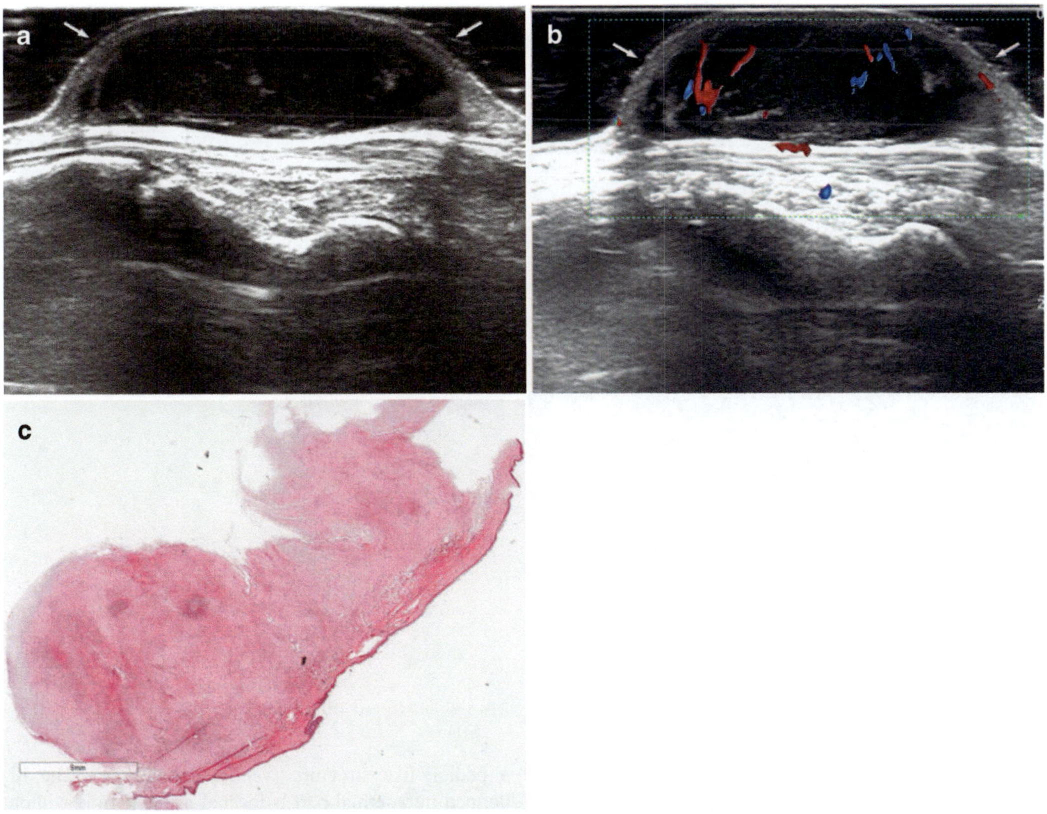

Fig. 5.34 Elevated neurofibroma. (**a**) Gray-scale ultrasound shows a regular, semicircular, elevated, well-defined, and homogeneous hypoechoic lesion (arrows) located in the dermis (size: 31.2 mm × 25.7 mm; thickness: 7.5 mm). The bottom is located in the dermis/subcutaneous tissue junction (Frequency: 22 MHz). (**b**) Color Doppler ultrasound shows rich blood flow signals in the lesion (arrows) (Frequency: 22 MHz). (**c**) Histopathology (HE staining, panoramic scanning): The well-defined lesion is located in the dermis without capsule. The tumor is composed of a large number of cells with short fusiform nuclei and lightly stained cytoplasm, as well as a few mast cells

with concentric sign in the transverse section. There is rare cystic change, necrosis, and hemorrhage. The above features are helpful to differentiate the two entities. However, it is still difficult to differentiate them in daily clinical work, and biopsy is required to confirm the diagnosis.

Hemangioma

When the internal blood flow signals of neurofibroma are rich, it needs to be differentiated from hemangioma. On gray-scale ultrasound, spongiform or honeycomb anechogenicity is visible in the hemangioma, and hyperechoic phleboliths are visible in some lesions. However, anechoic areas and hyperechoic structures are rare in the neurofibromas.

On color Doppler ultrasound, when the pressure from the transducer is quickly relieved, the transient increase of blood flow signal is observed, then returns to the status before pressurization. This phenomenon is a characteristic feature of hemangioma, caused by blood flowing in and out the hemangioma rapidly. The feature is helpful to differentiate the two entities.

5.1.12.4 Diagnosis Clues

1. Neurofibromas are often located in the neck and extremities. Patients often present with elevated painless nodules. Cafe-au-lait spots on the skin are helpful for the diagnosis of neurofibromatosis.
2. On ultrasound, neurofibroma mainly appears as a round or oval, elevated, well-defined, and

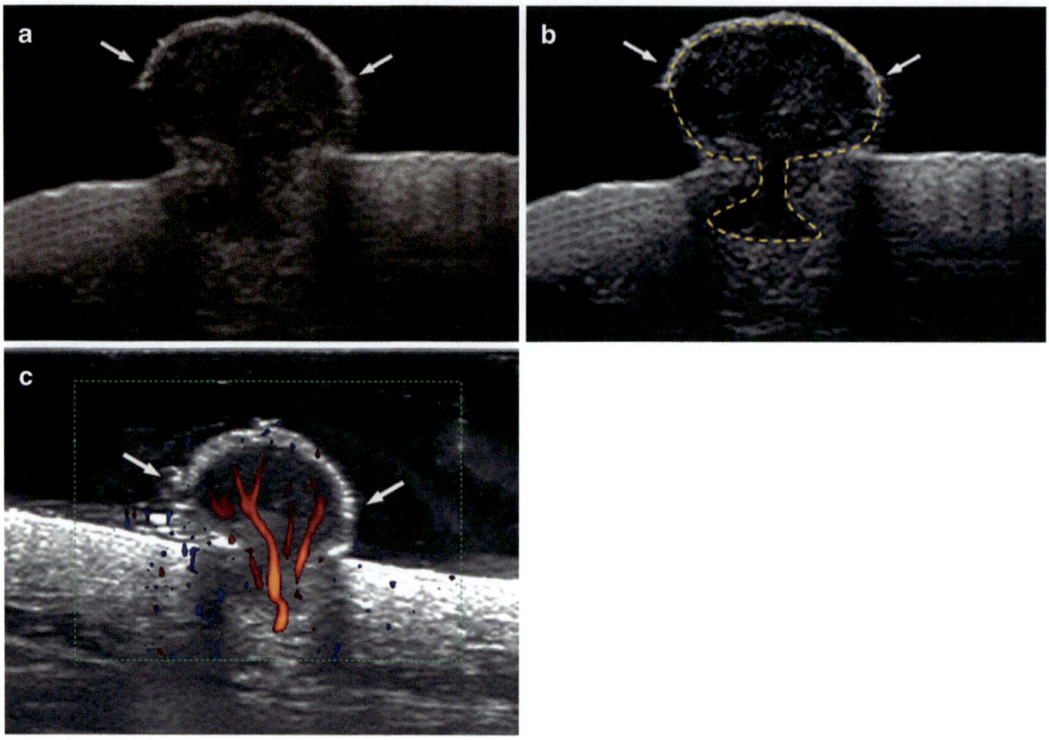

Fig. 5.35 Fungoides type neurofibroma. (**a**) Gray-scale ultrasound shows an irregular, fungiform, ill-defined, obviously elevated, and heterogeneous lesion (arrows) (size: 8.6 mm × 8.8 mm; thickness: 7.6 mm). The bottom is located in the dermis (Frequency: 22 MHz). (**b**) The lesion is divided into an extradermal elevated part and an intradermal basal part, and the two parts are connected by a pedicle-like structure (yellow dotted line). The ill-defined intradermal part is located in the dermis without space-occupying effect. (**c**) Power Doppler ultrasound shows abundant blood flow signals in the lesion, which shows nourishing vessels arising from the basal part into the elevated part through the pedicle-like structure (arrows) (Frequency: 22 MHz)

homogeneous hypoechoic lesion located in the dermis and/or subcutaneous tissue. Sometimes fungoides type lesion shows a pedicle-like structure and nourishing vessel. Due to the extremely fine nerve branches in the dermis, the lesion usually does not show a rat tail sign.

Key Points

- Neurofibroma is a common benign tumor, originated from peripheral nerve. The single type is called solitary neurofibroma, and the multiple type is called neurofibromatosis type I, which is an autosomal dominant pattern of inheritance.
- Ultrasound findings are divided into elevated and fungoides types according to the shape of the lesion, of which the fungoides type is more characteristic. The blood flow signals are usually rich.

5.1.13 Schwannoma

5.1.13.1 Clinical Manifestation and Pathology

Schwannoma, also known as neurilemmoma, is a benign tumor that originates from Schwann cells of the peripheral nerve sheath, with low malignant potential. The disease often occurs in the middle-aged people without obvious gender difference. Its etiology is uncertain and it may be related to trauma or stimulation. It is usually single, occasionally multiple.

Most schwannomas are located in the extremities, trunk, head, and neck. Most patients present with regular, smooth, and skin-colored bumps, usually accompanied with pain, especially paroxysmal pain. When the lesion compresses the nerve, patients may have symptoms such as local soreness and numbness. Dyskinesia is rare. Sometimes the disease is accompanied with multiple neurofibromas.

5.1.13.2 Ultrasound Manifestation

Gray-Scale Ultrasound

Schwannoma often appears as an oral or spindle-shaped, well-defined, and homogeneous hypoechoic lesion with capsule located in the intermuscle, subcutaneous tissue, or muscular layer. Dot-like or patchy hyperechogenicity and irregular anechogenicity are characteristically visualized inside some lesions, which are caused by cystic change, necrosis, and hemorrhage.

The lesion mainly grows eccentrically along the nerve. Sometimes, the two ends are connected to the hypoechoic nerve, forming the "rat tail" sign. Meanwhile, most lesions are accompanied with arteries and veins.

Color Doppler Ultrasound

There are rare or no blood flow signals in most of the lesions (Fig. 5.36).

5.1.13.3 Differential Diagnosis

Neurofibroma

The deeply located neurofibromas should be differentiated from schwannomas. On gray-scale ultrasound, sometimes both of the two diseases show "rat tail" sign, which is difficult to differentiate from each other.

However, schwannoma mainly grows eccentrically along the nerve. Cystic change, necrosis, and hemorrhage are common in the lesion. Neurofibroma grows surrounded the nerve, with concentric sign in the transverse section. There is rare cystic change, necrosis, and hemorrhage. The above features are helpful to differentiate the two diseases. However, it is still difficult to differentiate them in daily clinical work, and biopsy is required to confirm the diagnosis sometimes.

Superficial Lymph Node

Superficial lymph nodes are the most commonly palpable superficial masses, and gray-scale ultrasound shows a subcutaneous hypoechoic lesion with a lymphatic hilum. Color Doppler ultrasound shows "portal type" blood flow signals.

However, schwannoma does not have the above features. On ultrasound, dot-like or patchy hyperechogenicity and irregular anechogenicity are characteristically visualized inside some lesions. The lesion mainly grows eccentrically

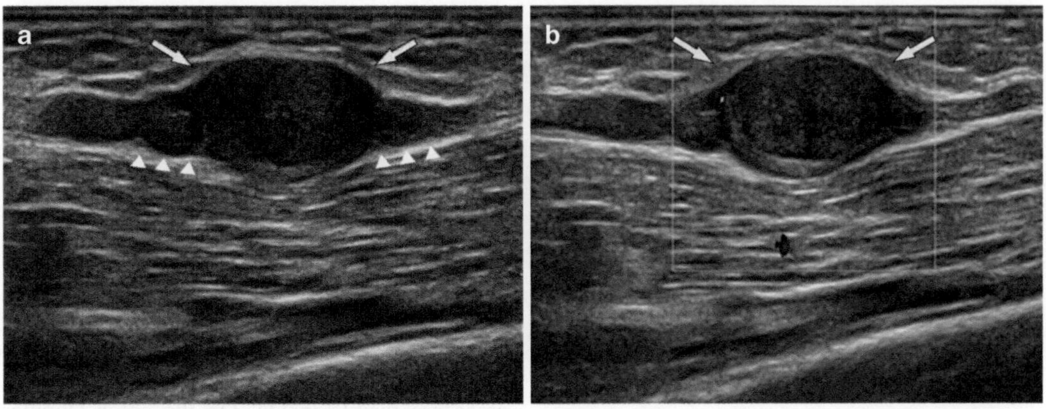

Fig. 5.36 Schwannoma. Female, 69 years of age. (**a**) Gray-scale ultrasound shows an oval, well-defined. and homogeneous hypoechoic lesion (arrows) with capsule located in the subcutaneous tissue (size: 18.5 mm × 17.4 mm; thickness: 9.9 mm). Patchy hyperechogenicity is visualized in the lesion. The two ends are connected to the hypoechoic nerve, forming the "rat tail" sign (△) marks the nerve (Frequency: 15 MHz). (**b**) Color Doppler ultrasound shows rare blood flow signals in the lesion (arrows) (Frequency: 15 MHz)

along the nerve showing the "rat tail" sign. The above features can be used to differentiate the two entities.

5.1.13.4 Diagnosis Clues

1. Schwannoma often occurs in the middle-aged people and is located in the extremities, trunk, head, and neck. Most patients present with regular, smooth, and skin-colored bumps, usually accompanied with pain, especially paroxysmal pain.
2. On high-frequency ultrasound, dot-like or patchy hyperechogenicity and irregular anechogenicity in the lesion are characteristic features. The lesion mainly grows eccentrically along the nerve, forming the "rat tail" sign.

Key Points

- Schwannoma is a benign tumor that originates from Schwann cells of the peripheral nerve sheath, with low malignant potential. It often occurs in the middle-aged people.
- On ultrasound, dot-like or patchy hyperechogenicity and irregular anechogenicity in the lesion are characteristic features. The "rat tail" sign is often observed.
- It should be differentiated from neurofibroma and superficial lymph node.

5.1.14 Angioleiomyoma

5.1.14.1 Clinical Manifestation and Pathology

Angioleiomyoma is a rare benign tumor of soft tissue. The disease originates from smooth muscle cells in the inner wall of arterioles or venules and is composed of blood vessels and smooth muscle. Mature smooth muscle bundles in tumors are located around or interspersed among blood vessels.

The diseases are classified into three types in histology:

1. Solid type: There are many slit-like thick-walled blood vessels of different sizes intertwined with peripheral smooth muscle bundles in the tumor.
2. Venous type: A smooth muscle nodule forms based on a large venous wall.
3. Spongiform type: Most portion of the lesion is composed of dilated vascular lumens and less smooth muscle components. This type is rare in clinic.

The disease often occurs in adult women, mostly in the lower extremities. The lesion is often single, firm, small, and has no significant changes in the skin. Most of the patients have spontaneous pain.

5.1.14.2 Ultrasound Manifestation

Gray-Scale Ultrasound

Angioleiomyoma often appears as a single, small, regular, and well-defined lesion located in the subcutaneous tissue. Usually, there is no obvious abnormality on the surface of the lesion.

Most of the lesions appear as hypoechogenicity and a few appear as mixed echogenicity. There is hyperechogenicity inside some lesions.

Color Doppler Ultrasound

There are rich blood flow signals in most lesions and rare blood flow signals in a few lesions (Figs. 5.37 and 5.38).

5.1.14.3 Differential Diagnosis

Glomus Tumor

For the two diseases, patients may have pain where the lesion is located. Glomus tumor is mostly located under the nail. The surface is mostly bluish-purple or black. While angioleiomyoma is mostly located in the lower extremities and has a normal surface. The lesion is firm.

On gray-scale ultrasound, glomus tumor appears as an oval or round and heterogeneous hypoechoic lesion in the subungual or subcutaneous tissue. The strip or honeycomb anechoic areas are visible inside. On the color Doppler ultrasound, rich blood flow signals are visible in the lesion. When the probe is pressurized, the blood flow signals are significantly increased, looking like a "color-ball".

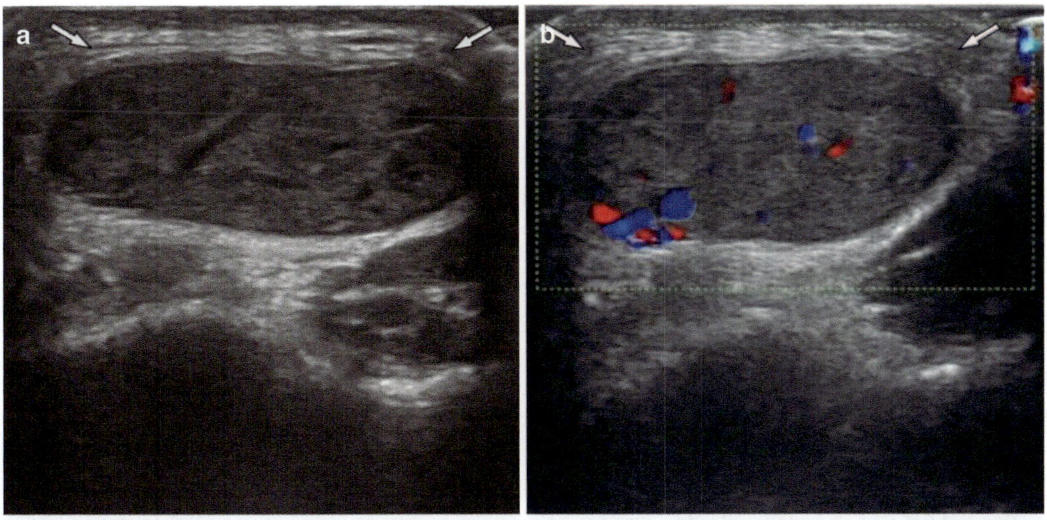

Fig. 5.37 Angioleiomyoma. (**a**) Gray-scale ultrasound shows an oval and well-defined hypoechoic lesion (arrows) located in the subcutaneous tissue (size: 15.2 mm × 16.2 mm; thickness: 8.4 mm). Strip anechoic areas are visible in the lesion (Frequency: 15 MHz). (**b**) Color Doppler ultrasound shows rare blood flow signals in the lesion (arrows) (Frequency: 15 MHz)

Epidermoid Cyst

Epidermoid cysts are often soft and some are palpable fluctuating. On gray-scale ultrasound, epidermoid cysts are round mixed echogenic lesions, showing characteristic anechoic or hypoechoic "fissures" with posterior acoustic enhancement. Sometimes the lesion is connected to the surface of skin through the sinus tract. On color Doppler ultrasound, there are often no blood flow signals in the lesion.

While angioleiomyomas mostly are small and firm nodules, ultrasound shows a homogeneous hypoechoic lesion without posterior acoustic enhancement. Color Doppler ultrasound shows blood flow signals in the lesion.

5.1.14.4 Diagnosis Clues

1. The disease often occurs in women. It is considered angioleiomyoma firstly if a slow-growing and firm nodule is found in the lower extremities accompanied with spontaneous pain.
2. On high-frequency ultrasound, angioleiomyomas mainly show oval, well-defined, and homogeneous hypoechoic lesions located in the subcutaneous tissue. Blood flow signals are generally rich. High-frequency ultrasound findings are not specific and need to be comprehensively assessed combining with clinical symptoms.

Key Points

- Angioleiomyoma is a rare benign soft tissue tumor that often occurs in women. It is often located in the lower extremities and grows slowly with spontaneous pain.
- Ultrasound findings are characteristics of benign cutaneous tumors but are non-specific. Diagnosis needs to be combined with clinical symptoms.
- It should be differentiated from glomus tumor and epidermoid cyst.

5.1.15 Poroma

5.1.15.1 Clinical Manifestation and Pathology

Poroma was first reported in 1956 by Goldman et al. This disease is a rare benign tumor arising from the terminal sweat gland duct. The majority are small in size and usually less than 10.0 mm in

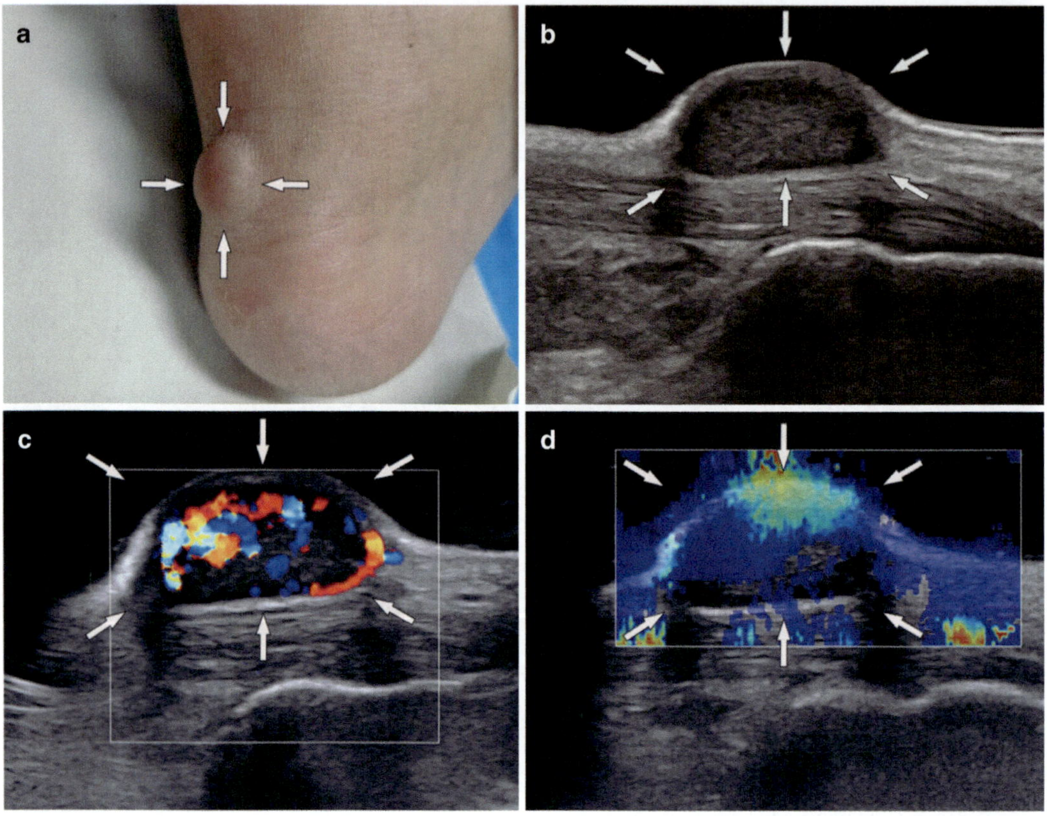

Fig. 5.38 Angioleiomyoma. Female, 34 years of age. (**a**) Visual observation shows a skin-colored hemispherical bump on the left heel (arrows), the size of which is about 10.0 mm in diameter. (**b**) Gray-scale ultrasound shows an oval, well-defined, and homogeneous hypoechoic lesion (arrows) in the subcutaneous tissue (size: 12.2 mm × 10.2 mm; thickness: 5.6 mm). And the lesion is elevated from the surface (Frequency: 15 MHz). (**c**) Color Doppler ultrasound shows rich blood flow signals in the lesion (arrows) (Frequency: 15 MHz). (**d**) The lesion is not fully covered with color on two-dimensional SWE image (arrows). The majority is covered by blue, indicating a soft tissue, with mean elastic modulus of 97.1 kPa and maximum elastic modulus of 285.2 kPa

diameter. The lesion is often single and mostly appears as a grayish black or skin-colored hemispherical nodule with a smooth surface. The disease often occurs in the head, face, palms, and feet. It occurs at any age.

Histologically, poroma is a well-defined homogeneous mass of cells that commonly extend from the basal layer into the dermis. According to the different layers of tumor cell infiltration, it is divided into 4 subtypes:

1. Hidroacanthoma simplex: The lesion is completely located in the epidermis;
2. Eccrine poroma: The lesion involves the epidermis and dermis;
3. Dermal ductal tumor: The lesion is completely located in the dermis;
4. Clear cell hidradenoma: The lesion is located in the dermis and sometimes is connected to the epidermis.

The most common subtype is eccrine poroma.

5.1.15.2 Ultrasound Manifestation

Gray-Scale Ultrasound

Gray-scale ultrasound shows a nodular, well-defined, elevated, and heterogeneous hypoechoic lesion located in the epidermis and/or dermis, usually without abnormal keratinization.

Color Doppler Ultrasound

There are rich blood flow signals in the lesion (Figs. 5.39 and 5.40).

5.1.15.3 Differential Diagnosis

Porocarcinoma

Porocarcinoma is derived from malignant transformation of poroma. High-frequency ultrasonography shows poroma has a regular shape and well-defined boundary. If the lesion grows rapidly and the boundary is ill-defined, the possibility of malignant transformation of the lesion should be alerted.

Both entities show rich blood flow signals, so color Doppler ultrasound is difficult to differentiate the two diseases.

Nodular Basal Cell Carcinoma (BCC)

The nodular BCC appears as a brown or pearl-like papule and some are patches. The poromas mostly appear as grayish black papules.

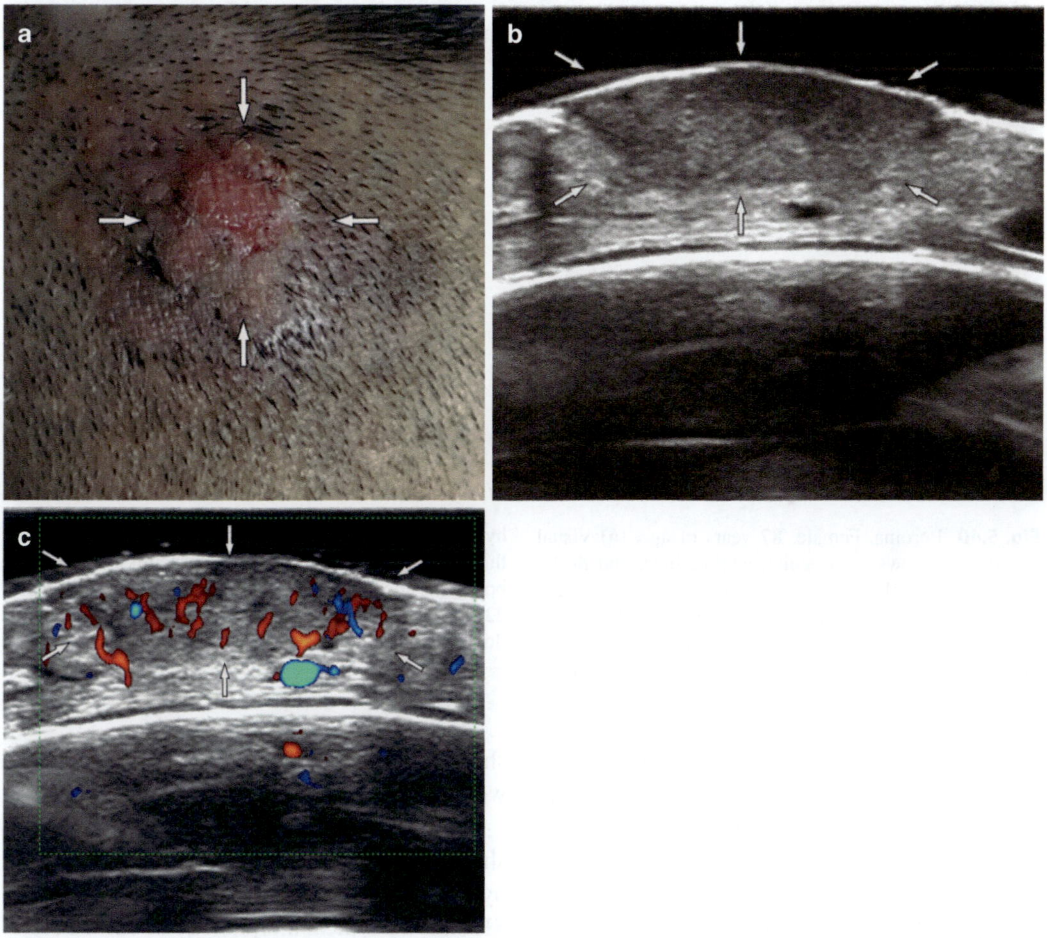

Fig. 5.39 Poroma. Male, 65 years of age. (**a**) Visual observation shows a dark red and well-defined hemispherical lesion on the right scalp (arrows), the size of which is about 10.0 mm in diameter. The surface is granular-like with slight exudates and scab. (**b**) Gray-scale ultrasound shows a nodular, well-defined, elevated, and heterogeneous hypoechoic lesion (arrows) located in the epidermis and dermis (size: 23.1 mm × 21.4 mm; thickness: 7.3 mm) (Frequency: 22 MHz). (**c**) Color Doppler ultrasound shows rich blood flow signals in the lesion (arrows) (Frequency: 22 MHz)

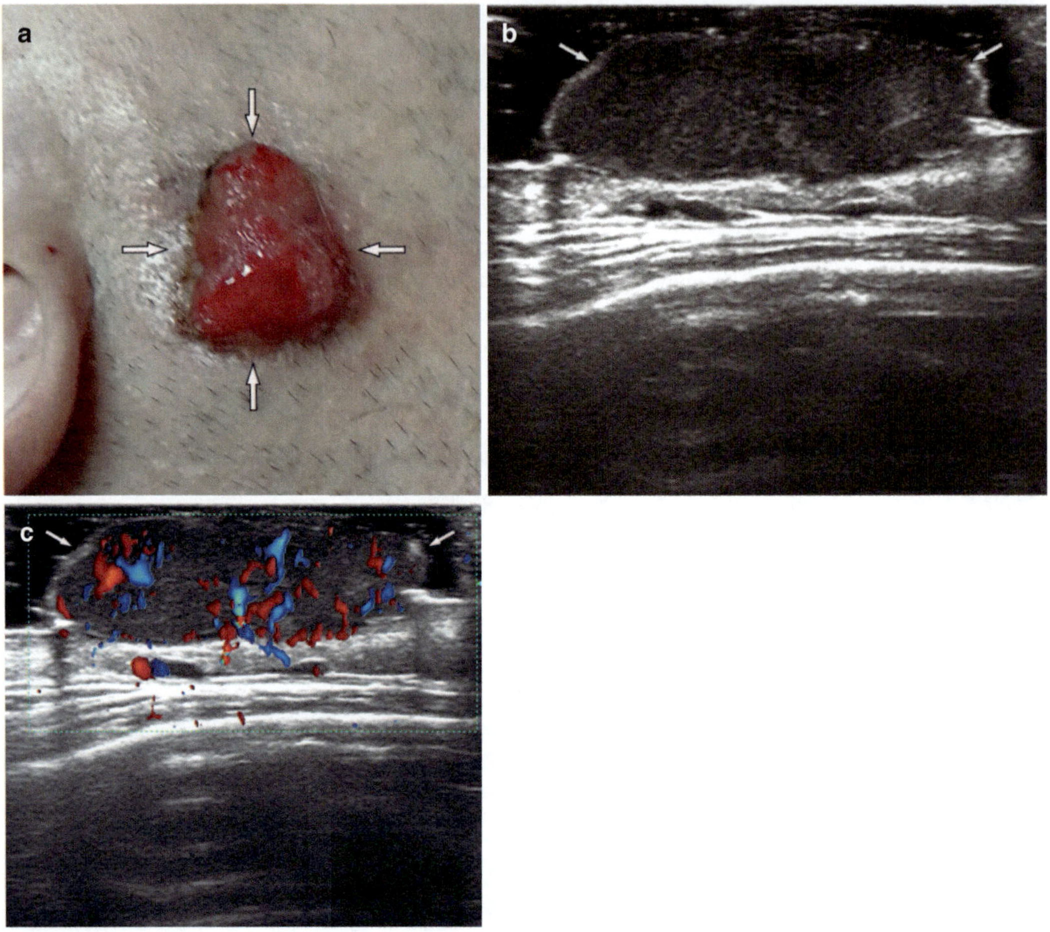

Fig. 5.40 Poroma. Female, 87 years of age. (**a**) Visual observation shows an irregular, well-defined, and fleshy red lesion in the left temporal region, with a little bleeding, without exudates (arrows), the size of which is about 24.0 mm × 26.0 mm. (**b**) Gray-scale ultrasound shows a nodular, elevated, well-defined, and homogeneous hypoechoic lesion (arrows) (size: 26.2 mm × 20.8 mm; thickness: 8.5 mm). The stratum corneum is absent. The bottom is located in the superficial dermis (Frequency: 22 MHz). (**c**) Color Doppler ultrasound shows rich blood flow signals in the lesion (arrows) (Frequency: 22 MHz)

On gray-scale ultrasound, sometimes both nodular BCC and poroma appear as regular and well-defined hypoechoic lesions located in the epidermis and dermis. However, hyperechoic spots and/or anechoic areas are visualized in most of nodular BCC, which is used as a differential point between the two entities.

Seborrheic Keratosis (SK)

The visual appearance of the two diseases may look like black nodules, but sometimes SK shows characteristic "cerebriform-like" appearance of hyperkeratosis, while the surface of poroma shows ulcer or bleeding, which is usually smooth without abnormal keratinization.

On high-frequency ultrasound, both of them show elevated, nodular, and well-defined hypoechoic lesions in the epidermis. However, SK shows a typical morphology of curved elevation with hyperechogenicity on the surface and various degrees of posterior acoustic shadowing, which disturbs the visualization of blood flow signals. However, there is no linear hyperechogenicity on the surface of poroma, and the internal structure and blood flow signals are clearly visualized.

5.1.15.4 Diagnosis Clues

Ultrasound findings of poroma are non-specific and it is easily confused with BCC and SCC with keratin shedding. The lesions mainly involve into the epidermis or dermis and usually do not break through the dermal base. The shape is regular and boundary is well-defined. The visual appearance of the lesion is helpful for the diagnosis, mostly showing red, blue, or black nodules, and some showing bleeding and ulceration on the surface.

Key Points

- Poroma is a rare benign tumor arising from the terminal sweat gland duct, which is small and often occurs in the head, face, palms, and feet.
- Ultrasound findings are characteristics of benign cutaneous tumors but are non-specific. Diagnosis needs to be combined with clinical features.
- It should be differentiated from porocarcinoma, BCC, and SK.

5.1.16 Abdominal Wall Endometriosis

5.1.16.1 Clinical Manifestation and Pathology

Abdominal wall endometriosis is one of the complications of uterine surgery, especially cesarean section. At present, it is believed that the disease is caused by the active endometrial tissue implanted in the subcutaneous tissue of the abdominal wall during surgery. Abdominal wall endometriosis is a benign lesion, but it is similar to malignant tumors biologically and can undergo implantation, infiltration, and recurrence, with the risk of malignant transformation.

The clinical incidence ranges from 0.03% to 0.45% and the disease is common in women of child-bearing period. Patients mostly present with firm, painful, and palpable mass at or around the abdominal incision, which is closely related to the menstrual cycle.

5.1.16.2 Ultrasound Manifestation

Gray-Scale Ultrasound

Abdominal wall endometriosis usually appears as a hypoechoic lesion located in the subcutaneous tissue under the abdominal wall incision and may involve into the fascia or deep muscle.

Most lesions are irregular and a few are oval. The lesion is ill-defined and even crabfoot-like or burr-like without a capsule. For some lesions, there are anechoic areas inside and hyperechoic halo in the periphery. In a word, the ultrasound findings of this disease are similar to that of typical breast cancer.

Color Doppler Ultrasound

There are no blood flow signals in most of the lesions, and dotted and strip blood flow signals are visible in some lesions (Figs. 5.41 and 5.42).

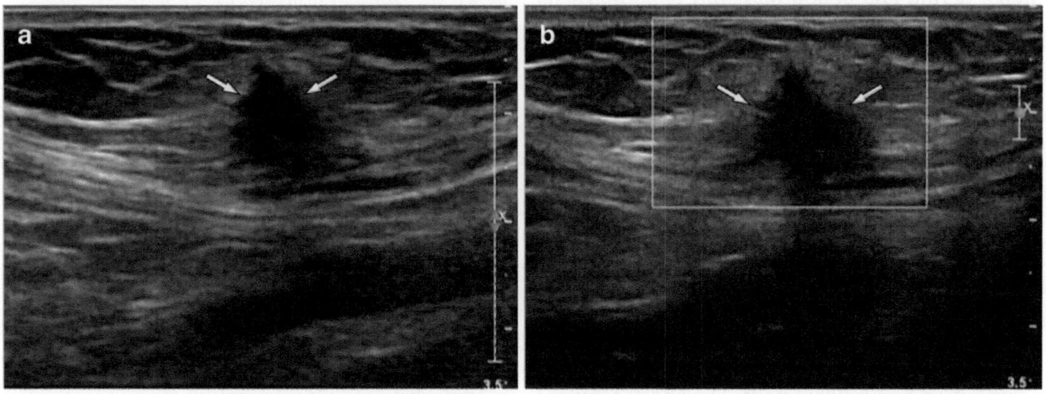

Fig. 5.41 Abdominal wall endometriosis. (**a**) Gray-scale ultrasound shows an irregular, ill-defined, and homogeneous hypoechoic lesion (arrows) located in the subcutaneous tissue of the abdominal wall (size: 13.2 mm × 10.2 mm; thickness: 11.4 mm), with posterior acoustic shadowing. The bottom is deep to the fascia. There are burr-like changes in the periphery (Frequency: 15 MHz). (**b**) Color Doppler ultrasound shows no blood flow signals in the lesion (arrows) (Frequency: 15 MHz)

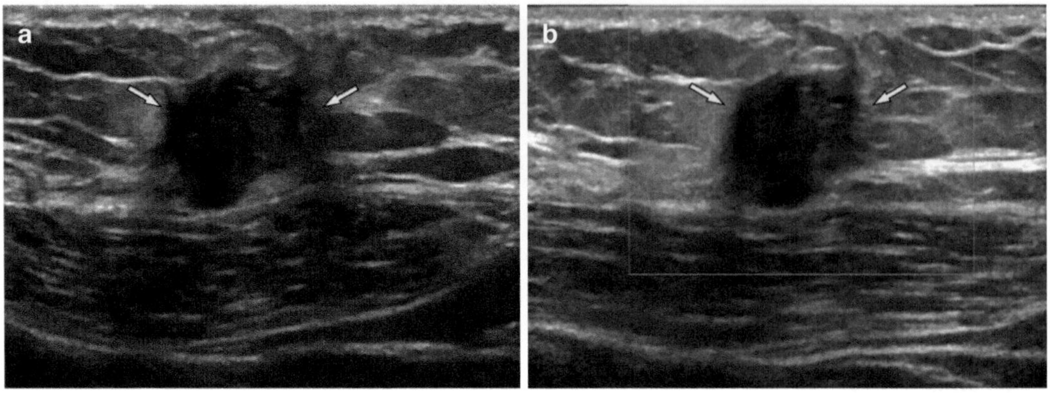

Fig. 5.42 Abdominal wall endometriosis. (**a**) Gray-scale ultrasound shows an irregular, ill-defined, and heterogeneous hypoechoic lesion (arrows) located in the subcutaneous tissue of the abdominal wall (size: 15.2 mm × 12.5 mm; thickness: 10.6 mm), with posterior acoustic shadowing. The bottom is deep to the fascia. There are crabfoot-like changes in the periphery (Frequency: 15 MHz). (**b**) Color Doppler ultrasound shows no blood flow signals in the lesion (arrows) (Frequency: 15 MHz)

5.1.16.3 Differential Diagnosis

Abdominal Incisional Hernia

The visual appearances of the both entities are masses in the abdominal incision, which need to be differentiated.

Gray-scale ultrasound finding of incisional hernia shows a mixed echogenic lesion (omentum or bowel) in the subcutaneous tissue under the surgical incision, with hyperechogenicity formed by intestinal gas. The connection between the mixed echogenic structure and the abdominal cavity is visualized.

The gray-scale ultrasound findings of incisional hernia and abdominal wall endometriosis are completely different and easy to differentiate from each other.

Scar at Abdominal Incision

Gray-scale ultrasound shows an irregular and ill-defined hypoechoic lesion in the subcutaneous tissue with posterior acoustic shadowing. It is similar to the ultrasound findings of abdominal wall endometriosis. However, sometimes the lesion in the subcutaneous tissue is connected to scars on the body surface. Most patients with scars have no significant pain. The above features are different from endometriosis and are helpful to differentiate the two entities.

Hematoma under Abdominal Incision

The patient's clinical symptoms are helpful to differentiate the two entities. When hematoma is located under the incision, the patient may present with persistent pain and discomfort, regardless of the menstrual cycle.

In addition, the gray-scale ultrasound findings of hematomas are various according to the time of formation. They appear as regular and well-defined hypoechogenicity or anechogenicity. There is no blood flow signals in the lesion on color Doppler ultrasound. The above findings are significantly different from those of abdominal wall endometriosis.

5.1.16.4 Diagnosis Clues

1. The patient has a history of cesarean section, with firm and palpable mass at the abdominal incision, accompanied by menstrual pain.
2. On ultrasound, abdominal wall endometriosis often appears as an irregular, ill-defined, and heterogeneous hypoechoic lesion in the subcutaneous tissue under the abdominal wall incision. The margin shows crabfoot-like or burr-like changes, similar to the typical breast cancer.
3. There are no or rare blood flow signals in the lesion on color Doppler ultrasound.

Key Points

- Abdominal wall endometriosis is a benign lesion and can undergo implantation, infiltration, and recurrence, with the risk of malignant transformation.
- The patient has a history of cesarean section, with firm and palpable mass under the abdominal incision, usually accompanied by menstrual pain.
- Gray-scale ultrasound shows an irregular, ill-defined, and heterogeneous hypoechoic lesion in the subcutaneous tissue with posterior acoustic shadowing. The margin shows crabfoot-like or burr-like changes.

5.1.17 Glomus Tumor

5.1.17.1 Clinical Manifestation and Pathology

Glomus tumor is a rare soft tissue tumor arising from the glomus apparatus of small arteriovenous anastomosis. It often occurs in the extremities, especially in the subungual region, occasionally in the kidneys, rectum, and other parts. The tumor is often single, occasionally multiple. The tumor is usually small.

The tumor is benign and rarely become malignant. The disease is more common in the young adults and slightly more common in women. Clinically, glomus tumors in the subungual region are characterized by subungual blue-purple spotty or nodular changes, typically with a specific pain triad of paroxysmal pain, tenderness, and cold sensitivity.

Pathologically, glomus tumors are mainly composed of mutated vascular smooth muscle cell at the arteriovenous anastomosis. There are globular cells and a small amount of smooth muscle and nerve fibers in the tumor.

5.1.17.2 Ultrasound Manifestation

Gray-Scale Ultrasound

Gray-scale ultrasound of subungual glomus tumor shows a regular, oval, well-defined, and heterogeneous hypoechoic lesion under the nail. Its bottom is adjacent to the phalangeal surface. Patient with the tumor has significantly tenderness under the transducer compression.

Color Doppler Ultrasound

Most lesions show rich blood flow signals on color Doppler ultrasound, appearing as a "color ball." For a few lesions, there are rare blood flow signals (Fig. 5.43).

5.1.17.3 Differential Diagnosis

Nail Papilloma

Nail papilloma mostly occurs in the thumb and is mainly characterized by longitudinal, brown,

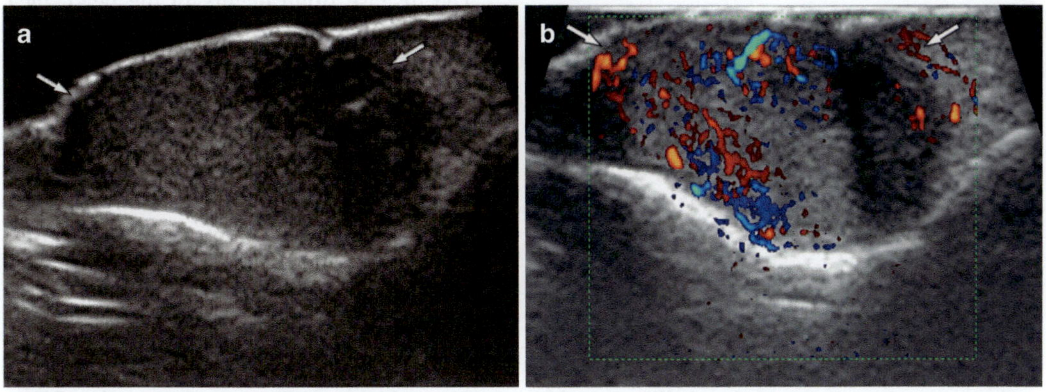

Fig. 5.43 Subungual glomus tumor. Female, 35 years of age. (**a**) Gray-scale ultrasound shows a regular, oval, well-defined, and heterogeneous hypoechoic lesion (arrows) located in the subungual region (size: 11.8 mm × 10.9 mm; thickness: 6.6 mm), with tiny posterior acoustic shadowing (Frequency: 15 MHz). (**b**) Color Doppler ultrasound shows rich blood flow signals in the lesion (arrows) (Frequency: 15 MHz)

white, or black bands on the deck, which is accompanied with deck separation. Patients mostly have no significant discomfort. While subungual glomus tumors mostly appear as subungual blue-purple spots or nodules, and patients are mostly accompanied by pain triad.

On gray-scale ultrasound, nail papilloma shows a regular and ill-defined hypoechoic lesion under the nails. Color Doppler ultrasound shows no or rare blood flow signals in the lesion. However, subungual glomus tumors are mostly clearly demarcated from the surrounding tissues, and it appears as a "color ball" on color Doppler ultrasound.

Nevi of the Nail Matrix

Nevi of the nail matrix are a type of nevus. Most of the diseases appear as longitudinal black bands or patchy change on the nail plate, and it may develop into melanoma. Patients have no obvious discomfort. Most subungual glomus tumors show subungual blue-purple spots or nodules and patients have pain triad.

On gray-scale ultrasound, nevus of the nail matrix shows an irregular and ill-defined hypoechoic lesion under the nails. Color Doppler ultrasound shows no or rare blood flow signals in the lesion. However, subungual glomus tumors are mostly oval and well-defined, and patients with the tumor are significantly tender under the transducer compression, and the lesion appears as a "color ball" on color Doppler ultrasound.

5.1.17.4 Diagnosis Clues

1. Visual appearance is helpful for the diagnosis of subungual glomus tumors. Most of the lesions appear as subungual blue-purple spots or nodules, and most patients present with pain triad of paroxysmal pain, tenderness, and cold sensitivity.
2. Gray-scale ultrasound shows an oval and well-defined hypoechoic lesion under nails. Patients with the tumor have significantly tenderness under the probe compression, and the lesion appears as a "color ball" on color Doppler ultrasound.

Key Points

- Glomus tumors often occur in the extremities, especially under the nail. It is more common in young adults. Most patients are associated with a specific pain triad of paroxysmal pain, tenderness, and cold sensitivity.
- Patients with the tumor have significantly tenderness under the transducer compression, and the lesion appears as a "color ball" on color Doppler ultrasound. Subungual glomus tumors should be differentiated from nail papilloma and nevi of the nail matrix.

5.2 Precancerous Skin Tumors

5.2.1 Actinic Keratosis

5.2.1.1 Clinical Manifestation and Pathology

Actinic keratosis (AK) is also known as senile keratosis. AK is an epithelial tumor characterized by varying degrees of atypical hyperplasia of keratinocytes. The classification of AK is still controversial, and some scholars believe that it is a premalignant lesion and some scholars believe that it is an early squamous cell carcinoma (SCC). Studies have reported that AK has a higher risk to develop into invasive SCC than Bowen's disease (BD), and is considered to be the most common precursor of SCC. So once diagnosed, it should be treated as early as possible.

The disease often occurs in the head, face, and dorsum of the hands in middle-aged and elderly people, which may be related to ultraviolet exposure. The visual appearances of AK are diverse, and typical lesions present with reddish-brown, black, or skin-colored dry papules in the early stage, with a smooth surface, well-defined borders, without blush at the bottom, which are often misdiagnosed as seborrheic keratosis (SK) at this time. In the late stage, some lesions appear as firm and rough papules with significant keratinization and scale on the surface, which are often misdiagnosed as BD or BCC (Fig. 5.44).

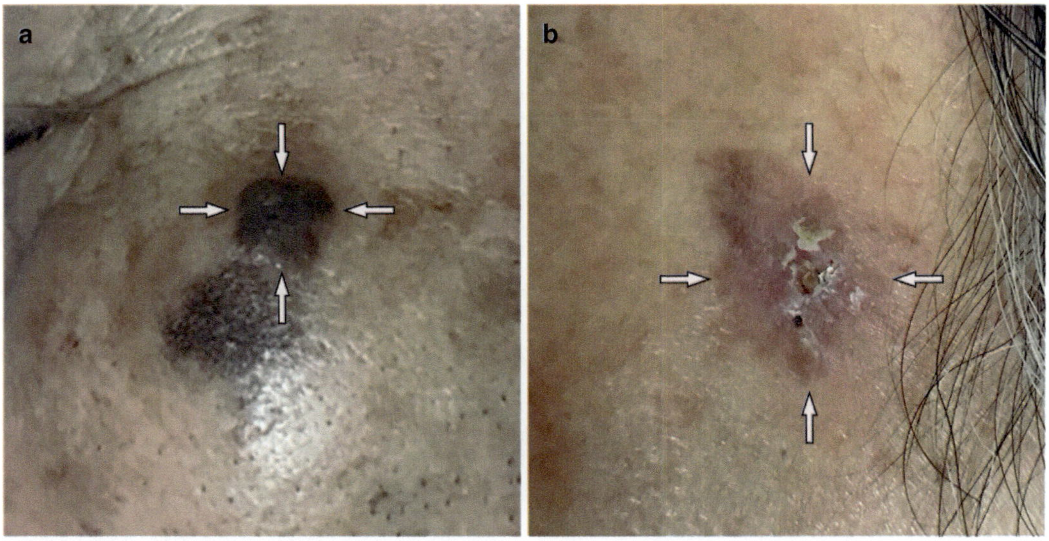

Fig. 5.44 Visual appearance of actinic keratosis. (**a**) A small, flat, well-defined, and black patch is located in the left cheek, with a smooth surface (arrows), the size of which is about 15.0 mm × 7.0 mm. Visual appearance of the lesion is similar to the early stage of SK. (**b**) A well-defined and reddish-brown patch is located in the left temporal, with a firm, rough, and scaly surface (arrows), the size of which is about 11.0 mm × 9.0 mm. Visual appearance of the lesion is similar to BD

Clinically, patients may present with pruritus and pain locally or without obvious symptoms. According to the histopathology, AK is classified into six types: atrophic, hypertrophic, bowenoid, acantholytic, lichenoid, and proliferative.

5.2.1.2 Ultrasound Manifestation

Gray-Scale Ultrasound

The ultrasound findings of this disease are diverse, and the lesions have various morphologies such as nodular, crawling, or irregular. The lesions are often confined to the epidermis. Due to solar elastosis and a mild inflammatory infiltration in the superficial dermis, the bottom shows irregular, so the lesions seem to reach the superficial dermis.

The degree of surface hyperkeratosis is milder than that of BD and SCC, so the internal structure is displayed. Some lesions of early AK are extremely thin and thus cannot be clearly visualized by ultrasound. As the disease progresses, the lesions gradually become thickened.

Color Doppler Ultrasound

Rich blood flow signals can be showed in some lesions, but due to the obstruction of acoustic shadowing produced by hyperkeratosis on the surface, some lesions show no or rare blood flow signals (Figs. 5.45 and 5.46).

5.2.1.3 Differential Diagnosis

SK

In the early stage, both entities appear as a small and black patch, which is difficult to distinguish by the naked eyes. As the disease progressing, SK may show scharacteristic “cerebriform-like” appearance, which is helpful to differentiate them.

On gray-scale ultrasound, the two diseases appear as hypoechoic lesions within the epidermis with abnormal keratinization. SK is obviously elevated, and the hyperechogenicity of the surface is serrated or lobulated, and the bottom is flat. However, the bottom of AK is ambiguous, and it seems to reach the superficial dermis. The

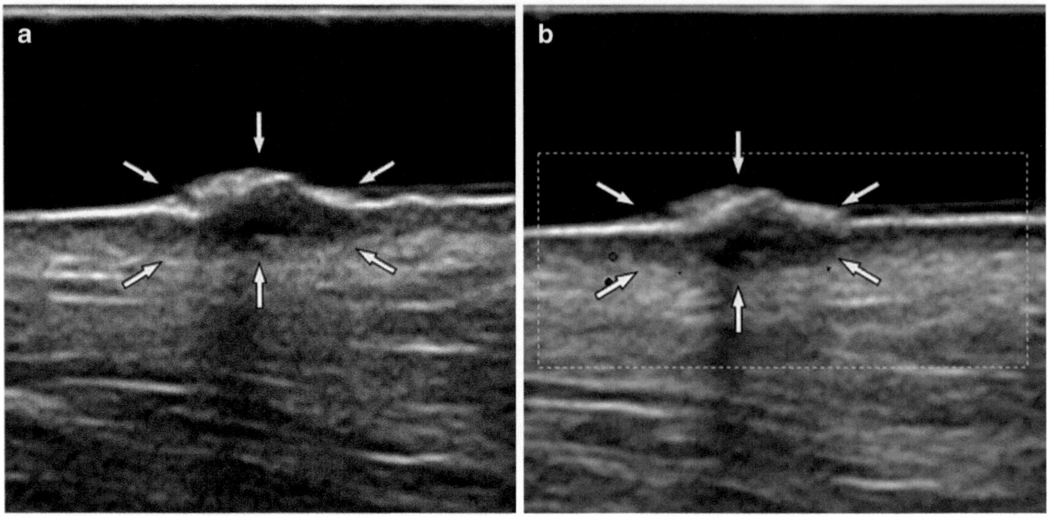

Fig. 5.45 Actinic keratosis. Female, 89 years of age. (**a**) Gray-scale ultrasound shows a slightly elevated, irregular, ill-defined, and homogeneous hypoechoic lesion (arrows) located in the epidermis (size: 9.3 mm × 6.4 mm; thickness: 1.3 mm). The surface appears as linear hyperechogenicity with tiny posterior acoustic shadowing (Frequency: 22 MHz). (**b**) Color Doppler ultrasound shows no blood flow signals in the lesion (arrows) (Frequency: 22 MHz)

lesion is elevated in a low degree, and the hyperechogenicity of the surface is heterogeneous and irregular.

BD

The two diseases have similar visual appearances and sometimes it is difficult to differentiate the two entities. The lesions are all reddish-brown patches with a rough surface accompanied by scales.

On gray-scale ultrasound, the two diseases appear as crawling hypoechoic lesions within the epidermis with abnormal keratinization on the surface. However, BD is mostly single, confined to the epidermis. The bottom is flat and demarcated from the dermis clearly. The degree of abnormal keratinization of the surface is more severe. AK is multiple, the degree of abnormal keratinization of the surface is mild and regular. Sometimes the bottom of AK is ambiguous, and it seems to reach the superficial dermis.

Superficial BCC

On ultrasound, both of them may appear as crawling hypoechoic lesions located on the epidermis. However, the surface of superficial BCC is flat, without abnormal keratinization, and the bottom is well-defined. On the other hand, the surface of AK shows different degrees of abnormal keratinization with posterior acoustic shadowing. The bottom is more ambiguous than that of superficial BCC. The abnormal keratinization on the surface and the clarity of the bottom are used as the main differential clues between the two diseases.

5.2.1.4 Diagnosis Clues

1. AK often occurs in the head and face of the elderly and is often multiple.
2. On the gray-scale ultrasound, the lesions are confined to the epidermis. Sometimes the bottom of some lesions is ambiguous and seems to reach the superficial dermis. The surface of the lesion shows varying degrees of abnormal keratinization with diverse morphology.
3. Blood flow signals are visualized in some lesions on color Doppler ultrasound.

5.2.1.5 Clinical Significance

Although it is still controversial that AK should be defined as a premalignant lesion or early SCC, it should be treated as early as possible once it is diagnosed clinically. High-frequency ultrasound features, including the involvement layer, the bottom condition, and internal blood flow signals, are helpful to differentiate AK from other

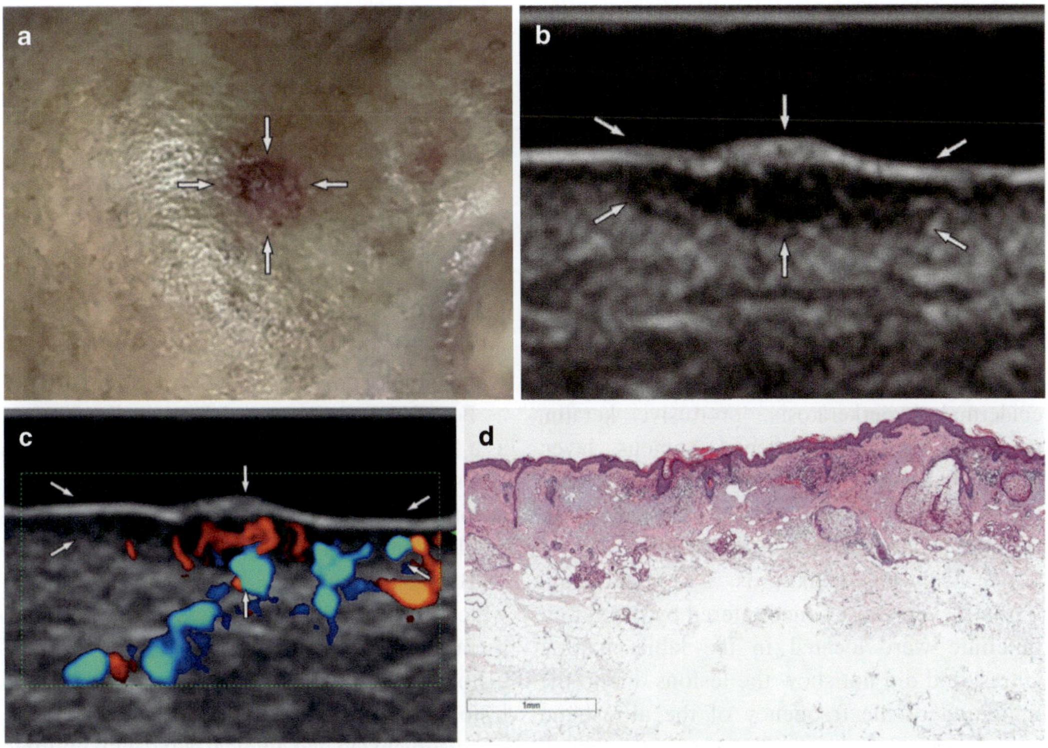

Fig. 5.46 Actinic keratosis. Female, 67 years of age. (**a**) Visual observation shows a well-defined and reddish-brown patch located in the right cheek, with no ulceration or exudates on the surface (arrows), the size of which is about 5.0 mm × 5.0 mm. (**b**) Gray-scale ultrasound shows an irregular, well-defined, and homogeneous hypoechoic lesion (arrows) located in the epidermis (size: 5.0 mm × 4.8 mm; thickness: 1.0 mm). The surface appears as fine linear hyperechogenicity without posterior acoustic shadowing (Frequency: 22 MHz). (**c**) Color Doppler ultrasound shows rich blood flow signals in the lesion (arrows) (Frequency: 22 MHz). (**d**) Histopathology (HE staining, panoramic scan) shows that the corneum layer exhibits alternating parakeratosis and hyperkeratosis. The basal layer shows bud-like hyperplasia into the dermis, and the cells in the deep spinosum layer are disorganized and mildly atypical. Superficial dermis shows solar elastosis with mild perivascular inflammatory infiltration

skin diseases with abnormal keratinization. It provides the evidence for the preoperative diagnosis of AK.

Key Points

- AK is an epithelial tumor characterized by various degrees of atypical hyperplasia of keratinocytes. Some scholars believe that it is a premalignant lesion and some scholars believe that it is an early SCC.
- AK often occurs in the head and face of the elderly. On the ultrasound, the lesions are confined to the epidermis. The bottoms of some lesions are ambiguous and seem to reach the superficial dermis. The surface of the lesion shows abnormal keratinization with diverse morphology.
- It should be mainly differentiated from SK, BD, and superficial BCC.

5.2.2 Leukoplakia

Leukoplakia is a white keratinizing disease with a tendency to develop into squamous cell carcinoma (SCC). Its etiology is uncertain and it may be related to endocrine disorders and diabetes. The disease often occurs in the mucosa of the oral cavity, vulva, or other parts. Oral leukoplakia is more common in the middle-aged and elderly men, whereas vulvar leukoplakia is more common in postmenopausal women, a very small number of men can be seen glans leukoplakia. The disease clinically appears as punctate, patchy, or strip keratotic patch, which is grayish or milky white. The surface of the lesion is milky white in the early stage, showing reticular changes. Sometimes the surface forms a firm white membrane, which may bleed when it is forcibly peeled. At present, the disease is mainly treated with local or systemic drugs in clinical practice. Malignant change may occur if the disease is not treated timely or prolonged. Patients with suspicious lesions should be operated early and usually have a better prognosis.

Leukoplakia is histologically characterized by epidermal hyperkeratosis, protrusive keratin, parakeratosis, and thickened spinous layer. Meanwhile, there are lightly stained balloon cells with pyknotic macronucleus in the upper part of the spinous layer under parakeratosis.

Mucosal leukoplakia is a premalignant lesion. Several cases encountered by the author in clinic were located in the labia majora. Ultrasound did not show the lesions due to the limitation of the frequency of the ultrasound transducer and the special location of the lesion. And there is no literature on the ultrasound diagnosis of mucosal leukoplakia. The author speculated that the thickness of the disease is extremely thin and 20 ~ 50 MHz high-frequency ultrasound is difficult to show the lesion. It needs higher frequency ultrasound equipment for examination. At present, the diagnosis of mucosal leukoplakia mainly depends on its location and typical visual appearance.

Key Points

- Leukoplakia is a white keratinizing disease with a tendency to develop into SCC.
- Ultrasound is usually difficult to visualize the lesion.

5.3 Malignant Skin Tumors

5.3.1 Bowen's Disease

5.3.1.1 Clinical Manifestation and Pathology

Bowen's disease (BD), also known as squamous cell carcinoma in situ (SCC in situ), is an early cutaneous carcinoma in situ that develops and is confined to the epidermis. This disease was originally described by Bowen in 1912. Its etiology is uncertain, most of the disease results from sunlight exposure, carcinogens (such as arsenic), immunosuppression, and viral infection.

The disease often occurs in the middle-aged and elderly people. It occurs throughout the body and mainly on sun-exposed sites. Usually, the course of the disease is long with slow progress. Most studies suggested a risk of invasive carcinoma of about 3% ~ 5% for typical SCC in situ, with a potential risk for metastasis of up to 10%.

For visual appearance, BD typically presents as a slowly enlarging, well-demarcated, erythematous hyperkeratotic plaque, which may be accompanied by scab, crusts, ulcerations, and exudates (Fig. 5.47).

BD has different types of histological changes, which may present as psoriasiform, atrophic, verrucous hyperkeratotic, and irregular types. These histological types are often mixed in the same lesion. Histopathology shows epidermal acanthosis, disorganized and atypical cells, with multiple mitotic figures and dyskeratosis. BD is characterized by full-thickness epidermal dysplasia, and dense lymphocytic infiltrations are seen in the superficial dermis.

5.3.1.2 Ultrasound Manifestation

Gray-Scale Ultrasound

Gray-scale ultrasound shows a crawling hypoechoic lesion located in the epidermis with a slightly elevated surface, which presents abnormal keratinization and sometimes shows the characteristic of "wave-sign" (wave sign: crumpled surface with linear hyperechogenicity). The bottom of the lesion is distinct and flat without destruction to dermo-epidermal junction. The lesion is homogeneous. The visualization of the bottom may be disturbed by posterior acoustic shadowing resulting from abnormal keratinization, but sometimes it can be visualized through gaps or edges of abnormal keratinization by adjusting the transducer.

Color Doppler Ultrasound

The lesions show rich blood flow signals, but sometimes they show no or rare blood flow signals

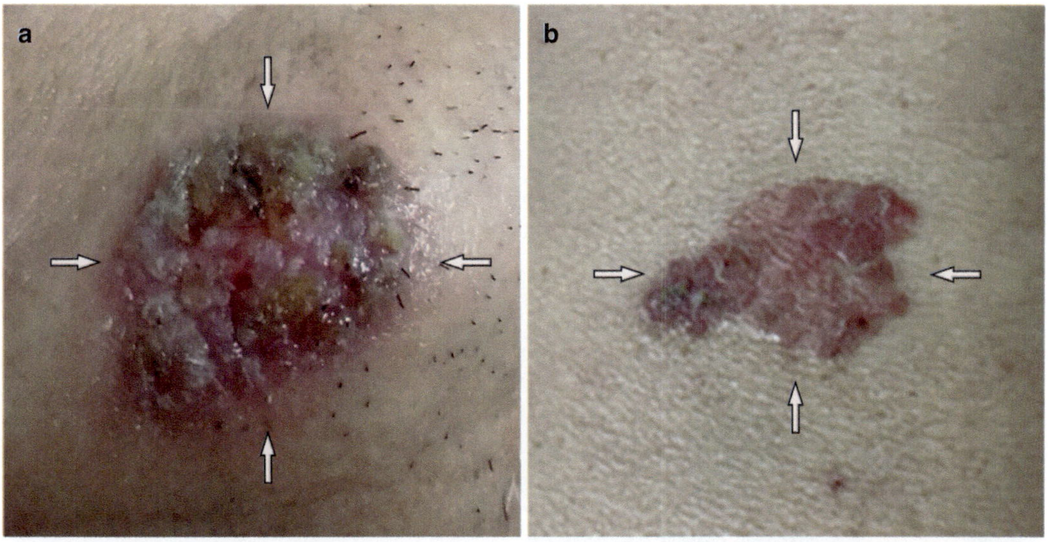

Fig. 5.47 Visual appearance of Bowen's disease. (**a**) Visual observation shows a dark red patch with crusts in the right lower jaw (arrows). (**b**) Visual observation shows a dark red, irregular, and well-defined patch observed in the left back (arrows), with repeated crust detachment, locally covered with brown or gray thick scab

due to posterior acoustic shadowing caused by abnormal keratinization (Figs. 5.48 and 5.49).

5.3.1.3 Differential Diagnosis

Superficial Basal Cell Carcinoma (Superficial BCC)

Both of them have similar visual appearance as dark red and scaly patches. On gray-scale ultrasound, both entities appear as crawling and hypoechoic lesions located in the epidermis. However, some superficial BCCs involve dermis. The surfaces are flat without hyperechogenicity of abnormal keratinization.

In contrast, BD is confined to the epidermis and presents a crumpled hyperkeratotic surface with posterior acoustic shadowing. The hyperechogenicity on the surface and the layers of involvement are key factors to differentiate them.

AK

Both of them sometimes have similar appearance, thus it is difficult to differentiate them. Most of them appear as reddish-brown and scaly patches with a rough surface.

On gray-scale ultrasound, both the diseases appear as crawling and hypoechoic lesions within the epidermis with abnormal keratinization. BD is mostly single, while AK is multiple. Besides that, the bottom of BD is flat, and the surface shows more severe and crumpled abnormal keratinization. However, the bottom of AK is ambiguous, and it seems to reach the superficial dermis. The surface shows relative slight and regular abnormal keratinization.

SK

Both of the diseases are confined to the epidermis and their bottoms are clearly demarcated from the dermis. The surface shows different degrees of keratinization with posterior acoustic shadowing. However, SK is elevated, while BD is mostly crawling. Color Doppler ultrasound is helpful for differentiating the two entities, and the blood flow signals of BD are richer than SK. In addition, BD appears as a reddish or dark red scaly papule or patch. SK shows a small, flat, yellow, or brown patch in the early stage, and characteristics of "cerebral like" in the later stage.

5.3.1.4 Diagnosis Clues

1. Clinically, BD typically presents as a erythematous hyperkeratotic patch or plaque,

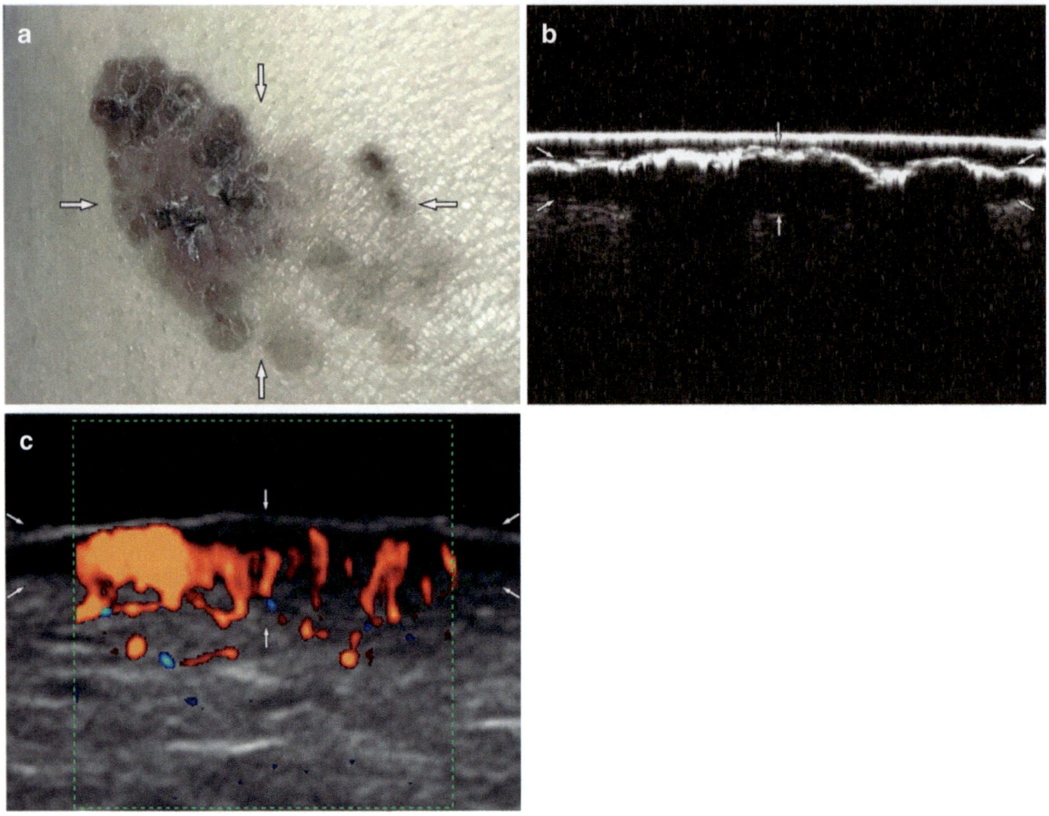

Fig. 5.48 Bowen's disease. Female, 63 years of age. (**a**) Visual observation shows a dark red and scaly plaque on the back (arrows), covered with brown scab on the surface, and without exudates (size: 55.0 mm × 23.0 mm). (**b**) Gray-scale ultrasound shows a crawling hypoechoic lesion (arrows) in the epidermis (thickness: 1.1 mm). The hyperkeratotic surface presents as linear hyperechogenicity with posterior acoustic shadowing. The bottom is flat with a well-defined demarcation from the dermis. The lesion is homogeneous (Frequency: 50 MHz). (**c**) Color Doppler ultrasound shows rich blood flow signals inside the lesion (arrows) (Frequency: 22 MHz)

which may be accompanied by scabs, crusts, ulcerations, and exudates.

2. Gray-scale ultrasound shows a crawling and hypoechoic lesion confined to the epidermis, with a "wave sign" surface, accompanied by posterior acoustic shadowing. The bottom is well-defined and flat with a clear demarcation from the dermis.
3. Color Doppler ultrasound shows rich blood flow signals.

5.3.1.5 Clinical Significance

The visual appearances of BD are too diverse to diagnose accurately, while high-frequency ultrasound shows the structure and vascularity of the lesion in detail. One of our previous study summarized the ultrasound features of 29 cases of BD, and the results demonstrated that the typical ultrasound features are "confined to the epidermis" and "wave sign," which are better visualized by ultrasound biomicroscopy than by high-frequency ultrasound (Table 5.1). The diagnostic accuracy of ultrasound biomicroscopy is significantly higher than that of high-frequency ultrasound (86.2% vs. 51.7%), so ultrasound biomicroscopy is recommended preferentially in the diagnosis of BD.

Key Points

- BD, also known as SCC in situ, develops and is confined to the epidermis. It often occurs in the middle-aged and elderly people and has a long course of disease with slow progress.

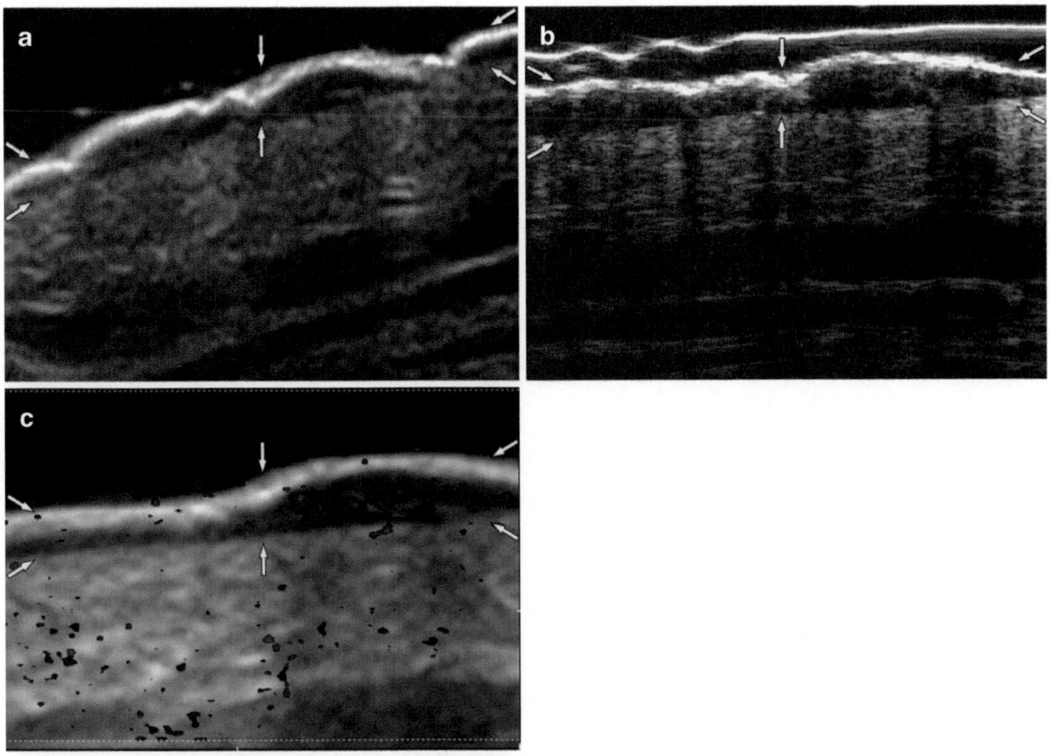

Fig. 5.49 Bowen's disease. Male, 69 years of age. (**a**) Gray-scale ultrasound shows a crawling and hypoechoic lesion (arrows) in the epidermis (thickness: 1.2 mm). The surface is crumpled with thick linear hyperechogenicity and tiny posterior acoustic shadowing. The bottom has a well-defined demarcation from the dermis. The lesion is homogeneous (Frequency: 22 MHz). (**b**) Ultrasound biomicroscopy shows the layers of involvement more clearly (Frequency: 50 MHz). (**c**) Color Doppler ultrasound shows rare blood flow signals inside the lesion (arrows) (Frequency: 22 MHz)

Table 5.1 The high-frequency ultrasound (HFUS) and ultrasound biomicroscopy (UBM) characteristics for BD

Characteristics	HFUS ($n = 29$)	UBM ($n = 29$)	P value
Confined to the epidermis (yes/no)	15 (51.7%)/14 (48.3%)	25 (86.2%)/4 (13.8%)	0.002
"Wave sign" on the surface (present/absent)	6 (20.7%)/23 (79.3%)	17 (58.6%)/12 (41.4%)	0.001

- Gray-scale ultrasound shows a crawling and hypoechoic lesion in the epidermis. A crumpled and hyperkeratotic surface is accompanied by posterior acoustic shadowing. The bottom is flat with a clear demarcation from the dermis.
- It should be mainly differentiated from superficial BCC, AK, and SK.

5.3.2 Basal Cell Carcinoma

5.3.2.1 Clinical Manifestation and Pathology

Basal cell carcinoma (BCC), also known as basal cell epithelioma, is caused by abnormal proliferation of pluripotent basal-like cells, which originates from the basal layer cells of epidermis. BCC is the most common skin malignancy. Its etiology and pathogenesis are uncertain and may be related to the complex interaction between genes and the environment. At present, ultraviolet radiation is considered to be the most important risk factor for BCC, and other risk factors include arsenic, coal tar derivatives, radiation, scars, chronic inflammation, ulcers, and immunodeficiency, etc.

BCC is rarely fatal. It usually occurs in exposed areas such as the head, nose, eyelids, and lips. Most

BCCs damage cosmetically, even psychosocially and mentally upon patients. Although BCC rarely metastasizes, there is a risk of invasion to deeper tissues, such as muscles, cartilage, and bones.

In clinic, BCC is mainly classified into three types: nodular, superficial, and morpheaform. The nodular type grows slowly, appearing as a brown papule or nodule and is prone to bleeding or ulceration after minor trauma. The superficial type appears as a flat and well-defined patch. The morpheaform appears as scar-like morphea with an indistinct boundary (Fig. 5.50).

Histologically, BCC consists of a fibrous stroma and islands of basaloid cells that are dependent cells, resembling basal cells of the epidermis and hair follicles.

Histologically, BCC is often divided into four subtypes: nodular, superficial, pigmented, and

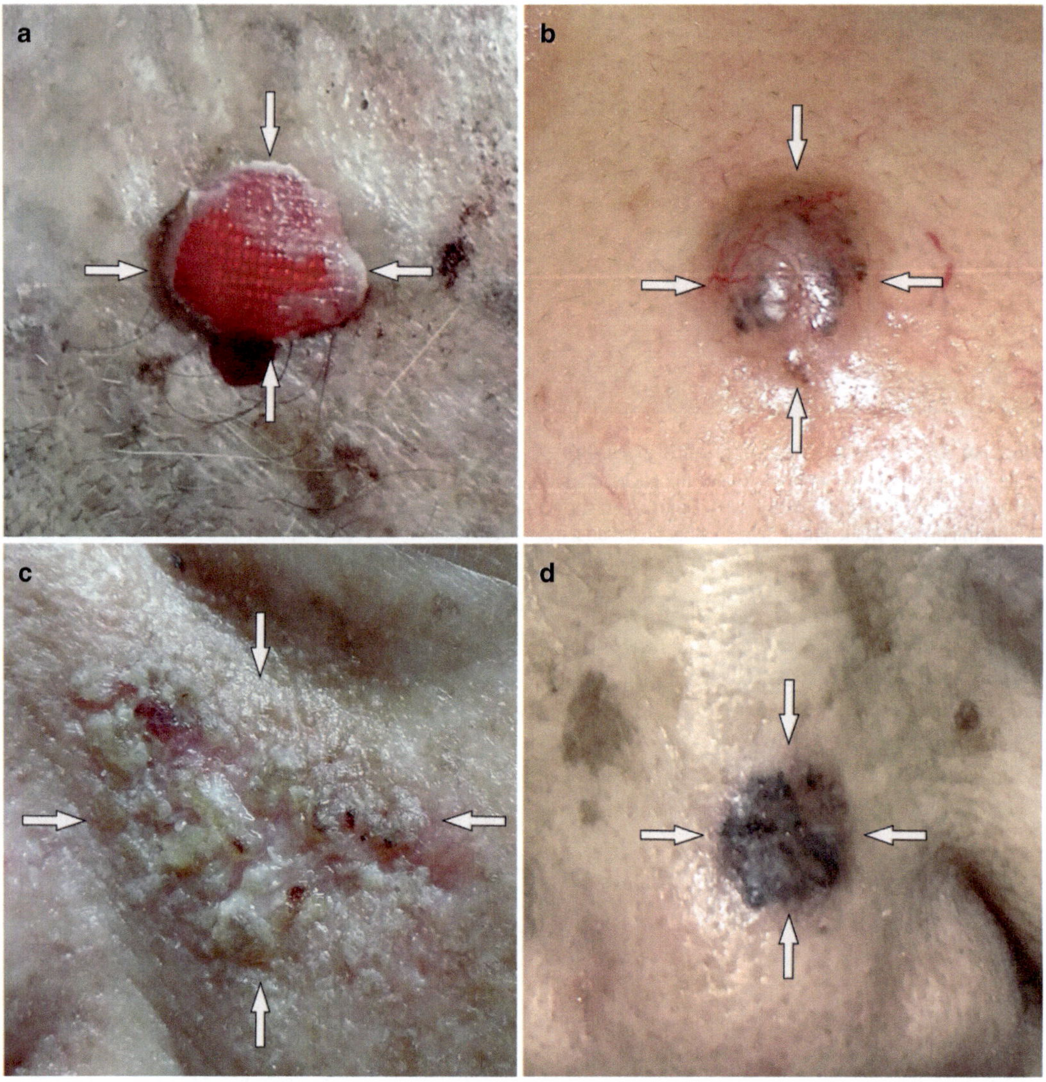

Fig. 5.50 Visual appearance of basal cell carcinoma. (**a**) nodular basal cell carcinoma at the right temporal region, appearing as a pearl-like papule with a bleeding surface (arrows) (diameter: 12.0 mm). (**b**) A nodular basal cell carcinoma on the left cheek, appearing as a well-defined light brown papule with a smooth surface (arrows) (diameter: 8.0 mm). (**c**) A superficial basal cell carcinoma on the left cheek, appearing as a flat and well-defined patch with a brownish-yellow scale (arrows) (diameter: 15.0 mm). (**d**) A morpheaform basal cell carcinoma in the middle of the nose, appearing as a round and well-defined black plaque with uneven pigment (arrows) (diameter: 10.0 mm)

morpheaform. There are also other rare histological types of BCC, such as fibroepithelioma, micronodular, infundibulocystic, infiltrative, morpheaform, and basosquamous subtypes. Multiple subtypes may occur simultaneously in one lesion. All the above subtypes of BCC are divided into two categories: non-invasive BCC and invasive BCC. Non-invasive BCC includes nodular, superficial, fibroepitheliomatous, and infundibulocystic BCC; while invasive BCC includes micronodular, morpheaform, pigmented, and basosquamous BCC.

For the grading and staging of BCC, the guidelines recommend the risk stratification system for BCC recurrence in the National Comprehensive Cancer Network (NCCN) (Table 5.2).

5.3.2.2 Ultrasound Manifestation

The ultrasound findings of different subtypes of BCC are various. The authors have summarized the ultrasound features of common subtypes of BCC as following on the basis of the cases from Shanghai Skin Disease Hospital.

Table 5.2 Risk stratification system for recurrence of BCC in NCCN

Characteristics	Low risk	High risk
Clinical		
Location/size	Area L, < 20 mm	Area L, ≥ 20 mm
	Area M, < 10 mm	Area M, ≥ 10 mm
	Area H, < 6 mm	Area H, ≥ 6 mm
Borders	Well defined	Poorly defined
Primary vs. recurrent	Primary	Recurrent
Immunosuppression	(−)	(+)
Tumor at the site with prior radiotherapy	(−)	(+)
Pathology		
Subtype	Nodular type, superficial [a]	Aggressive growth pattern [b]
Peripheral nerve involvement	(−)	(+)

Notes: L zone = trunk and extremities (excluding hands, nail units, pretibial, ankles, feet); M zone = cheeks, forehead, scalp, neck, and pretibial; H zone = "mask areas" of face (central face, eyelids, eyebrows, periorbital, nose, lips [cutaneous and vermilion], chin, mandible, preauricular and postauricular skin/sulci, temple, ear), genitalia, hands, and feet

[a]Low-risk histologic subtypes include nodular, superficial, and other non-aggressive growth patterns such as keratotic, infundibulocystic, and fibroepithelioma of Pinkus; [b] Having (mixed) infiltrative, micronodular, morpheaform, basosquamous, sclerosing, or carcinosarcomatous differentiation features in any portion of the tumor. In some cases basosquamous tumors may be prognostically similar to SCC; clinicopathologic correlation is recommended in these cases

Nodular BCC

It generally presents as a nodular, well-defined, and hypoechoic lesion in the epidermis and dermis. The surface is elevated without abnormal keratinization. However, the lesion often presents a thick hyperechoic surface with posterior acoustic shadowing due to the hemorrhagic crusts, which is similar to keratinization and needs to be differentiated by visual appearance. The multiple hyperechoic spots and cystic degeneration zones are visualized in some lesions, both of which are characteristic features of BCC. The lesion involves the epidermis in the early stage, as the disease progresses, it invades the dermis and subcutaneous tissues inferiorly in turn. Color Doppler ultrasound shows rich blood flow signals inside the lesion, sometimes with thick nourishing vessels (Figs. 5.51 and 5.52).

Superficial BCC

Superficial BCC is mostly located in the epidermis and also involves the dermis. Gray-scale ultrasound shows a crawling, well-defined, and homogeneous hypoechoic lesion. The surface is flat without abnormal keratinization. Color Doppler ultrasound shows no or rare blood flow signals in the lesion (Fig. 5.53).

Pigmented BCC

Its ultrasound features resemble that of the nodular type. The lesions are often hypoechoic areas located in the epidermis and dermis. The surface is elevated. The shape is oval or irregular with a well-defined boundary. Scattered or clustered hyperechoic spots are also presented in the lesion (Fig. 5.54).

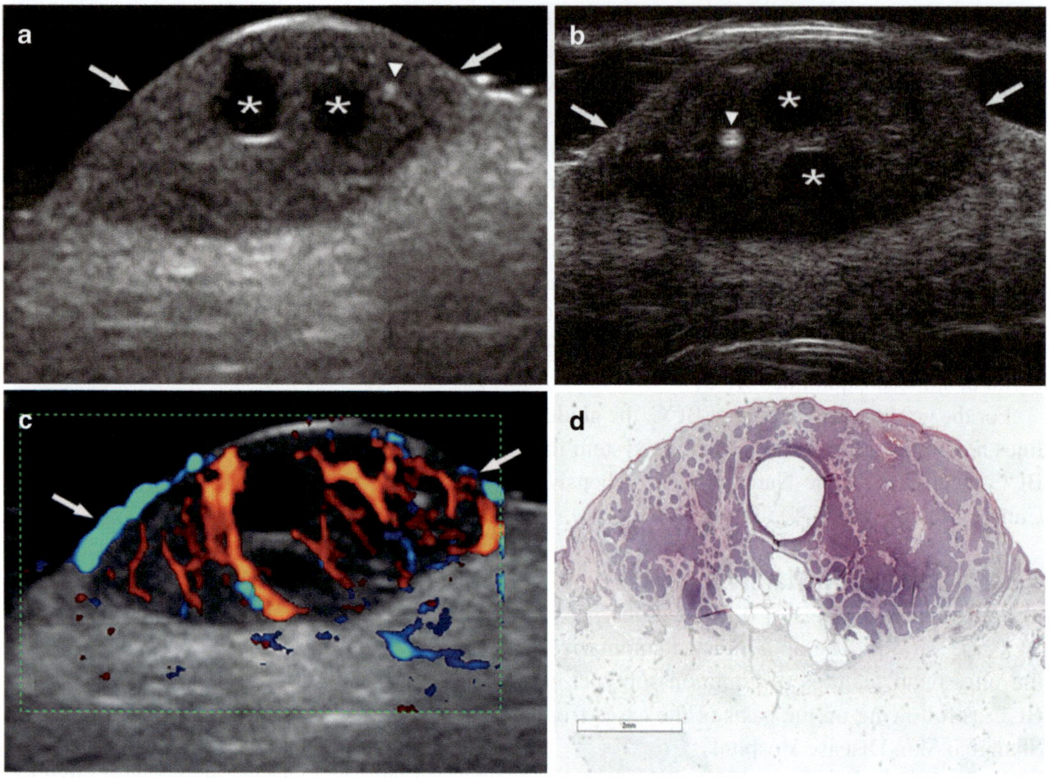

Fig. 5.51 Nodular basal cell carcinoma with cystic degeneration zones. Female, 63 years of age. (**a**) Gray-scale ultrasound shows a nodular, well-defined, and mixed echogenic lesion (arrows) in the epidermis and dermis (size: 9.0 mm × 7.1 mm; thickness: 4.6 mm). The surface is elevated without abnormal keratinization. Hyperechoic spots (▽) and cystic degeneration zones (*) are visualized in the lesion (Frequency: 22 MHz). (**b**) Ultrasound biomicroscopy clearly shows the cystic degeneration zones (*), hyperechoic spots (▽), and the bottom of the lesion (arrows) (Frequency: 50 MHz). (**c**) Color Doppler ultrasound shows rich blood flow signals inside the lesion (arrows) (Frequency: 22 MHz). (**d**) Histopathology (HE staining, panoramic scanning) shows a basophilic tumor mass in the dermis. The lesion is connected to the epidermis and consists of basaloid cells with a palisade arrangement, with a cleft surrounding a cell nest

Morpheaform BCC

The lesion mainly shows an irregular, well-defined, isoechoic, or hypoechoic area in the epidermis and dermis. The surface is flat without abnormal keratinization. The lesions are homogeneous or heterogeneous. Color Doppler ultrasound shows rich blood flow signals inside the lesion (Fig. 5.55).

5.3.2.3 Differential Diagnosis

Malignant Melanoma (MM)

Pigmented BCC needs to be differentiated from MM. First of all, MM often occurs in the lower extremities, while BCC often occurs in the head and face.

In addition, on gray-scale ultrasound, MM shows a hypoechoic or very hypoechoic lesion, with mostly lobulated shapes and posterior acoustic enhancement. Owing to the trend of downward-directed proliferation, MM often involves deep subcutaneous tissue. However, the shape of BCC is generally more regular, and mostly involves epidermis and dermis. The characteristic features of hyperechoic spots and cystic degeneration zones are visualized in BCC.

Cutaneous Squamous Cell Carcinoma (cSCC)

The clinical symptoms of BCC are mild or asymptomatic and the disease progresses slowly. BCC often presents as nodular papule or flat

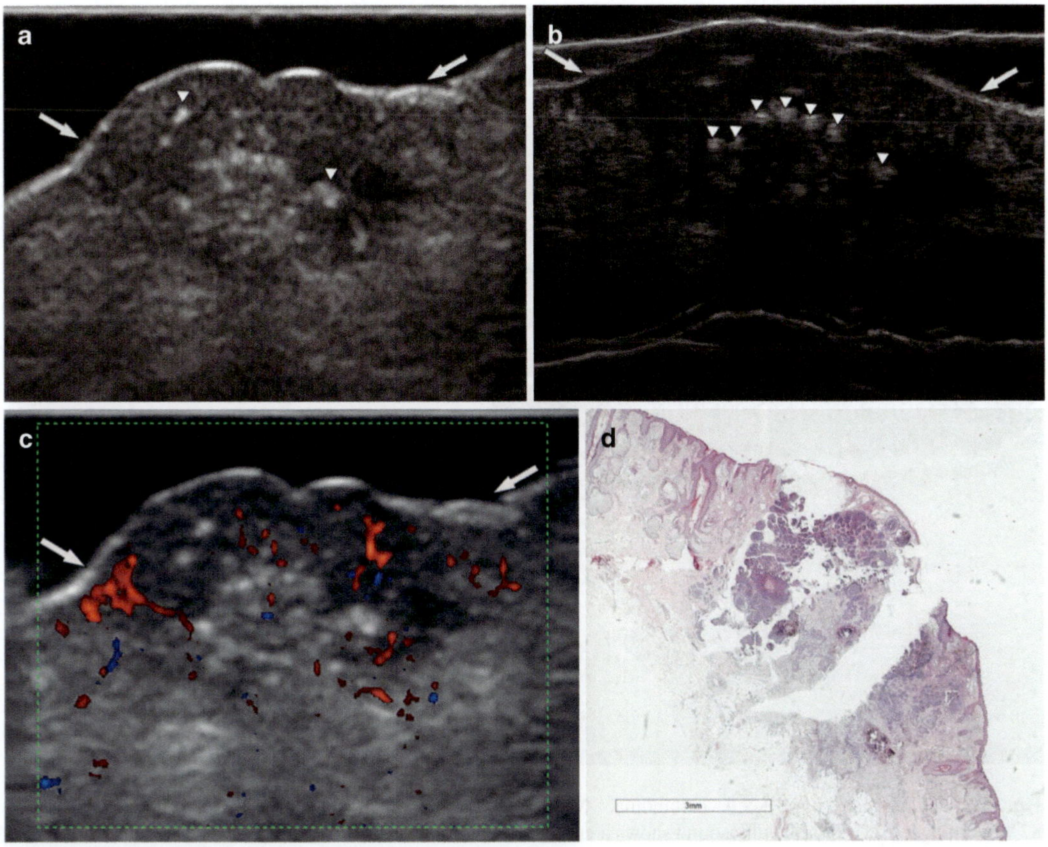

Fig. 5.52 Nodular basal cell carcinoma with multiple hyperechoic spots. Male, 77 years of age. (**a**) Gray-scale ultrasound shows an irregular, well-defined and hypoechoic lesion (arrows) in the epidermis and dermis (size: 8.7 mm × 8.1 mm; thickness: 5.5 mm). The surface is elevated without abnormal keratinization. The lesion is heterogeneous with multiple hyperechoic spots (▽) (Frequency: 22 MHz). (**b**) Ultrasound biomicroscopy clearly shows hyperechoic spots inside the lesion (▽), with the bottom located in the dermis (Frequency: 50 MHz). (**c**) Color Doppler ultrasound shows rich blood flow signals inside the lesion (arrows) (Frequency: 22 MHz). (**d**) Histopathology (HE staining, panoramic scanning) shows a basophilic tumor mass in the dermis. The lesion is connected to the epidermis and consists of basaloid cells with a palisade arrangement, with a cleft surrounding a cell nest

patch, and some lesions bleed on the surface after touching.

cSCC is prone to form central ulcers, and the margin is a cauliflower-like irregular elevation. Significant abnormal keratinization is visualized on the surface. On gray-scale ultrasound, due to the severe abnormal keratinization of the surface, heterogeneous acoustic shadowing of the lesion often obstructs sufficient visualization.

In contrast, BCC usually has no abnormal keratinization, its internal echogenicity is often clearly visualized, and the characteristics of hyperechoic spots and cystic degeneration zones are observed in the lesion.

5.3.2.4 Diagnosis Clues

1. The lesions often occur in the head and face. Clinically, the lesion appears as a painless papule, nodule, or patch. The surface of nodular lesions may be associated with hemorrhage.
2. On gray-scale ultrasound, nodular BCCs are mostly oval; pigmented and superficial BCCs are mostly crawling; and morpheaform type is mostly irregular. All types of lesions are mainly located in the epidermis and/or dermis, without abnormal keratinization on the surface. The boundary is well-defined, and the features of hyperechoic spots and cystic

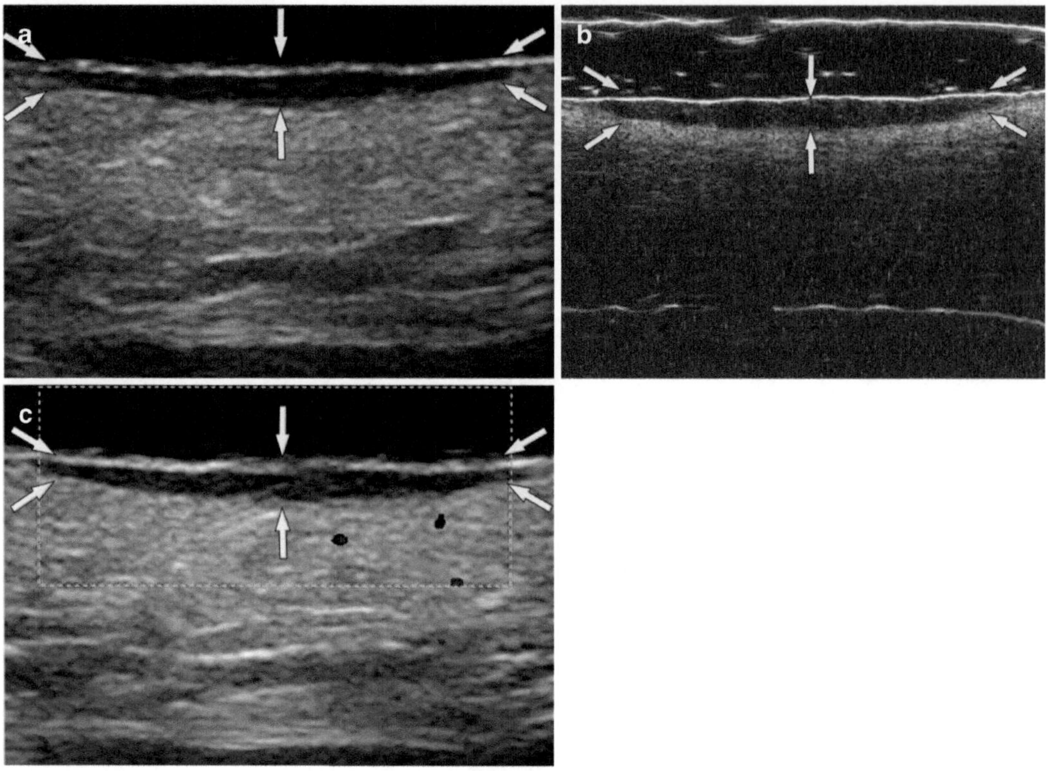

Fig. 5.53 Superficial basal cell carcinoma. Male, 87 years of age. (**a**) Gray-scale ultrasound shows a crawling and well-defined hypoechoic lesion (arrows) in the epidermis and superficial dermis (size: 13.4 mm × 11.2 mm; thickness: 1.1 mm). The surface is flat without abnormal keratinization. The bottom of lesion is located in the superficial dermis (arrows) (Frequency: 22 MHz). (**b**) Ultrasound biomicroscopy clearly shows that the lesion is located in the superficial dermis (arrows) (Frequency: 50 MHz). (**c**) Color Doppler ultrasound shows no blood flow signals inside the lesion (arrows) (Frequency: 22 MHz)

degeneration zones are characteristic ultrasound findings of BCC.

3. On color Doppler ultrasound, rich blood flow signals are observed in all types of lesions, and some with thick nourishing vessels.

5.3.2.5 Clinical Significance

Wortsman et al. reported that the number of hyperechoic spots inside the BCC lesion can be used to predict a high risk of recurrence, with a cut-off value of ≥7 hyperechoic spots, a sensitivity of 0.79, and a specificity of 0.53. Fernando et al. demonstrated that invasive BCC has stiffer margin than non-invasive BCC on elastography, and increased margin stiffness has a sensitivity of 0.89 and a specificity of 0.82 for the diagnosis of invasive BCC. Hernández-IbáñezC et al. suggested that the accuracy of high-frequency ultrasound in the diagnosis of BCC is 0.737, with a sensitivity of 0.745 and a specificity of 0.73; the sensitivity of diagnosing superficial BCC is 0.622, with a specificity of 0.982; and the sensitivity of diagnosing nodular BCC is 0.651, with a specificity of 0.805.

But the diagnostic performance for other subtypes of BCC has not yet been reported in the relevant literatures. Our study showed that three ultrasound features, including growth pattern, the layers of involvement, and distribution of intralesional hyperechoic spots, might play key roles in evaluating the invasiveness of BCC (Table 5.3). Invasive BCCs tended to be irregular in growth

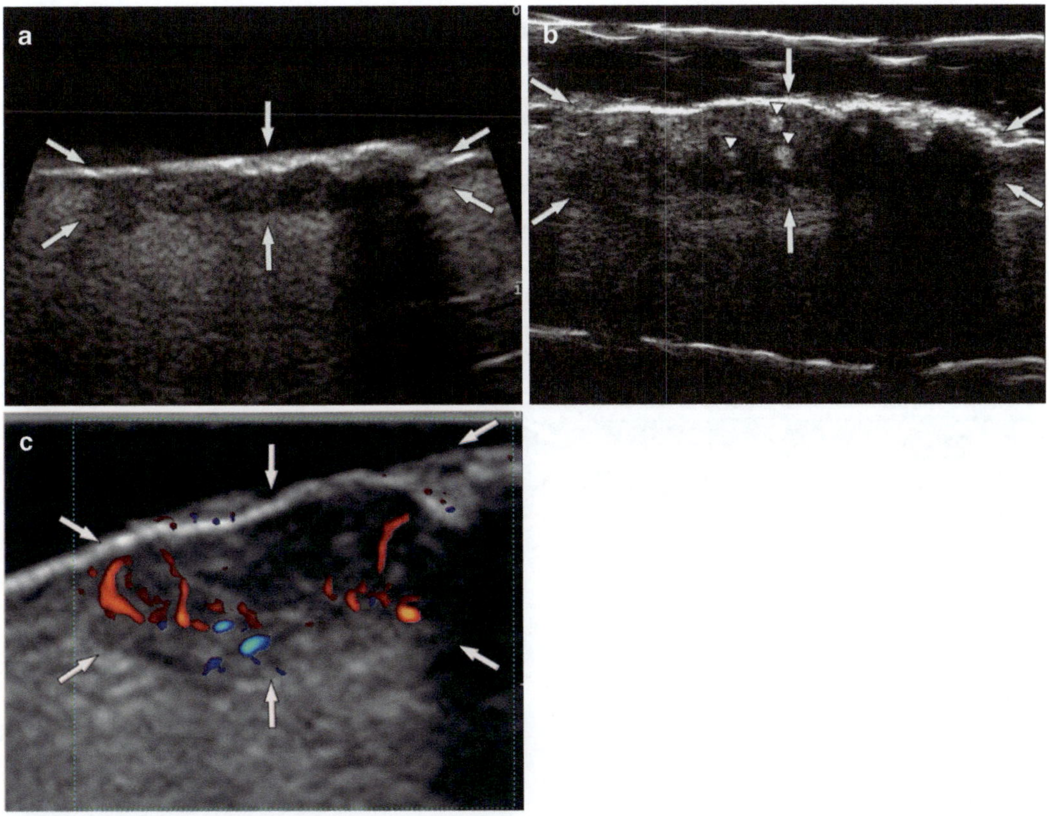

Fig. 5.54 Pigmented basal cell carcinoma. Female, 71 years of age. (**a**) Gray-scale ultrasound shows a crawling and well-defined hypoechoic lesion (arrows) in the epidermis and dermis (size: 11.3 mm × 7.6 mm; thickness: 2.5 mm). The surface is slightly elevated, with local hyperechogenicity (hemorrhagic crusts) and posterior acoustic shadowing. The lesions are homogeneous (Frequency: 22 MHz). (**b**) Ultrasound biomicroscopy clearly shows hyperechoic spots inside the lesion (▽) (Frequency: 50 MHz). (**c**) Color Doppler ultrasound shows rich blood flow signals inside the lesion (arrows) (Frequency: 22 MHz)

pattern, whereas most of the non-invasive BCCs were nodular or crawling. Almost all invasive BCCs broke through the dermis, whereas rare non-invasive BCC involved the subcutaneous tissue. For invasive BCCs, intralesional hyperechoic spots distribution tended to be clustered, whereas it was more likely to be absent or scattered in non-invasive BCCs.

According to the author's experience, ultrasound biomicroscopy sometimes reveals hyperechoic spots that cannot be visualized by high-frequency ultrasound, and the combination of the two techniques is expected to improve the accuracy of BCC diagnosis.

Key Points

- BCC is a common malignant tumor of the skin. It is rarely fatal and metastatic. Histologically, it is often divided into four subtypes: nodular, superficial, pigmented, and morpheaform.
- On ultrasound, BCC is mainly located in the epidermis and/or dermis, without abnormal keratinization on the surface. The boundary is well-defined, and hyperechoic spots and cystic degeneration zones are characteristic features of BCC.
- It should be differentiated from melanocytic nevi, MM, and cSCC.

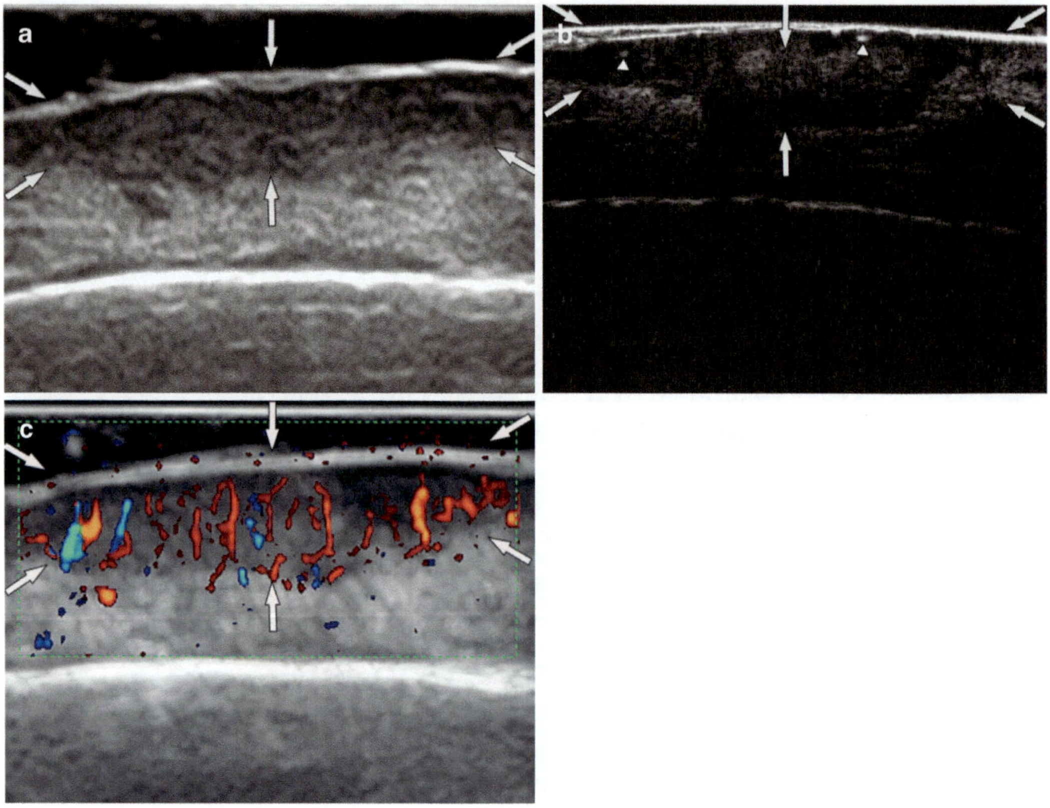

Fig. 5.55 Morpheaform basal cell carcinoma. Female, 76 years of age. (**a**) Gray-scale ultrasound shows an irregular, ill-defined, and hypoechoic lesion (arrows) in the epidermis and dermis (size: 13.8 mm × 12.6 mm; thickness: 2.8 mm). The surface is flat without abnormal keratinization. The lesions are homogeneous (Frequency: 22 MHz). (**b**) Ultrasound biomicroscopy clearly shows the hyperechoic spots within the lesion near the epidermis (▽) (Frequency: 50 MHz). (**c**) Color Doppler ultrasound shows rich blood flow signals inside the lesion (arrows) (Frequency: 22 MHz)

Table 5.3 Sensitivity and specificity of ultrasound features for evaluating the invasiveness of BCC

Ultrasound features	Sensitivity	Specificity	PPV	NPV	Accuracy
Growth pattern	0.605	0.895	0.813	0.750	0.770
Involvement layers	0.953	0.596	0.641	0.944	0.750
Distribution of intralesional hyperechoic spots	0.558	0.912	0.828	0.732	0.760
All three features	0.814	0.860	0.814	0.860	0.840

PPV: Positive predictive value
NPV: Negative predictive value

5.3.3 Cutaneous Squamous Cell Carcinoma

5.3.3.1 Clinical Manifestation and Pathology

Cutaneous squamous cell carcinoma (cSCC) is a cutaneous malignancy originating from keratinocytes of the epidermis or appendages. In Europe and the United States, the incidence of cSCC in cutaneous malignancies is second only to BCC. However, studies in China have found that the incidence of cSCC is ranking first in nonmelanoma skin tumors, and the incidence is increasing year by year. Among cutaneous malignancies, cSCC is secondary to malignant melanoma in the degree of malignancy.

Some cSCCs involve the epidermis, dermis, and subcutaneous tissues simultaneously, causing significant disfigurement in appearance so as to affect the patients' mental health and social adaptability seriously. Lymph node metastasis may occur in advanced stages of the disease which is fatal in severe cases. The risk of lymph node metastasis in cSCC is reported to be 4% and the risk of death is 1.5%.

Like BCC, its etiology and pathogenesis are uncertain, but ultraviolet exposure is recognized as the most important pathogenic factor of cSCC. Other risk factors include infection with human papillomavirus, chemical carcinogens, and immunodeficiency.

cSCC commonly occurs in areas with scaly epithelium, such as mouth, lips, perineum, etc. The visual appearance of cSCC is diverse, mainly manifested as infiltrative morphea in the early stage, which gradually develops into plaques and nodules. Some lesions appear as cauliflower-like bumps, and some lesions have central ulcers, often with necrotic tissues and hemorrhagic secretions. The extent of the disease expands as the disease progresses (Fig. 5.56).

Clinically, cSCC is mainly divided into four subtypes: nodular ulcer type, pigmented type, fibrotic type, and superficial type, of which nodular ulcer type is the most common. Histopathologically, based on the classification

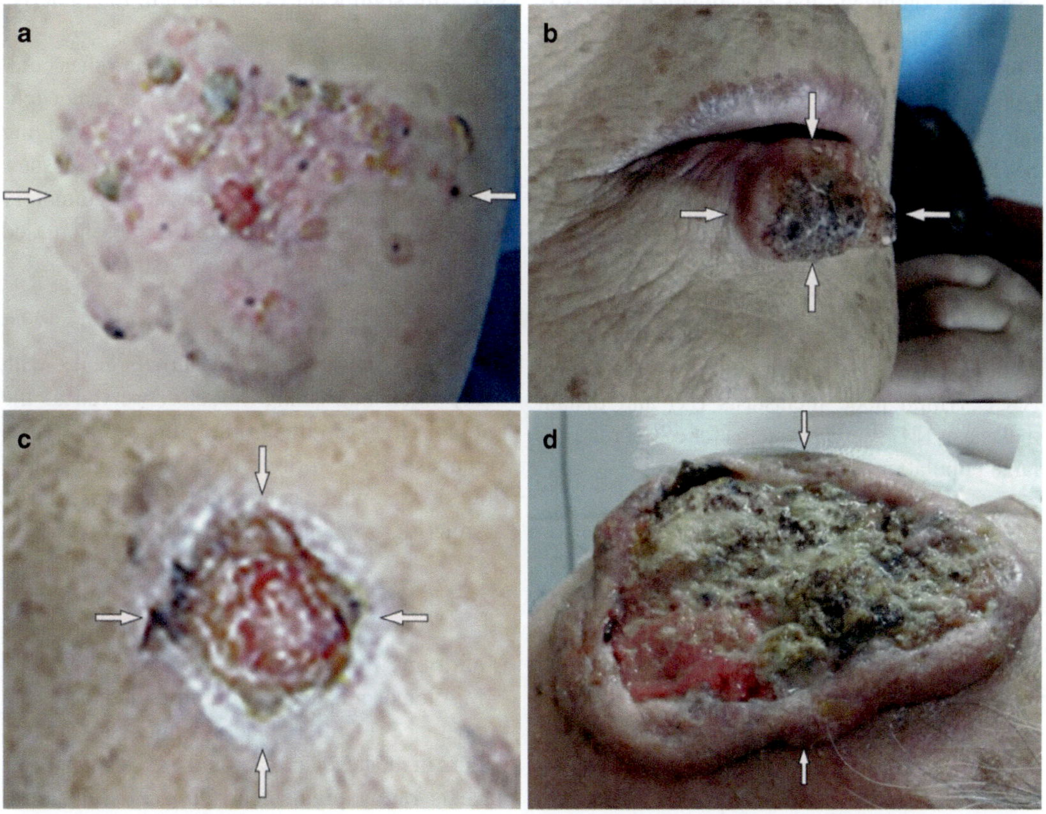

Fig. 5.56 Visual appearance of cutaneous squamous cell carcinoma. (**a**) A reddish plaque on the right hypochondrial region with scattered papular nodules and poor demarcation from the surrounding tissues (arrows) (size: about 80.0 mm × 130.0 mm). The surface is rough and covered with scales and hemorrhagic crusts. (**b**) A reddish patch on the vermilion of the lower lip, with the lower margin involving the vermilion border of the lip (arrows) (size: about 30.0 mm × 20.0 mm). The surface of the lesion shows papillomatous hyperplasia without ulceration or erosion. The boundary is well-defined. (**c**) An ulcer on the scalp, with oozing exudate and brown crust on the surface, slight redness and swelling in the periphery of the lesion (arrows) (size: about 30.0 mm × 25.0 mm). (**d**) A lesion of about 60.0 mm in diameter in the scalp presenting a necrotic center and prominent rim, with hemorrhagic secretions (arrows)

Table 5.4 BWH staging criteria for cSCC

Stage	
T1	0 high-risk factors
T2a	1 high-risk factor
T2b	2 ~ 3 high-risk factors
T3	4 high-risk factors

Risk factors include: tumor diameter ≥ 20.0 mm, poorly differentiated histology, perineural invasion, and tumor invasion beyond the subcutaneous fat (excluding bone, which automatically upgrades to T3). BWH: Brigham and Women's Hospital

of borders, cSCC is classified as: grade I (well differentiated), grade II (moderately differentiated), grade III (poorly differentiated), and grade IV (undifferentiated).

The American Academy of Dermatology (AAD) recommends the classification of cSCC using the classification method in the NCCN, which is divided into two categories: low-risk and high-risk. For staging of cSCC, there is no universally accepted staging system for cSCC, and BWH (Brigham and Women's Hospital) staging system is recommended for AAD (Table 5.4).

Since lymph node metastasis or distant metastasis of primary cSCC is very rare, the American Joint Committee on Cancer (AJCC) is also limited to tumors at stages N0 and M0 in the updated eighth edition of the guidelines. Validation of AJCC lymph node metastasis (N) and distant metastasis (M) staging systems for cSCC requires large population-based cohort studies.

5.3.3.2 Ultrasound Manifestation

Gray-Scale Ultrasound

The surface of cSCC is uneven and appears as thick linear hyperechogenicity resulted from hyperkeratosis, with various degrees of posterior acoustic shadowing, which is an important characteristic of cSCC. Sometimes the visualization of the lesion is disturbed by posterior acoustic shadowing resulting from abnormal keratinization, but it is occasionally visualized through gaps or edges of abnormal keratinization and the periphery of the lesion by adjusting the direction of the transducer. It is not recommended to remove the abnormal keratinized surface deliberately with the intention to facilitate ultrasound examination, which may cause unnecessary damage and bleeding.

In addition, cSCC is highly susceptible to ulcer formation and shows a crater-like elevation around the ulcer. On gray-scale ultrasound, the lesion appears as a depressed morphology and loses local stratum corneum.

Sometimes the hyperkeratotic area may have been removed because of natural detachment or other intervention. At this time, the visualization of ultrasound features of the lesion can be easily achieved. The lesion shows a hypoechoic area that breaks through the dermo-epidermal junction or even infiltrates into the subcutaneous tissue. The lesion is heterogeneous, mostly presenting an irregular shape and lobulated margin, with significant extension into the underlying tissues.

In general, cSCCs are larger than other cutaneous malignancies and have a significant tendency to invade deeply, frequently involving subcutaneous tissues and surrounding tissues. Peripheral soft tissues may show inflammatory findings such as thickened soft tissue, increased echogenicity, and disorganized distribution.

Color Doppler Ultrasound

The lesion shows rich blood flow signals, with many thick nourishing vessels observed at the bottom. However, due to the influence of hyperkeratosis, many lesions only show rare blood flow signals, which cannot reflect the vascularity in true (Figs. 5.57 and 5.58).

5.3.3.3 Differential Diagnosis

Malignant Melanoma (MM)

MM often occurs in the extremities and the visual appearance is often black, while cSCC often occurs in the head and face and the visual appearance is rarely pigmented. On gray-scale ultrasound, there is no abnormal keratinization of MM, which is significantly different from cSCC.

BCC

BCC often appears as a nodular papule or flat patch, and some lesions have bleeding on the surface. However, the cSCC lesions are prone to

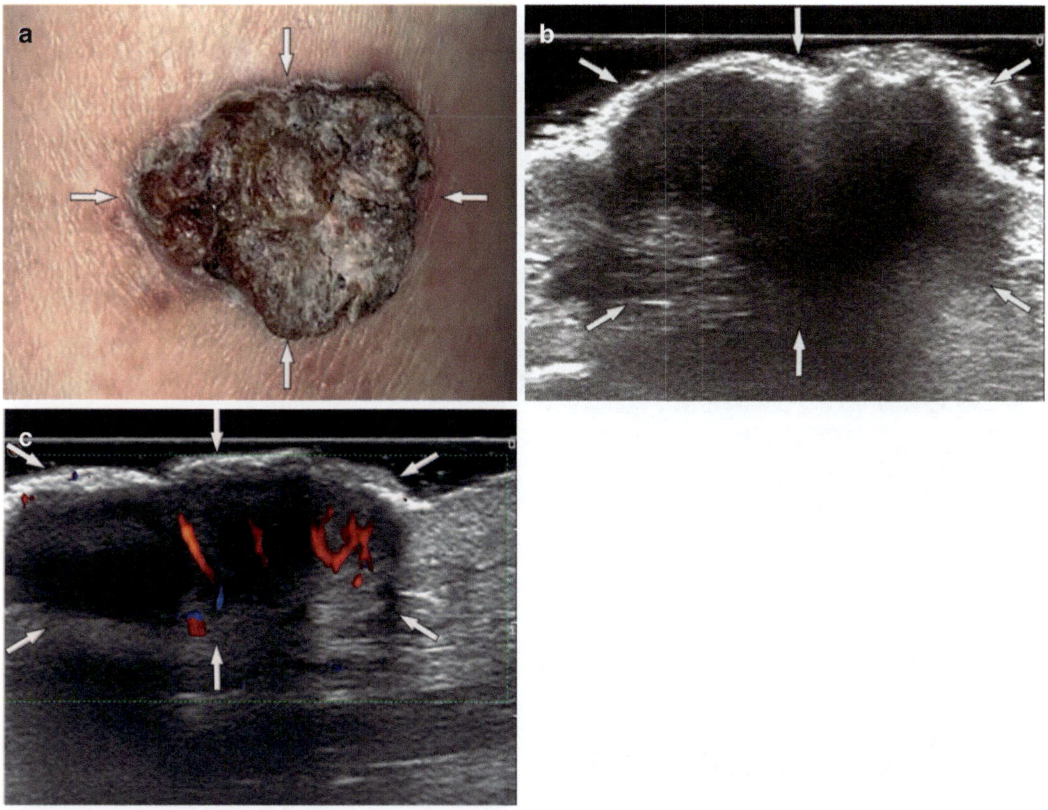

Fig. 5.57 Cutaneous squamous cell carcinoma. Male, 80 years of age. (**a**) Visual observation shows a gray and well-defined verrucous plaque at the right medial malleolus, with a rough surface, no ulceration or exudates (arrows) (size: 25.0 mm × 32.0 mm; thickness: 4.9 mm). (**b**) Gray-scale ultrasound shows an irregular and ill-defined hypoechoic lesion (arrows) that involves the epidermis, dermis, and subcutaneous tissue. The surface is irregularly elevated, appearing thick linear hyperechogenicity with posterior acoustic shadowing. The internal ultrasound features of the lesion could not be visualized due to the posterior acoustic shadowing. The layers of involvement of the lesion are roughly observed (Frequency: 22 MHz). (**c**) Color Doppler ultrasound shows rare blood flow signals inside the lesion through an abnormally keratinized gap (arrows) (Frequency: 22 MHz)

form central ulcers, and the margins may be cauliflower-like irregular elevations. On gray-scale ultrasound, the surface of cSCC appears as thick linear hyperechogenicity formed by hyperkeratosis, with various degrees of posterior acoustic shadowing, which even leads to insufficient visualization of the lesion. In contrast, BCC usually has no abnormal keratinization so that its internal ultrasound features are often clearly visualized, and hyperechoic spots and anechoic areas are frequently observed.

5.3.3.4 Diagnosis Clues

1. Clinically, most cSCC shows an infiltrative morphea in the early stage, which gradually develops into plaques and nodules. Some lesions appear as cauliflower-like bumps, and some lesions have central ulcers, often with necrotic tissues and hemorrhagic secretions.
2. Gray-scale ultrasound shows an irregular hypoechoic lesion involving the epidermis or dermis, even subcutaneous tissue. The surface is irregularly elevated, appearing thick linear hyperechogenicity due to hyperkeratosis and accompanied by posterior acoustic shadowing. The demarcation from the surrounding tissue is not clear, and the bottom of the lesion shows a significant tendency to invade into the deep layer.

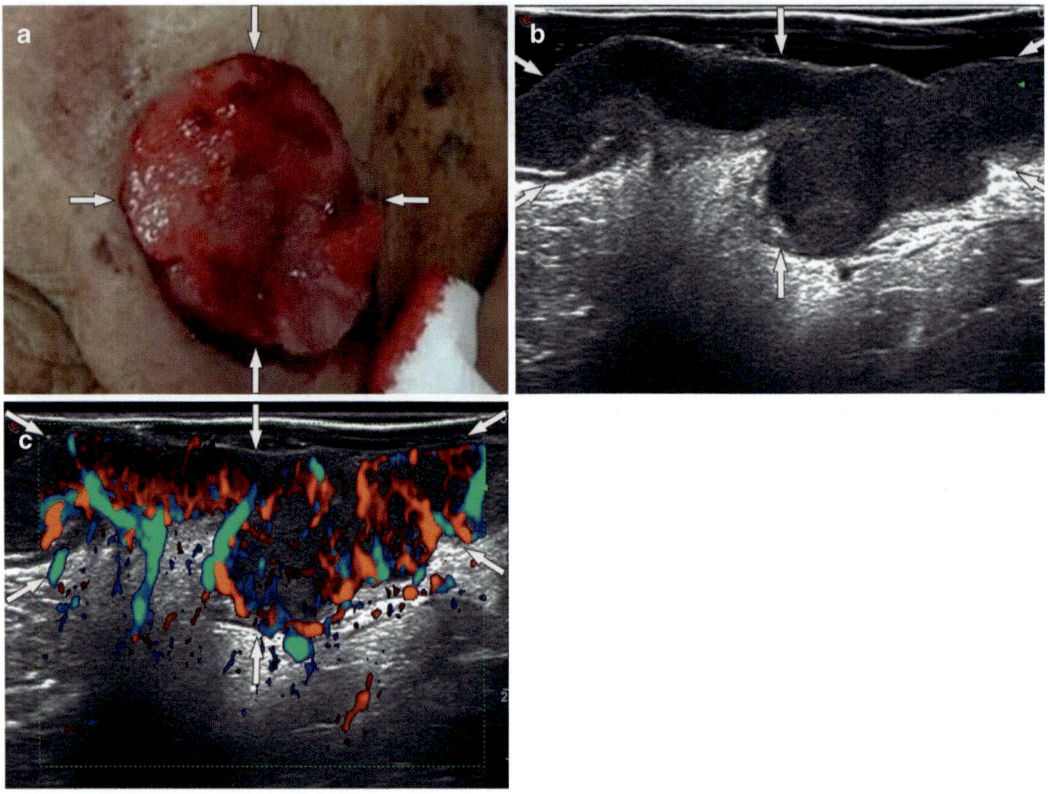

Fig. 5.58 Cutaneous squamous cell carcinoma. Female, 90 years of age. (**a**) Visual observation shows a red exophytic lesion on the left face, without adhesion to the surrounding tissues and satellite lesion. Ulceration and bleeding are presented on the surface (arrows). The shape of the lesion is regular and the bottom is wide (size: 50.0 mm × 40.0 mm). (**b**) Gray-scale ultrasound shows an irregular hypoechoic lesion (arrows) involving the epidermis, dermis, and subcutaneous tissue (thickness: 15.0 mm of the thickest part). The surface is elevated without thick linear hyperechogenicity (the epidermis is absent). It is lobulated with significant extension into the underlying tissues. The lesion is homogeneous. (Frequency: 22 MHz). (**c**) Color Doppler ultrasound shows rich blood flow signals inside the lesion (arrows) (Frequency: 22 MHz)

3. Color Doppler ultrasound shows rich blood flow signals inside most lesions with many thick nourishing vessels.

5.3.3.5 Clinical Significance

At present, many studies considered AK (precancerous lesions), BD (squamous carcinoma in situ), and invasive SCC as a disease continuum. cSCC typically manifests as a spectrum of progressively advanced malignancies, ranging from a precursor AK to BD (SCC in situ), and invasive cSCC in normal skin under the continuous ultraviolet exposure. As a form of intraepidermal keratinocytic neoplasia, AK is the most common precursor of invasive SCC. Several studies have reported that the estimated rate of progression from AK to invasive SCC ranges from 0.1% to 20%, with a substantially higher risk in patients with multiple AK lesions. In general, it is about 3% ~ 5% that the risk of BD developing into invasive cancer (Fig. 5.59).

In our previous study, we retrospectively analyzed the features of ultrasound biomicroscopy and high-frequency ultrasound in 160 patients with AK, BD, or invasive SCC confirmed by pathology. The results indicated that high-frequency ultrasound showed irregular bottom and regular hyperkeratotic surface were helpful in the diagnosis of AK. On the other hand, flat bottom, crumple hyperkeratotic surface, and

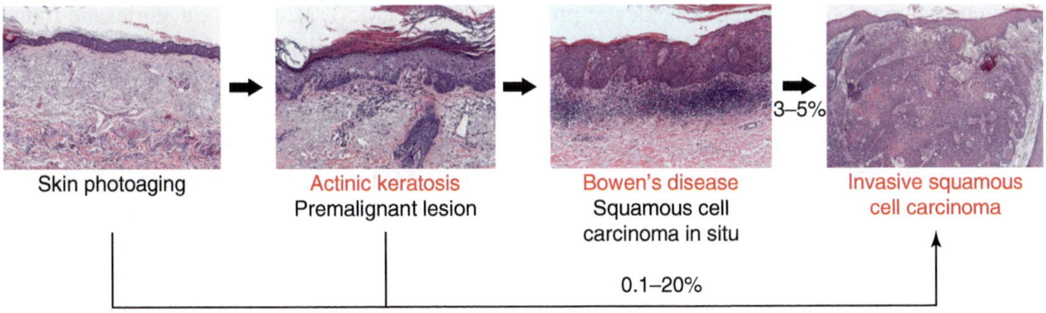

Fig. 5.59 The progression pathways of cSCC

Table 5.5 Diagnostic performance of high-frequency ultrasound for AK, BD, and invasive SCC

Ultrasound	Sensitivity (%)	Specificity (%)	AUROC
AK	85.3%	73.6%	0.879
BD	88.9%	84.9%	0.935
Invasive SCC	92.3%	88.0%	0.949

AUROC: area under the receiver operating characteristic curve

confined to the epidermis were helpful in diagnosing BD. In addition, irregular shape and a surface without thick linear hyperechogenicity help to diagnose invasive SCC. The findings suggested that high-frequency ultrasound is helpful in the differential diagnosis of AK, BD, and invasive SCC based on the features of surface, bottom, and layers involvement (Table 5.5).

Key Points

- The incidence of cSCC is higher than that of BCC in China, and the degree of malignancy is second only to MM. Lymph node metastasis and death occur in most severe cases. It is more common in the face, mouth, lips, and perineum.
- Gray-scale ultrasound shows irregular and hypoechoic lesions involving the epidermis or dermis, even subcutaneous tissue with hyperkeratotic surface appearing thick linear hyperechogenicity. The lesion is ill-defined, with a tendency of invasion into the deep layer. Color Doppler ultrasound shows rich blood flow signals inside the lesion.
- It should be mainly differentiated from MM and BCC.

5.3.4 Malignant Melanoma

5.3.4.1 Clinical Manifestation and Pathology

Malignant melanoma (MM) is a highly malignant tumor originating from melanocytes and most MM occurs in the skin and mucous membranes (respiratory tract, digestive tract, and other parts).

In the early stage, MM mostly appears as a black lesion on the skin, or developed from an original pigmented nevus enlarging and darkening in a short time. With the progression of the disease, the lesion may appear patchy or nodular, with ulceration and bleeding on the surface. Sometimes a halo of pigmentation or depigmentation appears around the lesions. If MM grows to the surrounding or subcutaneous tissues, satellite lesions or subcutaneous nodules may appear.

The pathogenesis of MM is associated with many factors such as malignant change of melanocytic nevi, genetics, ultraviolet radiation, trauma, and irritation.

According to the etiology and genetic background of MM, it is divided into four subtypes: mucosal type, acral type, chronic sun-damaged type, and non-chronic sun-damaged type. Histologically, MM is divided into four subtypes:

1. Acral lentiginous melanoma (ALM): It is the most common type of cutaneous MM in China and often occurs in hairless areas, such as the palms, soles, and nail beds. Histologically, it

is characterized by atypical melanocytic proliferation composed by nests of different sizes in the basal layer. This type has a poor prognosis.

2. Superficial spreading melanoma (SSM): It is common in Caucasians and often occurs in sites that are exposed intermittently to sunlight, such as the back and calf. Histologically, it is characterized by marked intraepidermal Pagetoid spread.
3. Lentigo maligna melanoma (LMM): It is common in the elderly people and often occurs at sites of long-term sunlight exposure. Histologically, it is characterized by lentiginous hyperplasia of atypical melanocytes.
4. Nodular melanoma: It refers to skin MM in vertical growth phase, surrounded by or without horizontal growth phase or MM in situ components. Visual appearance is a rapidly growing expansive papule or nodule. Histologically, it is characterized by nested, nodular, or diffuse atypical melanocytic hyperplasia in the dermis.

The staging and thickness of the tumor affect the prognosis of MM. In the literatures, the BRAF mutation rate in MM is 25.9%, of which V600E/CKIT being 87.3%/10.8%, respectively. Therefore, most studies suggest that CKIT and BRAF mutations are independent poor prognostic factors in cutaneous MM.

The American Joint Committee on Cancer (AJCC) updated the eighth edition of the staging of MM in 2018. TNM staging of the tumor is shown in Table 5.6.

Table 5.6 TNM staging of melanoma

Clinical staging of tumors	T	N	M
0	Tis	N0	M0
IA	T1a	N0	M0
IB	T1b, T2a	N0	M0
IIA	T2b, T3a	N0	M0
IIB	T3b, T4a	N0	M0
IIC	T4b	N0	M0
III	Any T	≥ N1	M0
IV	Any T	Any N	M1

The specific T, N, and M categories are found in the relevant guidelines of AJCC. Among them, T staging is mainly based on Breslow tumor thickness (vertical tumor thickness) and the presence of primary tumor ulceration. The Breslow depth in MM without ulceration refers to the histologic depth of the tumor from the granular layer of the epidermis to the deepest point of invasion; while the Breslow thickness in ulcerated MM refers to the histologic depth of the tumor from the ulcer bottom to the deepest point of invasion. On gray-scale ultrasound, Breslow thickness is approximately assessed by measuring the vertical distance from the top of the lesion to the bottom (Fig. 5.60).

Most patients with early stage (stage I and II) MM have a good prognosis. The prognosis of patients with stage III MM varies greatly. The MM has high tendency to spread to neighboring soft tissue (in the form of transit metastasis or satellite lesion), tumor draining lymph nodes, and distance organs, including liver, lung, even central nervous system. Thus, along with primary MM lesion scanning, surrounding soft tissue, tumor draining lymph nodes, and liver should also be included for examination (Fig. 5.61).

The overall prognosis of patients with stage IV MM is very poor. The degree of malignancy and mortality of MM rank first among cutaneous malignancies. In China, due to the lack of understanding of MM, most patients are already in the advanced stage of the tumor at the time of being found (Fig. 5.62). According to relevant literatures, the 5-year survival rate of MM patients in China is less than 20%. Based on the authors' experience, patients with MM in our hospital are mostly recurrent and received medical intervention before obtaining a definite preoperative diagnosis.

5.3.4.2 Ultrasound Manifestation

Gray-Scale Ultrasound

In the early stage, the lesion is small, involving the epidermis and dermis, with a nodular or crawling shape and a well-defined boundary. As the disease progresses, the lesion increases in size and infiltrates deeply, involving the subcuta-

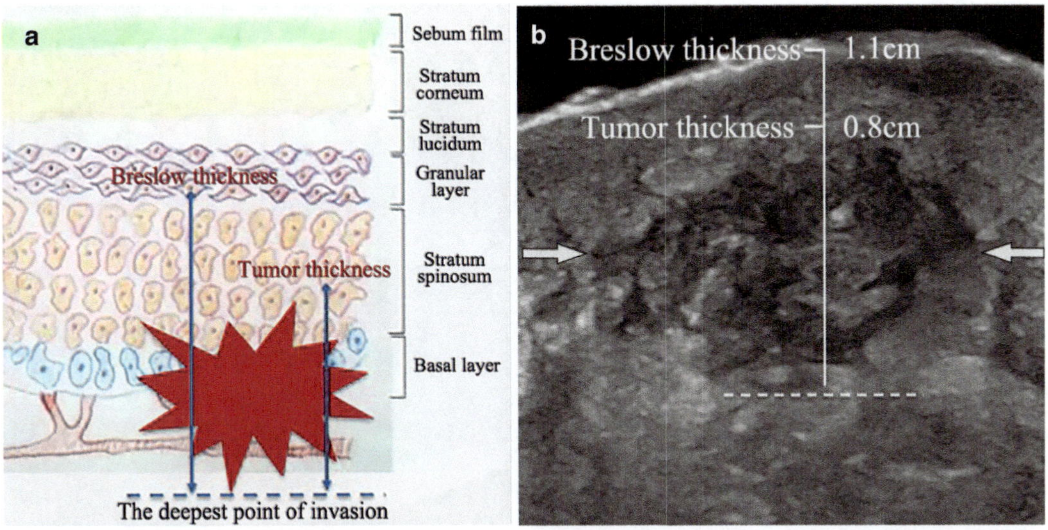

Fig. 5.60 Measurement of Breslow thickness. (**a**) Schematic diagram shows that Breslow thickness was measured from the granular layer to the bottom of the malignant melanoma (red part). While, the thickness of tumor is measured from the top to the bottom of the lesion's main body. (**b**) On gray-scale ultrasound, Breslow thickness of an malignant melanoma (arrows) is 1.1 cm. However, the thickness of its main body is only 0.8 cm (Frequency: 22 MHz)

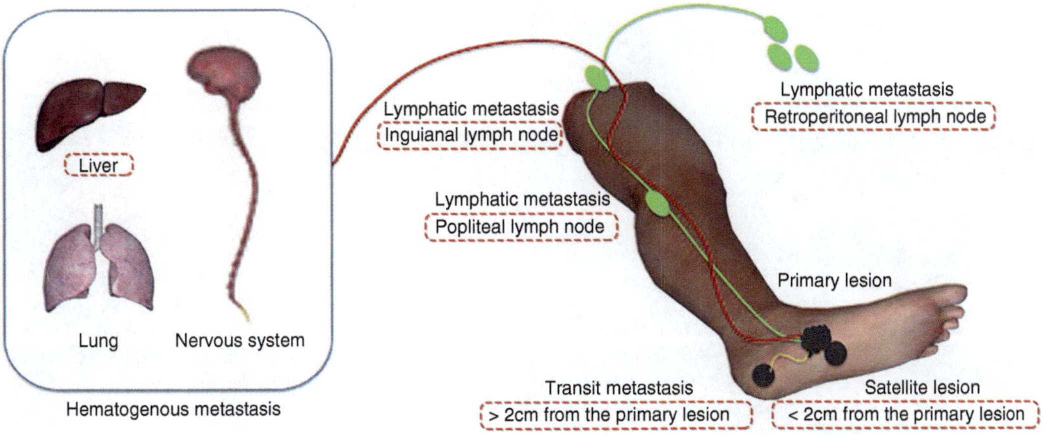

Fig. 5.61 Schematic diagram of the metastasis of malignant melanoma

neous tissue or even the muscles and bones, with an irregular shape and an ill-defined boundary. Sometimes in-transit and satellite metastases can appear. In the late stage, lymph node metastasis and distant metastasis occur. The lesion is homogeneous or heterogeneous.

Color Doppler Ultrasound

The lesion shows rich blood flow signals (Figs. 5.63, 5.64, and 5.65).

5.3.4.3 Differential Diagnosis

Melanocytic Nevus

The visual observations of MM in the early stage and melanocytic nevus are similar. Most of MM originates from the malignant change of melanocytic nevus. If the original melanocytic nevus grows rapidly, and shows uneven or increased pigmentation, and irregular margin, the malignant change of melanocytic nevus should be

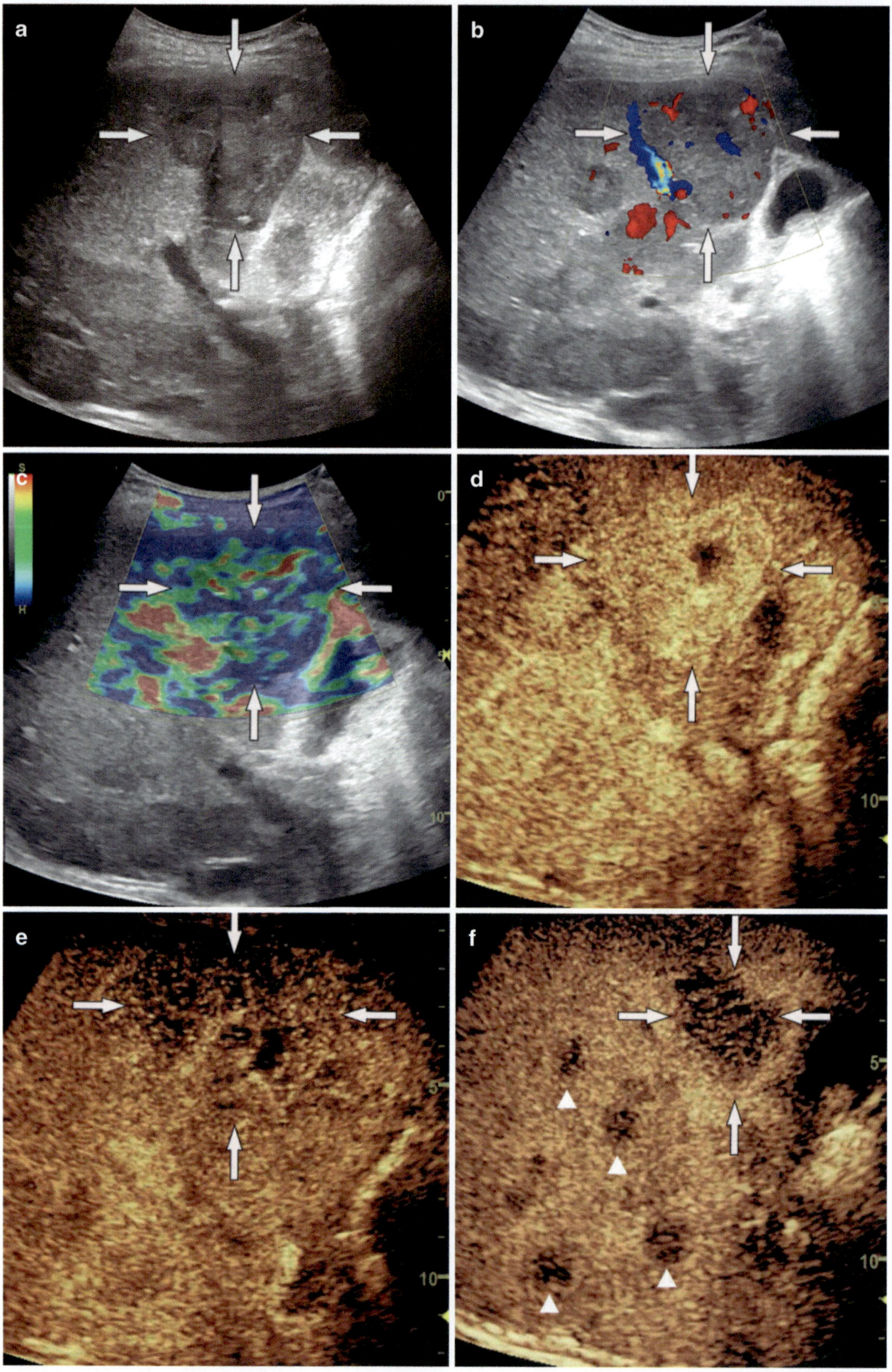
a
b
c
S
H
d
e
f
10
5
10

Fig. 5.62 Liver metastasis of malignant melanoma. Female, 59 years of age. (**a**) Gray-scale ultrasound shows an irregular and heterogeneous hypoechogenic lesion in the right anterior lobe of liver (size: 91 mm × 70 mm) (Frequency: 3.5 MHz). (**b**) Color Doppler ultrasound shows rich blood flow signals in and around the lesion (Frequency: 3.5 MHz). (**c**) Strain elastography shows that the stiffness distribution in the lesion is uneven (Frequency: 3.5 MHz). (**d**) Arterial phase (22 sec) on contrast-enhanced ultrasound shows that the lesion is heterogeneous, slight hyper-enhancement in comparison with adjacent liver tissue (Frequency: 3.5 MHz). (**e**) Portal phase (40 sec) shows that the lesion turns to hypo-enhancement gradually (Frequency: 3.5 MHz). (**f**) Late venous phase shows the significant hypo-enhancement in the lesion. Meanwhile, more than 5 hypo-enhancement areas are detected (△), which are suspected of metastasis (Frequency: 3.5 MHz). (**g**) The biopsy sample of the live metastasis lesion of MM (1.8 cm in length) appears black, and is similar to the primary lesion. Arrows point to lesions

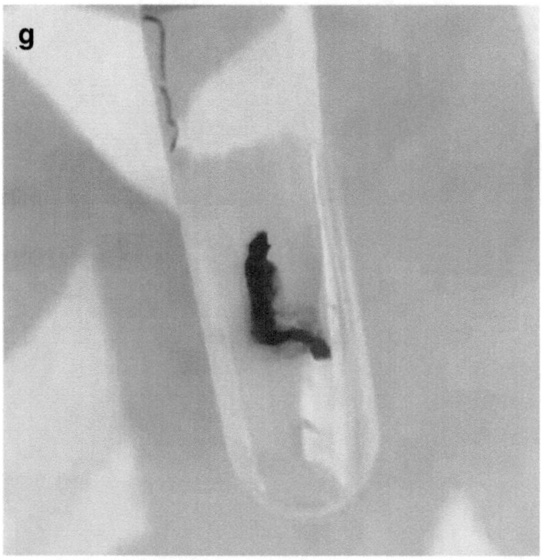

Fig. 5.62 (continued)

highly suspected. Also, if the lesion appears as an irregular, ill-defined, and heterogeneous area with rich blood flow signals on ultrasound, the diagnosis of MM is a high priority.

Hemangioma

In terms of visual appearance, hemangioma typically presents as a red-blue patch on the skin surface, while MM is often black. On ultrasound, hemangiomas show hypoechoic, hyperechoic, or mixed echogenic. Hypoechoic hemangiomas need to be differentiated from MM. Although the blood flow signals inside the lesions are both rich, they can be differentiated by "squeeze test." Hemangioma is soft, and the compression of transducer causes the deformation of the lesion. When the transducer rapidly squeezes the lesion, the blood flow signals increased transiently on color Doppler ultrasound, followed by decrease or even disappearance of blood flow signals in the lesion. However, MM is firm, and the compression of transducer has no significant effect on the morphology and internal blood flow signals of MM.

cSCC

Both of them are highly aggressive, and can involve the whole layer of the skin. The lesions both can appear as irregular, ill-defined, and heterogeneous hypoechoic lesions. However, different degrees of hyperkeratosis are observed on the surface of cSCC, with posterior acoustic shadowing, while there is generally no abnormal keratinization on the surface of MM.

In addition, the location and visual appearance of the lesions can also be used as differential clues between the two diseases. cSCC often occurs on the head and neck. Most lesions appear as infiltrative morphea in the early stage, and gradually develop into plaques and nodules. Some lesions appear as cauliflower-like bumps, and some lesions have central ulcers, often with necrotic tissues and hemorrhagic secretions. MM, on the other hand, often occurs at the extremities in Chinese, and is usually black in appearance.

5.3.4.4 Diagnosis Clues

1. MM is usually black in appearance and often occurs at the extremities in Chinese, particularly on the toes or soles of the feet. It is similar to melanocytic nevus in the early stage and is easily misdiagnosed. With the rapid progression of the disease, the lesion usually appears as a patch or nodule, with ulceration and bleeding on the surface. Sometimes a halo

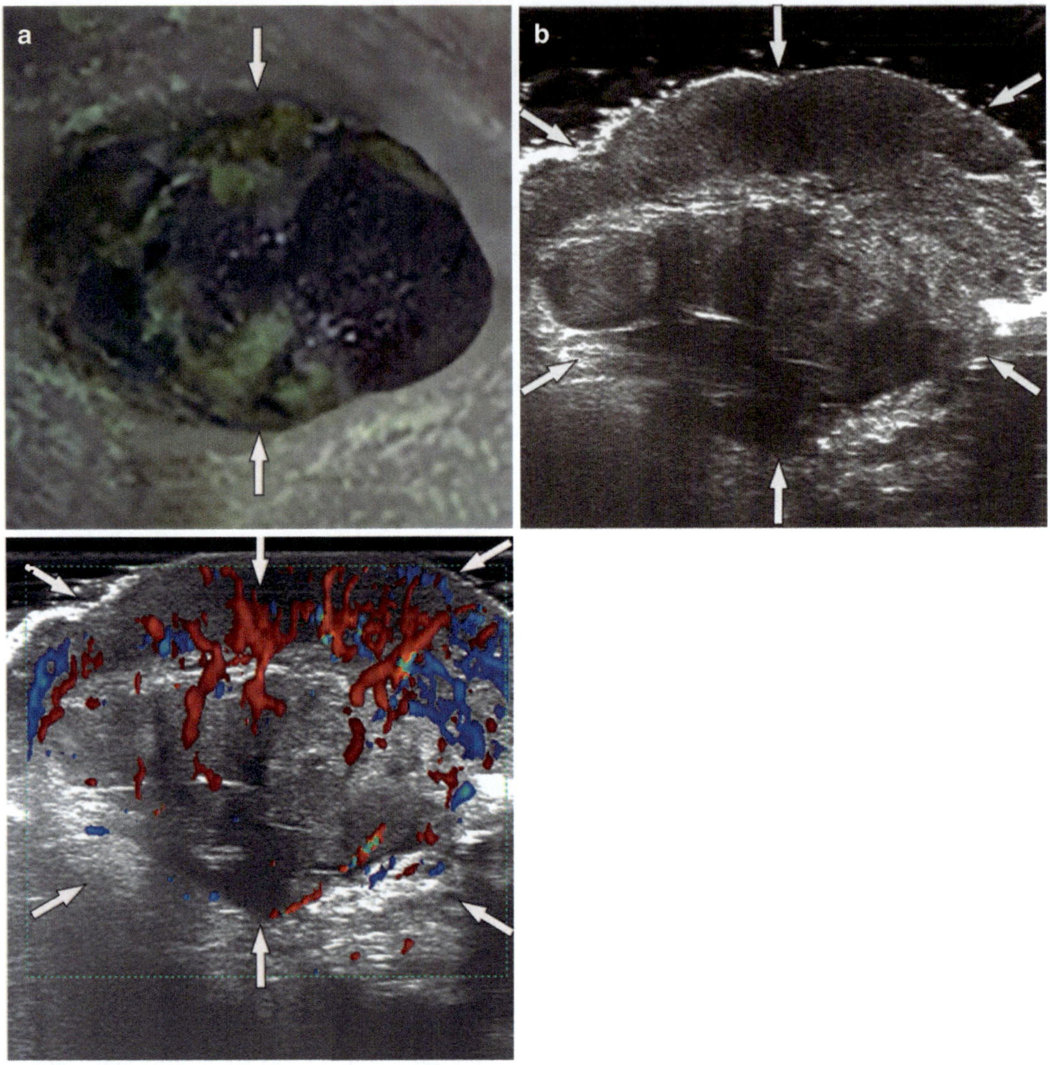

Fig. 5.63 Malignant melanoma. Male, 70 years of age. (**a**) Visual observation shows a dark brown and well-defined lesion in the left heel, with ulceration and slight exudates on the surface (arrows) (size: 36.0 mm × 34.0 mm). (**b**) Gray-scale ultrasound shows an irregular and ill-defined hypoechoic lesion (arrows) involving the epidermis, dermis, and subcutaneous tissue (size: 35.0 mm × 32.0 mm; thickness: 27.0 mm). The surface is elevated without abnormal keratinization. The lesion is heterogeneous (Frequency: 22 MHz). (**c**) Color Doppler ultrasound shows rich blood flow signals inside the lesion (arrows) (Frequency: 22 MHz)

of pigmentation or depigmentation appears around the lesions. Lymph node metastasis and distant metastasis occur in the late stage of the disease.

2. Gray-scale ultrasound shows an irregular and ill-defined hypoechoic lesion in the skin layers with an elevated surface and no abnormal keratinization. Color Doppler ultrasound shows rich blood flow signals inside the lesions. The lesion shows a significant tendency to invade deeply, which may involve the whole layer of the skin, even the muscles and bones. Sometimes in-transit and satellite metastases appear. Lymph node metastasis and distant metastasis in the late stage of the disease have corresponding ultrasound features.

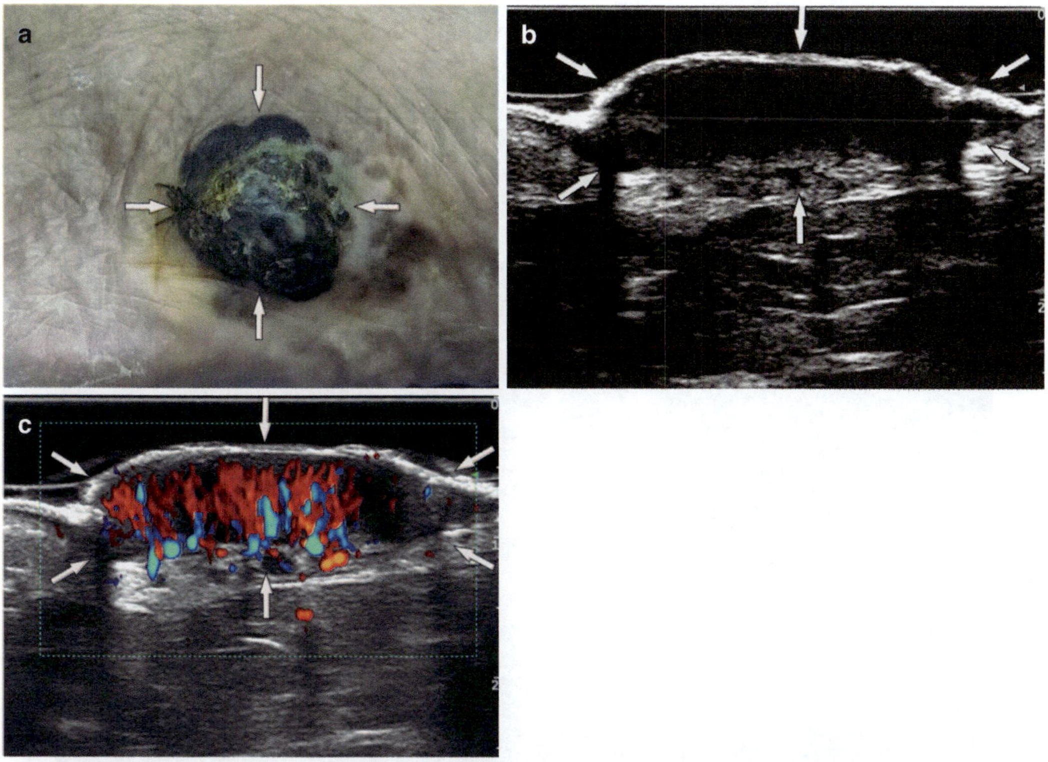

Fig. 5.64 Malignant melanoma. Male, 75 years of age. (**a**) Visual observation shows a black and well-defined lesion in the left heel with slight exudates on the surface (arrows) (size: 45.0 mm × 37.0 mm). (**b**) Gray-scale ultrasound shows a regular hypoechoic lesion (arrows) in the epidermis and dermis (size: 45.0 mm × 34.0 mm; thickness: 7.6 mm). The surface is elevated without abnormal keratinization. The bottom of the lesion is ill-defined, and reaches the dermis/subcutaneous tissue junction. The lesion is homogeneous (Frequency: 22 MHz). (**c**) Color Doppler ultrasound shows rich blood flow signals inside the lesion (arrows) (Frequency: 22 MHz)

5.3.4.5 Clinical Significance

Gray-scale ultrasound features in early MM are not specific. Advanced MM invades subcutaneous tissue and even the muscles and bones, which can be assessed by ultrasound. However, according to literatures, the diagnostic performance of PET-CT, MRI, CT, and ultrasound for regional lymph node metastasis is unsatisfactory. Dinnes reported a sensitivity of 35.4% and a specificity of 93.9% for ultrasound assessment of regional lymph node metastasis before sentinel lymph node biopsy in patients with MM. The results of the multicenter study conducted by Thompson et al. demonstrated that ultrasound had a sensitivity of 6.6% and a specificity of 98% for assessing regional lymph node metastasis, and concluded that preoperative ultrasound did not provide reliable lymph node staging for MM patients. Future studies should consider the effect of different imaging studies on the management of patients with MM.

Key Points

- MM ranks first in cutaneous malignancies in terms of the degree of malignancy and mortality. ALM is the most common type in China and often occurs in the palms, soles, and nail beds.
- On gray-scale ultrasound, the lesion appears as an irregular and ill-defined area. The surface is elevated without abnormal keratinization. Rich blood flow signals are observed inside the lesion. MM has a significant tendency to invade deeply, which may involve the

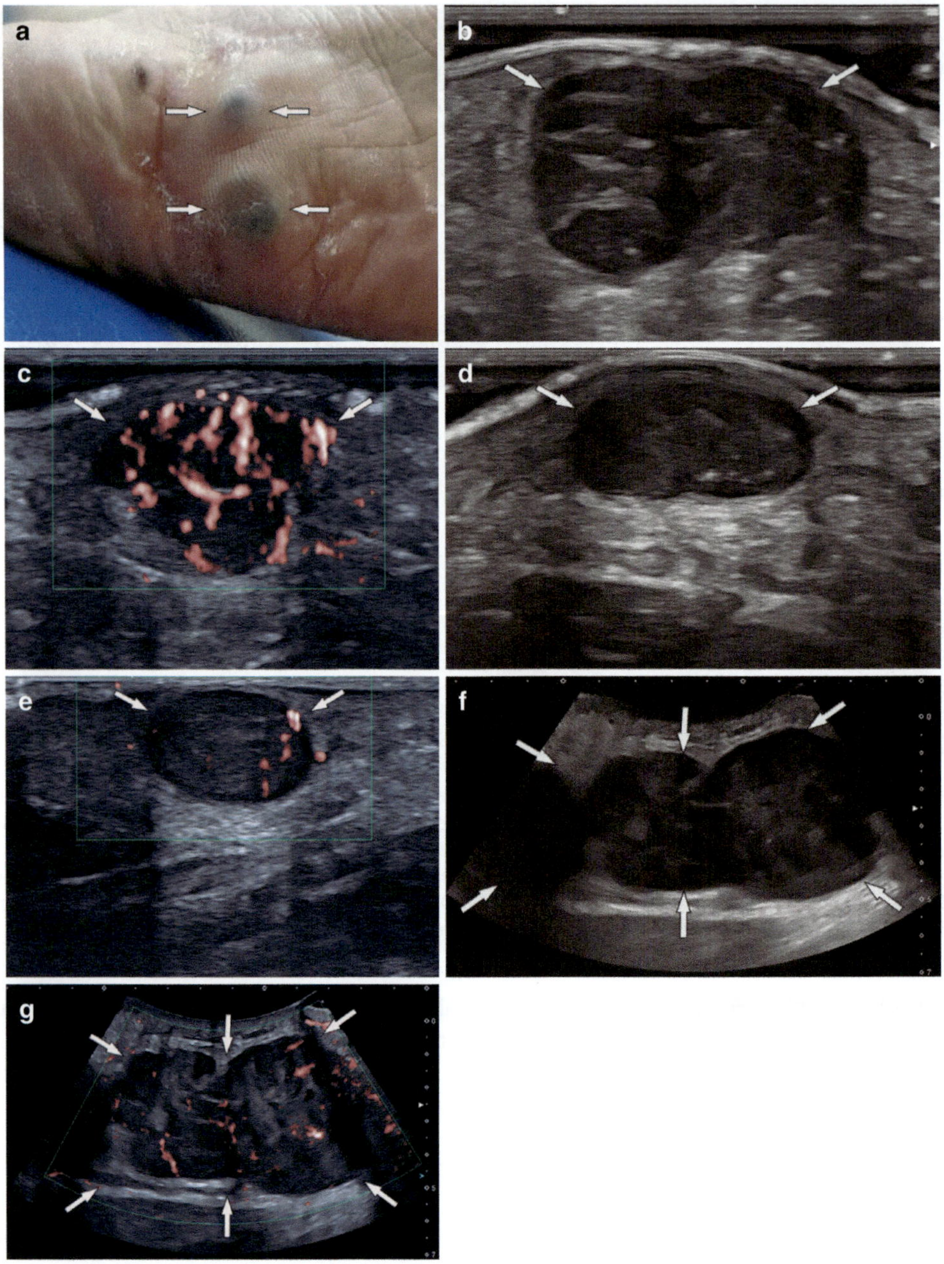

Fig. 5.65 Malignant melanoma. Male, 75 years of age. (**a**) Visual observation shows two dark brown and well-defined lesions in the sole of the left foot (arrows) (diameter: about 23.0 mm and 14.0 mm, respectively). (**b**) Gray-scale ultrasound shows an oval and heterogeneous hypoechoic lesion (arrows) in the dermis and subcutaneous tissue (size: 23.0 mm × 20.0 mm; thickness: 18.3 mm). The bottom of the lesion is well-defined. (Frequency: 24 MHz). (**c**) Color Doppler ultrasound shows rich blood flow signals inside the lesion (arrows) (Frequency: 24 MHz). (**d**) Gray-scale ultrasound shows another hypoechoic lesion (arrows) beside the above lesion, and the ultrasound feature is the same as the lesion described above (size: 14.0 mm × 16.0 mm; thickness: 9.1 mm) (Frequency: 24 MHz). (**e**) Color Doppler ultrasound shows blood flow signals inside the lesion (arrows) (Frequency: 24 MHz). (**f**) An irregular and heterogeneous hypoechoic lesion (arrows) in the medial aspect of the left thigh, with invisible lymphatic hilum and ill-defined corticomedullary demarcation, (MM lymph node metastasis confirmed by histopathology, diameter: 70.0 mm) (Frequency: 3.5 MHz). (**g**) Color Doppler ultrasound shows rich blood flow signals inside the lesion (arrows) (Frequency: 3.5 MHz)

whole layer of the skin, or even the muscles and bones. Sometimes in-transit and satellite metastases appear.
- It should be mainly differentiated from melanocytic nevus, hemangioma, and cSCC.

5.3.5 Extramammary Paget's Disease

5.3.5.1 Clinical Manifestation and Pathology

Extramammary Paget's disease (EMPD), also known as eczematoid carcinoma, is an uncommon skin malignancy. Its histological origin is controversial, and mainly has the following theories. (1) Apocrine sweat gland theory: It is based on the fact that the disease mainly occurs in the apocrine sweat gland site, which is the mainstream theory of the pathogenesis of the disease at present. (2) Migration theory: It is mainly based on the fact that EMPD may be associated with malignant tumors in its adjacent sites, such as skin appendages cancer and visceral organs tumors. (3) Evolutionary theory of pluripotential germinative cell: It is mainly based on the presence of ectopic EMPD, so some studies supposed that pluripotent stem cells are the origin of Paget cells.

In the Western populations, vulva is the most common site for EMPD. In the Eastern populations, on the other hand, EMPD occurs mostly in middle-aged and elderly men and is common in areas of apocrine sweat gland distributed such as the perineum, scrotum, penis, and groin. A few EMPD are ectopic, which can be observed in the axilla, chest, eyelids, auricle, etc.

EMPD clinically presents as a red eczematoid patch covered with scales and crusts on the surface, accompanied by pigmentation or hypopigmentation. The margin is slightly elevated. There may be exudates and erosion in the center of the lesion. With the progression of the disease, the lesion gradually develops into verrucous plaques or nodules (Fig. 5.66).

Patients with EMPD confined to the epidermis have an excellent prognosis. The disease develops slowly and is often misdiagnosed in the early

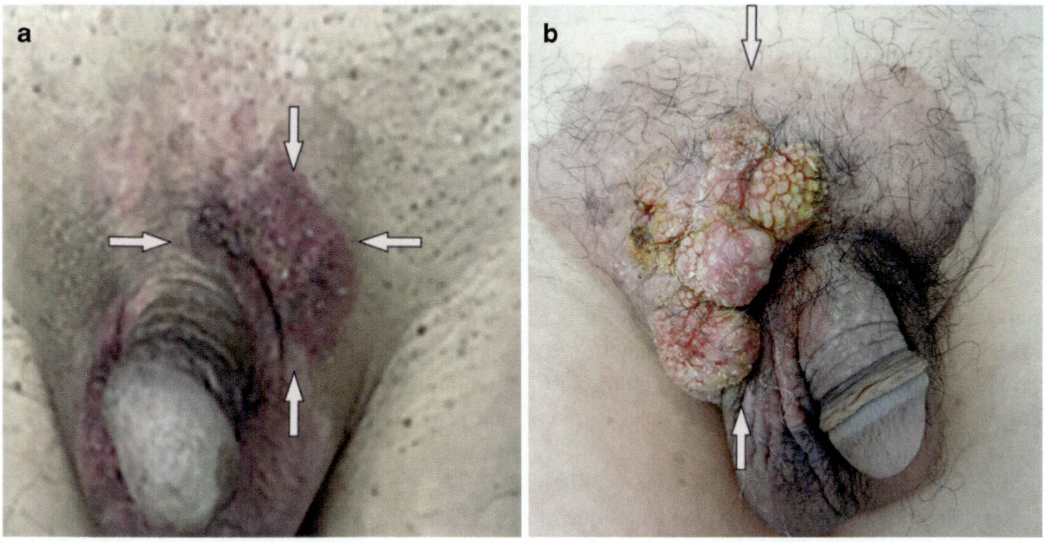

Fig. 5.66 Visual appearance of extramammary Paget's disease. (**a**) Visual observation shows eczematoid erythema in the perineum, with pigmentation and scab (arrows). (**b**) Visual observation shows verrucous nodules in the perineum with exuduates on the surface (arrows)

stage so as to be delayed in treatment. Approximately 20% of the lesions that are diagnosed as EMPD have already invaded the dermis, and some even have developed lymph node and distant metastases.

The thickness of lesion, the layers of involvement, the invasion of skin appendages, and the presence of lymph node metastasis are important factors in evaluating the disease.

Histopathologically, EMPD is typically characterized by thickened stratum spinosum and the presence of single or nests of Paget cells in the epidermis.

Paget cells are divided into two types. (1) Classical type (type A): The cells are large and round, with translucent cytoplasm, hyperchromatic nuclei, which were round and centered, and mitotic figures. (2) Signet ring type (type B): The cytoplasm contains a large amount of mucus.

The hyperchromatic nuclei are semilunar and squeezed by the cytoplasm to one side in a ring shape. Immunohistochemically, CK7 is usually positive and CK20 is negative in primary EMPD tumor cells, and the expression of GCDFP-15 is specific. CK7 and CK20 are usually negative in secondary EMPD tumor cells.

5.3.5.2 Ultrasound Manifestation

Gray-Scale Ultrasound

The lesion usually shows a crawling hypoechoic area in the epidermis. The surface is mostly flat and has abnormal keratinization, with various degrees of posterior acoustic shadowing. In the early stage, the bottom of the lesion is usually flat. With the progression of the disease, it can break through the dermo-epidermal junction to invade the dermis, appendages, and even the subcutaneous tissue. Lymph node metastasis may occur in the late stage.

Because the extent of the disease is often larger than that of the transducer, the technique of extended field of view can be conducted. On high-frequency ultrasound, if there is a "pseudopodia-like" hypoechogenicity extending to the deep tissue at the bottom of the lesion, the invasion of skin appendages should be considered.

Color Doppler Ultrasound

Most lesions show rich blood flow signals (Figs. 5.67 and 5.68).

5.3.5.3 Differential Diagnosis

BD

The location and appearance of the lesion can be helpful in differentiation. BD is mostly located in the face and trunk, showing local reddish-brown patches, with scales on the surface. EMPD, on the other hand, is mostly located in the perineum and shows eczematoid erythema, which is more extensive than BD. On gray-scale ultrasound, BD appears as a hypoechoic lesion confined to the epidermis, with thick linear hyperechogenicity of the surface due to abnormal keratinization. While EMPD can involve the whole layers of the skin, and the degree of abnormal keratinization on the surface is milder than Bowen's disease. Compared with BD, EMPD shows more rich internal blood flow signals.

In addition, EMPD should especially be differentiated from Paget-like BD, and the two entities show similar ultrasound features. Immunohistochemical examination is helpful to differentiate the two entities, the former tumor cells are often positive for CK7, and the latter tumor cells are negative for CK7 and CEA.

MM

The location and appearance of the lesion are helpful in differentiating the two entities. MM lesions are mostly located at the extremity and face, and often black. However, EMPD is mostly located in the perineum and shows eczematoid erythema. On gray-scale ultrasound, malignant melanoma appears irregular or nodular shape with a tendency to invade deeply, while EMPD is crawling.

5.3.5.4 Diagnosis Clues

1. EMPD occurs mostly in middle-aged and elderly people, and are mostly located in the perineum.
2. In visual appearance, the lesions appear as eczematoid erythemas, verrucous patches, or nodules.

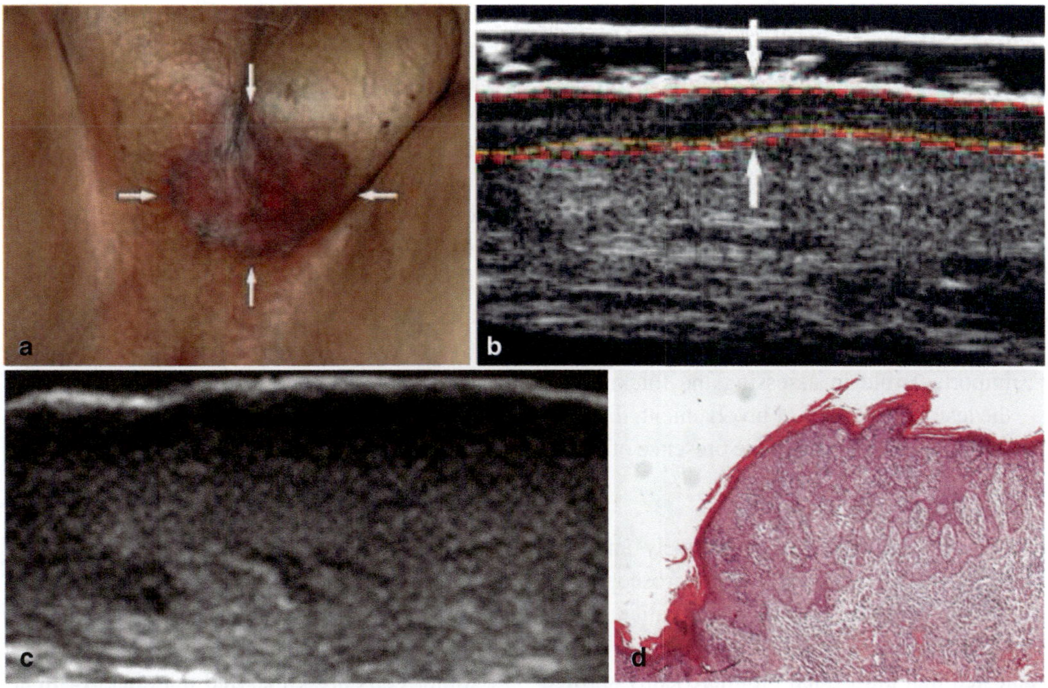

Fig. 5.67 Paget's disease in the perineum. Female, 67 years of age. (**a**) Visual observation shows eczematoid erythema with an area of pigmentation and erosion in the scrotum (arrows) (diameter: approximately 30.0 mm). (**b**) Gray-scale ultrasound shows a regular, crawling, and ill-defined hypoechoic lesion (arrows) located in the epidermis and dermis (thickness: 0.8 ~ 1.2 mm). The surface shows fine linear hyperechogenicity. The bottom of the lesion (yellow dotted line) reaches the junction of dermis/subcutaneous tissue (red dotted line). The surrounding subcutaneous tissue is thickened, with increased echogenicity. The lesions are homogeneous (Frequency: 50 MHz). (**c**) The ultrasound features are the same as that of the lesion described above (Frequency: 22 MHz). (**d**) Histopathology (HE staining, panoramic scan) shows nests of Paget cells [Image cited from Chen ST et al., J Ultrasound Med, 2019, 38 (12): 3229–3237]

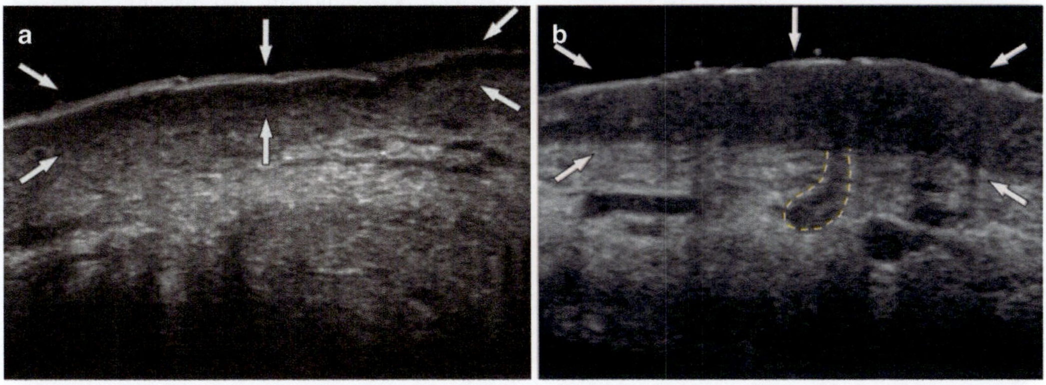

Fig. 5.68 Paget's disease with different invasion extent. (**a**) Male, 82 years of age. Gray-scale ultrasound shows a regular, crawling, ill-defined hypoechoic lesion (arrows) located in the epidermis and dermis (thickness: 0.8 ~ 1.6 mm). The surface appears as fine linear hyperechogenicity. The bottom is ill-defined but regular. The lesion was homogeneous (Frequency: 34 MHz). (**b**) Male, 79 years of age. Gray-scale ultrasound shows a regular, protrusive, ill-defined hypoechoic lesion (arrows) in the epidermis and dermis (thickness: 2.7 ~ 5.0 mm). The surface appears as fine linear hyperechogenicity. The bottom is ill-defined with the pseudopodia extending to the depth (yellow dotted line). The lesion is homogeneous in echo texture (Frequency: 34 MHz)

3. Gray-scale ultrasound shows a crawling hypoechoic lesion that involves the whole layers of the skin, with “pseudopodia-like” hypoechogenicity at the bottom of some lesions, suggesting the invasion of skin appendages.
4. Color Doppler ultrasound shows rich blood flow signals inside the lesion.

5.3.5.5 Clinical Significance

1. High-frequency ultrasound plays a very important role in assessing the thickness of the lesion, the layers of involvement, the invasion of appendages, and the presence of lymph node metastasis in EMPD.

Our previous study retrospectively analyzed the features of ultrasound biomicroscopy and high-frequency ultrasound in 17 patients with EMPD confirmed pathologically. The results indicated that ultrasound biomicroscopy showed the layers of involvement more clearly than high-frequency ultrasound (100% vs. 29.4%). However, high-frequency ultrasound showed rich blood flow signals in 11 lesions (64.7%), and inguinal lymph node metastasis was found in one lesion.

Ultrasound biomicroscopy provides detailed morphological information, while high-frequency ultrasound is prone to show lymph node metastasis. The combination of ultrasound biomicroscopy and high-frequency ultrasound can provide key information for the diagnosis of EMPD.

2. Among various factors related to the clinical risk of EMPD, the pathological invasion level is the most pivotal factor leading to poor prognosis. Therefore, according to the layers of involvement, EMPD is divided into 2 groups as follows: Lesions in situ in the epidermis and lesions invade into the dermis or subcutaneous tissue. Our previous study found that tumor growth pattern and infiltration depth were significantly different between the two groups, which could be used to assess the invasion extent of EMPD. With a cutoff value of 1.55 mm for infiltration depth, the AUROC was 0.833 (Table 5.7).
3. In addition, high-frequency ultrasound can also be used to monitor the effect of disease treatment. Skin defects, penile reconstruction, and functional effects after the surgery of EMPD are challenges to cure this disease. Photodynamic treatment (PDT) is performed by injecting patients with photosensitizers, which specifically accumulate in tumor tissue over a period of time. Then a specific wavelength of light is used to irradiate the skin lesions, so as to stimulate the photosensitizer to produce reactive oxygen species, thereby tumor cells are killed and the effect of treatment is achieved. PDT can be used as an important treatment for EMPD. In Shanghai Skin Disease Hospital, the treatment of recurrent EMPD by non-surgical methods uses a therapy combining 5-aminolevulinic acid photodynamic treatment (ALA-PDT) with holmium laser. After 9 sessions of treatment, the abnormal echogenicity in the original lesion area disappears on gray-scale ultrasound, and the process from presence to absence of the lesion is recorded.

Key Points

- EMPD, also known as eczematoid carcinoma, is a rare cutaneous malignancy. It is common in middle-aged and elderly people, and often located in the perineum.
- Gray-scale ultrasound shows a crawling hypoechoic lesion that can involve the whole

Table 5.7 High-frequency ultrasound features of EMPD of different pathological invasion levels

	IE Group (n = 42)	ID Group (n = 18)	P value
Lesion infiltration depth[a] (mm)	1.1 (0.6 ~ 1.5)	2.2 (1.6 ~ 3.9)	0.000
Tumor growth pattern (localized/invasive)	38 (90.5%)/4 (9.5%)	6 (33.3%)/12 (66.7%)	0.000

IE group: lesions in situ in the epidermis
ID group: lesions invade into the dermis or subcutaneous tissue
[a]Data are presented as median (25th, 75th)

layer of the skin, with "pseudopodia-like" hypoechogenicity at the bottom of some lesions, suggesting the invasion of skin appendages. Rich blood flow signals are observed inside the lesion.

- It should be mainly differentiated from BD and MM.
- Ultrasound can be used to assess the thickness of the lesion, the layers of involvement, the invasion of appendages, and the presence of lymph node metastasis in EMPD.

5.3.6 Dermatofibrosarcoma Protuberans

5.3.6.1 Clinical Manifestation and Pathology

Dermatofibrosarcoma protuberans (DFSP) originates from spindle cell in the dermis and is a cutaneous fibroblastic neoplasm with a low degree of malignancies. DFSP often occurs in the trunk, followed by the extremities, and rare in the head and neck. The lesions grow slowly and mostly present as painless subcutaneous nodules with a tendency to infiltrate, mostly involving the dermis and subcutaneous tissues.

Some lesions invade upwards into the epidermis or downwards into deeper tissue. When the epidermis is involved, the lesion appears as a brownish-red, reddish nodule with a slightly elevated surface and occasional ulceration and exudates. When the epidermis is not involved, most patients are asymptomatic except having palpable masses, which are easily misdiagnosed.

The etiology of DFSP is unknown. DFSP may occur congenitally, and some may relate to a history of surgery, trauma, local injection of drugs, or insect bites.

The main treatment of the disease is surgery, with high rates of recurrence (20% ~ 50%) and the average time for local recurrence is 32 months. If the surgical margin is negative, the patient has a good prognosis, with 2-year and 5-year survival rates of 97% and 92%, respectively. The metastasis rate of this disease is low, less than 5%, and occurs on the basis of multiple recurrences.

5.3.6.2 Ultrasound Manifestation

Gray-Scale Ultrasound

Most lesions show oval or lobulated, ill-defined mixed echogenic areas in the dermis and subcutaneous tissues, which are parallel to the skin. The disease specifically invades adipose tissue, that is, hypoechogenic pseudopodial-like protrusions extending into peripheral hyperechoic adipose tissue, which can form a characteristic of "whirlpool sign." The lesion is heterogeneous in echo texture, and banded hyperechogenicity and hypoechogenicity are observed inside, which is associated with mucinous degeneration of tumor cells and hyalinization of fibrous tissue. The lesion is firm, and the compression of transducer has no significant effect on the morphology of the lesion.

Color Doppler Ultrasound

Blood flow signals can be observed in the lesion, and the degree of vascularization varies from rare to rich, usually without nourishing vessels (Figs. 5.69 and 5.70).

5.3.6.3 Differential Diagnosis

DFSP appears to be benign lesion on ultrasound and is often misdiagnosed, so it needs to be differentiated from benign soft tissue tumors.

Lipoma

Lipomas appear as hyperechoic, isoechoic, or hypoechoic lesions in the subcutaneous fat layer on ultrasound. DFSP needs to be differentiated from hypoechoic lipomas. Both are palpable subcutaneous nodules, lipoma is generally skin-colored, while DFSP appears brownish-red or reddish when invading the epidermis.

On ultrasound, both can show banded hyperechoic septa inside. However, the hypoechoic lipoma appears regular and well-defined with capsule, which does not invade the surrounding tissue, and shows no blood flow signals inside. DFSP is ill-defined without capsule. The characteristic hypoechoic pseudopodia-like protrusions extend to adipose tissue in the periphery, forming a typical characteristic of "whirlpool sign," indi-

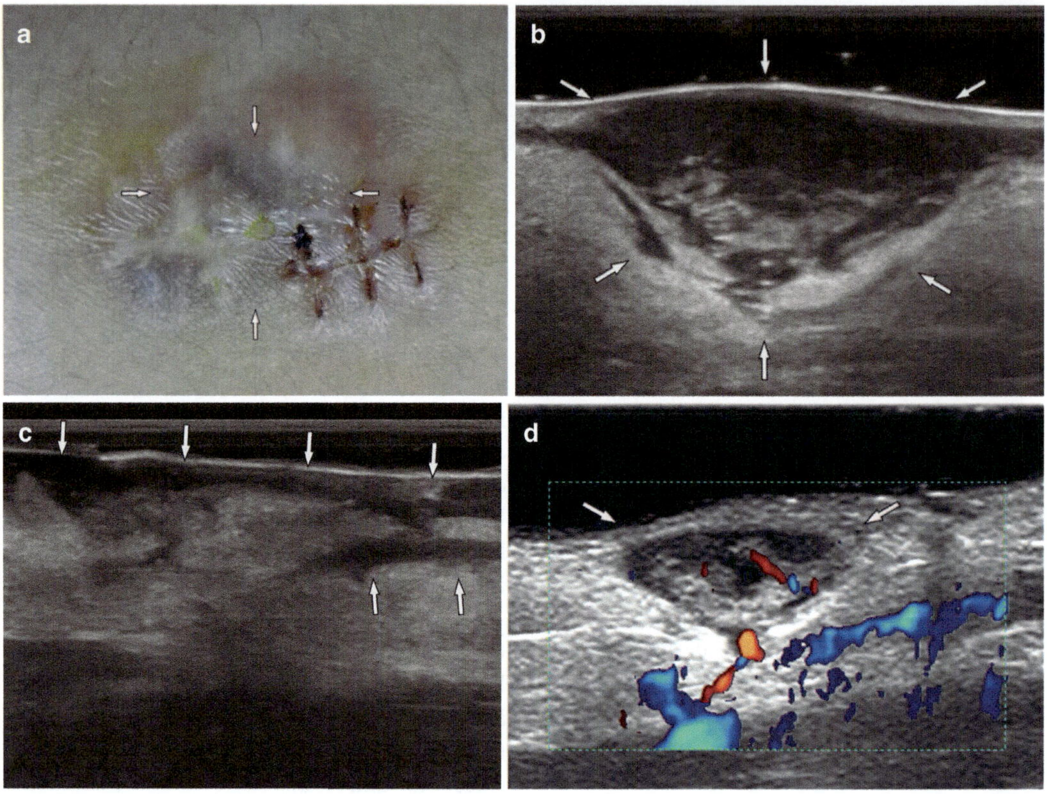

Fig. 5.69 Dermatofbrosarcoma protuberans. A 12-year-old girl underwent tumor resection in her right forearm 6 years ago. (**a**) Visual observation shows two bean-sized subcutaneous nodules at the surgical site, beside an incision (arrows). (**b**) Gray-scale ultrasound shows an irregular hypoechoic lesion (arrows) in the subcutaneous tissue, with multiple hypoechoic pseudopodia-like protrusions in the periphery (size: 28.0 mm × 26.0 mm; thickness: 10 mm). The lesion is heterogeneous, and banded hyperechogenicity and hypoechogenicity are observed inside (Frequency: 34 MHz). (**c**) Gray-scale ultrasound shows the pseudopodia-like protrusions extend into the peripheral adipose tissue (arrows) (Frequency: 34 MHz). (**d**) Color Doppler ultrasound shows rare blood flow signals in the periphery and interior of the lesion (arrows) (Frequency: 22 MHz)

cating the invasion of surrounding fat layer, and blood flow signals can be detected inside.

Keloid

This disease refers to exuberant scarring due to reactive proliferations produced by an abnormal healing process after skin trauma. Clinically, it appears as a red and elevated nodule with a smooth surface. While DFSP may present as a subcutaneous nodule and also as a reddish elevated nodule with a smooth surface. On gray-scale ultrasound, keloid shows significantly thickened dermis with plaque-like hypoechogenicity. The lesion has no space-occupying effect. However, DFSP shows the pseudopodia-like protrusions extending to adipose tissue in the periphery, forming a typical characteristic of "whirlpool sign".

Nodular Panniculitis

Both of the diseases locate in the subcutaneous adipose tissue. In contrast to DFSP, most nodular panniculitis is accompanied by pain. The ultrasound features of the two diseases are similar. Nodular panniculitis is characterized by increased echogenicity and thickened subcutaneous adipose tissue, with patchy hyperechoic and irregular hypoechoic areas in the lesion. The lesion is irregular and ill-defined with no space-occupying effect. However, DFSP is irregular and involves subcutaneous tissues mostly, with characteristic hypoechoic pseudopodia-like protrusions extend-

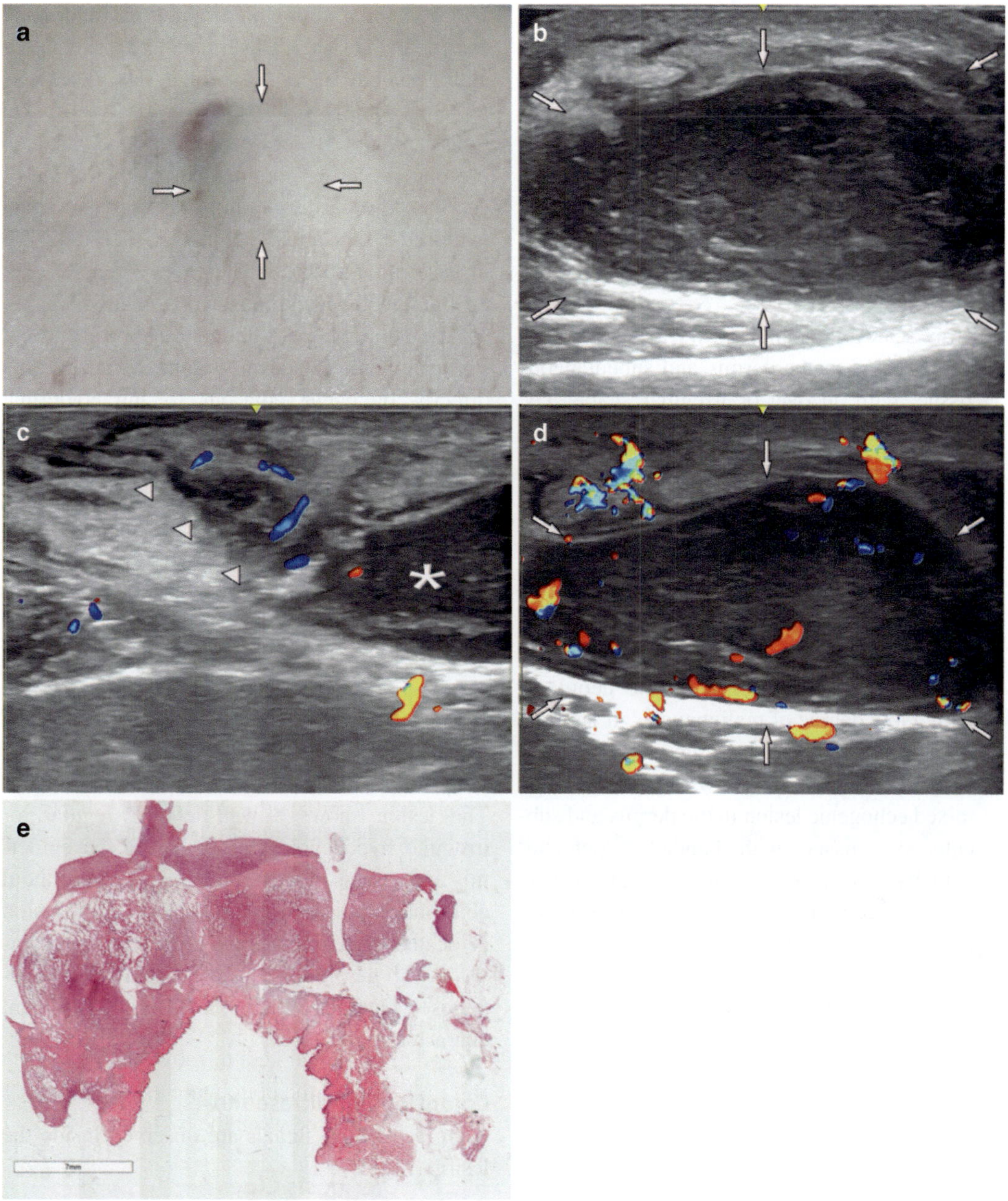

Fig. 5.70 Dermatofbrosarcoma protuberans. Male, 30 years of age. (**a**) Visual observation shows a subcutaneous nodule in the abdominal wall (size: 25.0 mm × 20.0 mm), and a reddish nodule in the periphery with an elevated surface (arrows). (**b**) Gray-scale ultrasound shows an oval and well-defined hypoechoic lesion (arrows) in the subcutaneous tissue (size: 24.4 mm × 20.2 mm; thickness: 11.2 mm). The lesion is heterogeneous, and banded hyperechogenicity and hypoechogenicity are observed inside (Frequency: 22 MHz). (**c**) Characteristic hypoechoic pseudopodia-like protrusions (△) are presented in the periphery of the lesion, emanating from the lesion (*) and extending to adipose tissue to form the "whirlpool sign". (**d**) Color Doppler ultrasound shows rich blood flow signals in the periphery and interior of the lesion (arrows) (Frequency: 22 MHz). (**e**) Histopathology (HE staining, panoramic scan) shows mild irregular hyperplasia of the epidermis. Diffuse proliferation of spindle cells is observed in the dermis and can be deep to the subcutaneous tissue. The tumor cells and collagen fibers are interwoven with storiform arrangement, involving the subcutaneous fat layer and shuttling between the interlobular septa. There are no obvious atypical cells and mitotic figures. Pigmentation can be observed in some areas

ing to adipose tissue in the periphery, forming a typical characteristic of "whirlpool sign".

5.3.6.4 Diagnosis Clues

1. Clinically, DFSP presents as a palpable, painless, and skin-colored subcutaneous nodule. When the lesion involves the epidermis, it shows a brownish-red or reddish nodule with a smooth surface and occasional ulceration and exudates.
2. Gray-scale ultrasound shows a mixed echogenic lesion in the dermis and subcutaneous tissue, with an oval or irregular shape. The lesion is heterogeneous with banded hyperechogenicity and hypoechogenicity.
3. Characteristic hypoechogenic pseudopodial-like protrusions extend into peripheral hyperechoic adipose tissue, which can form a characteristic of "whirlpool sign".

Key Points

- DFSP is a cutaneous fibroblastic neoplasm with a low degree of malignancies. It is prone to recurring and has a low rate of metastasis.
- Gray-scale ultrasound shows a heterogeneous mixed echogenic lesion in the dermis and subcutaneous tissue with banded hyperechogenicity and hypoechogenicity. Characteristic hypoechogenic pseudopodial-like protrusions extend into peripheral hyperechoic adipose tissue, which can form a characteristic of "whirlpool sign".
- The lesions appear to be benign lesions on ultrasound and are often misdiagnosed, which should be mainly differentiated from lipoma, keloid, and nodular panniculitis.

5.3.7 Porocarcinoma

5.3.7.1 Clinical Manifestation and Pathology

Porocarcinoma, also known as malignant eccrine poroma, is a malignant tumor originating from the eccrine ducts in the epidermis. This disease was first reported by Pinkus and Mehregan in 1963, when it was called epidermal endocrine carcinoma. In 1969, Mishima and Morioka officially named it eccrine poroma. The disease is rare, accounting for 0.005% to 0.01% of skin tumors. About 50% of porocarcinomas occur in prolonged eccrine poroma. The average time of eccrine poroma developing into porocarcinoma is reported to be about 8.5 years in literature. The disease often occurs in the elderly people, with an equal incidence in men and women.

The etiology and pathogenesis are uncertain. Porocarcinoma can develop from eccrine poroma directly or occur adjacent to intraepidermal eccrine poroma. The lesions are often located in the head and neck and lower extremities. The visual appearance is similar to that of eccrine poroma, which appears as red, blue, or black nodules, plaques, or ulcerative lesions. About 20% of this disease develops local metastasis and 10% develops distant metastasis, with a mortality rate of 67% if distant metastasis occurs.

5.3.7.2 Ultrasound Manifestation

Gray-Scale Ultrasound

The lesion shows a well-defined, regular, or irregular hypoechoic area involving the epidermis and dermis. The surface is elevated without abnormal keratinization. The bottom of the lesion is located in the dermis, and some extends downward with a cornu form. The lesion is homogeneous. Overall, there are no significant characteristic features.

Color Doppler Ultrasound

Rich blood flow signals are observed inside the lesion (Fig. 5.71).

5.3.7.3 Differential Diagnosis

Eccrine Poroma

Porocarcinoma originates from the malignant transformation of eccrine poroma. Eccrine poroma is regular and well-defined on gray-scale ultrasound. Color Doppler ultrasound shows rich blood flow signals in both of them, which is dif-

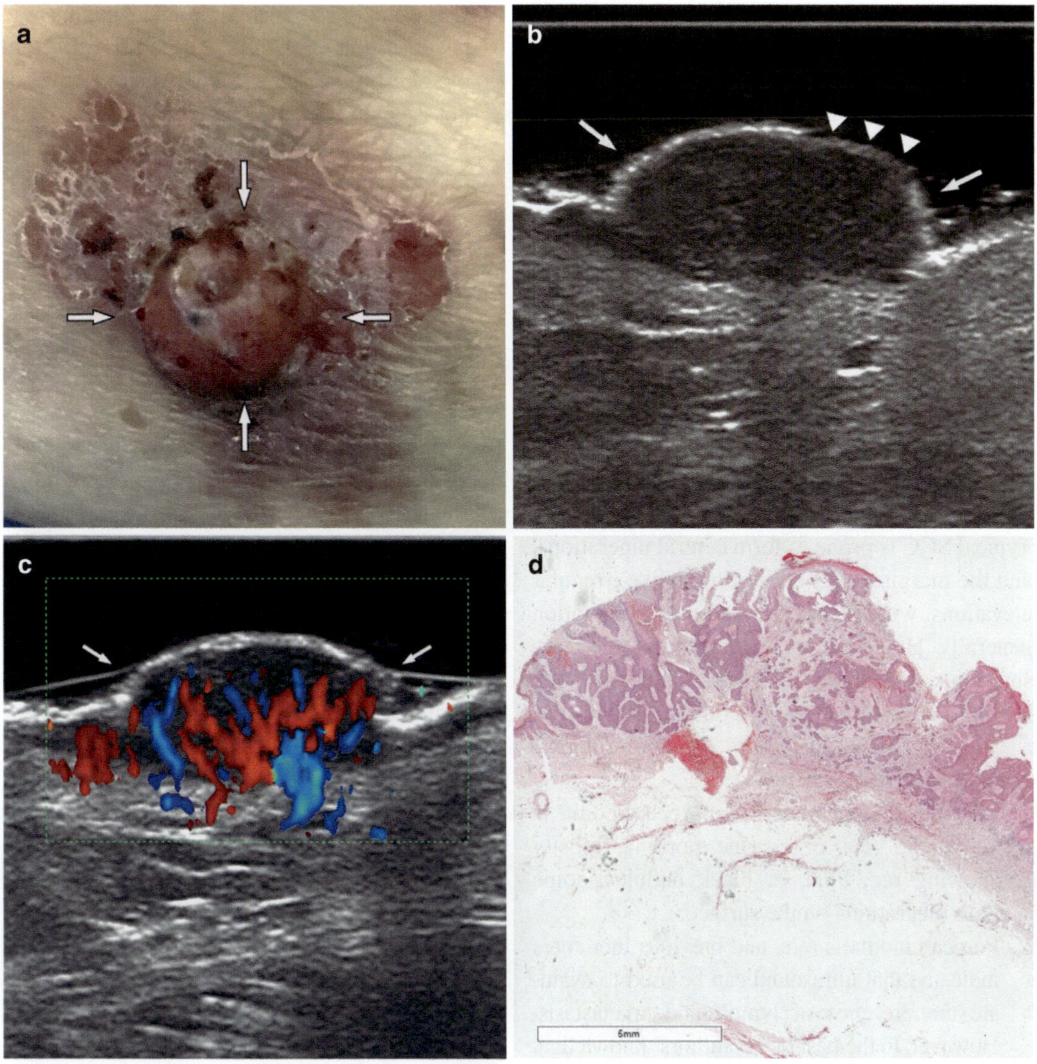

Fig. 5.71 Porocarcinoma. Female, 83 years of age. (**a**) Visual observation shows a hemispherical bump of about 15.0 mm in diameter in the right lower leg (arrows), with a mild ulceration and a small number of exudates on the surface. Dark red scaly patches are observed in the periphery of the lesion. (**b**) Gray-scale ultrasound shows an oval, well-defined, and homogeneous hypoechoic lesion (arrows) in the epidermis and dermis (size: 14.8 mm × 15.6 mm; thickness: 6.7 mm). The surface is elevated, with incomplete hyperechogenicity on the top of the lesion (the epidermis is absent locally) (△) (Frequency: 22 MHz). (**c**) Color Doppler ultrasound shows rich blood flow signals inside the lesion (arrows), with nourishing vessels observed at the bottom (Frequency: 22 MHz). (**d**) Histopathology (HE staining, panoramic scanning) shows that the epidermis is locally lost with ulceration. The lesion is connected to the epidermis and grows aggressively into the dermis. The tumor cell clumps are irregular in shape, with multiple foci of necrosis and duct-like differentiation. The tumor cells are small cuboidal, with increased mitotic figures and a large number of dyskeratotic cells. Collagen proliferation in the interstitium is accompanied by deposition of mucin-like material. Inflammatory cell infiltration, mainly plasma cells, is observed

ficult to differentiate. Some porocarcinomas are also difficult to differentiate pathologically due to the large cellular components of eccrine poroma. If eccrine poroma grows rapidly in a short time with an ill-defined boundary, the possibility of malignant transformation should be considered.

cSCC

The gray-scale ultrasound features of the two entities are similar, which show an ill-defined boundary and the tendency to infiltrate deep tissues. However, the invasion of SCC is deeper and wider, and the lesion usually shows more significant abnormal keratinization on the surface.

In addition, the appearance of the lesion can provide a diagnostic clue for differentiation. Typical SCC is prone to form central ulcerations, and the margin may be cauliflower-like irregular elevations, with a large size and no pigmentation generally. However, porocarcinoma is relatively small in size and appears as a red, blue, or black lesion, some with ulcerations on the surface.

5.3.7.4 Diagnosis Clues

1. The visual appearance of porocarcinoma is similar to that of eccrine poroma, mostly showing red, blue, or black nodules, some with ulcerations on the surface.
2. Porocarcinoma is rare, and previous literatures indicated that ultrasound can be used to evaluate the presence of lymph node metastasis. However, to the best of the authors' knowledge, there is no literature reporting the ultrasound features of porocarcinoma. The authors have summarized the ultrasound features of 5 porocarcinomas confirmed by pathology in Shanghai Skin Disease Hospital. The ultrasound features are non-specific and mainly show ill-defined hypoechoic lesions in the epidermis and dermis with rich blood flow signals inside.

Key Points

- Porocarcinoma is rare and originates from the eccrine ducts in the epidermis, mostly from the malignant change of poroma. It often occurs in the elderly people and located in the head, neck, and lower extremities. Metastasis may occur.
- Ultrasound shows an ill-defined hypoechoic lesion in the epidermis and dermis with rich blood flow signals inside, which is overall non-specific.
- It should be mainly differentiated from eccrine poroma and cSCC.

5.3.8 Sebaceous Gland Carcinoma

5.3.8.1 Clinical Manifestation and Pathology

Sebaceous gland carcinoma is a rare cutaneous malignancy accounting for 0.2% to 4.6% of cutaneous malignancies. Sebaceous gland carcinoma originates from the sebaceous glands of the eyelids, face, scalp, etc. Its etiology is uncertain. Sebaceous gland carcinoma has been found to be associated with smoke, exposure to organic compounds, local inflammatory irritation, radiation history around the eye, and partial gene mutations and deletions.

According to the location of the lesion, it is divided into periocular sebaceous gland carcinoma and extraocular sebaceous gland carcinoma. Periocular sebaceous gland carcinoma is common in the upper and lower eyelids and lacrimal caruncle, especially in the upper eyelids. Periocular sebaceous gland carcinoma accounts for about 3/4 of sebaceous gland carcinoma and is the second common eyelid malignancy after basal cell carcinoma in China, with poor differentiation. However, extraocular sebaceous gland carcinoma is relatively rare, accounting for about 1/4 of sebaceous gland carcinomas, commonly in the head and neck. The disease often occurs in middle-aged and elderly people. Periocular sebaceous gland carcinoma often presents as diffuse thick and stiff eyelid, or a single, yellow, and firm nodule without pain. However, most lesions have non-specific visual appearances and are often misdiagnosed as cysts, benign tumors, or inflammation of the eye. Sebaceous gland carcinoma is prone to metastasize, easy to recur after surgical resection, and has a poor prognosis with a mortality rate of 5% to 29%.

Histopathologically, it shows lobulated or papillary growth. Basaloid cells are segmented by the surrounding fibrous stroma into nests or cords, with a sharp boundary and an infiltrative growth pattern.

5.3.8.2 Ultrasound Manifestation

Gray-Scale Ultrasound

Gray-scale ultrasound features of sebaceous gland carcinoma are non-specific and resemble those of BCC. The authors summarized the ultrasound features of sebaceous gland carcinoma confirmed by pathology in Shanghai Skin Disease Hospital. On gray-scale ultrasound, sebaceous gland carcinoma mainly appears as an irregular and well-defined hypoechoic lesion involving the whole layer of the skin. The lesion is heterogeneous or homogeneous.

Color Doppler Ultrasound

Rich blood flow signals can be observed inside the lesion (Fig. 5.72).

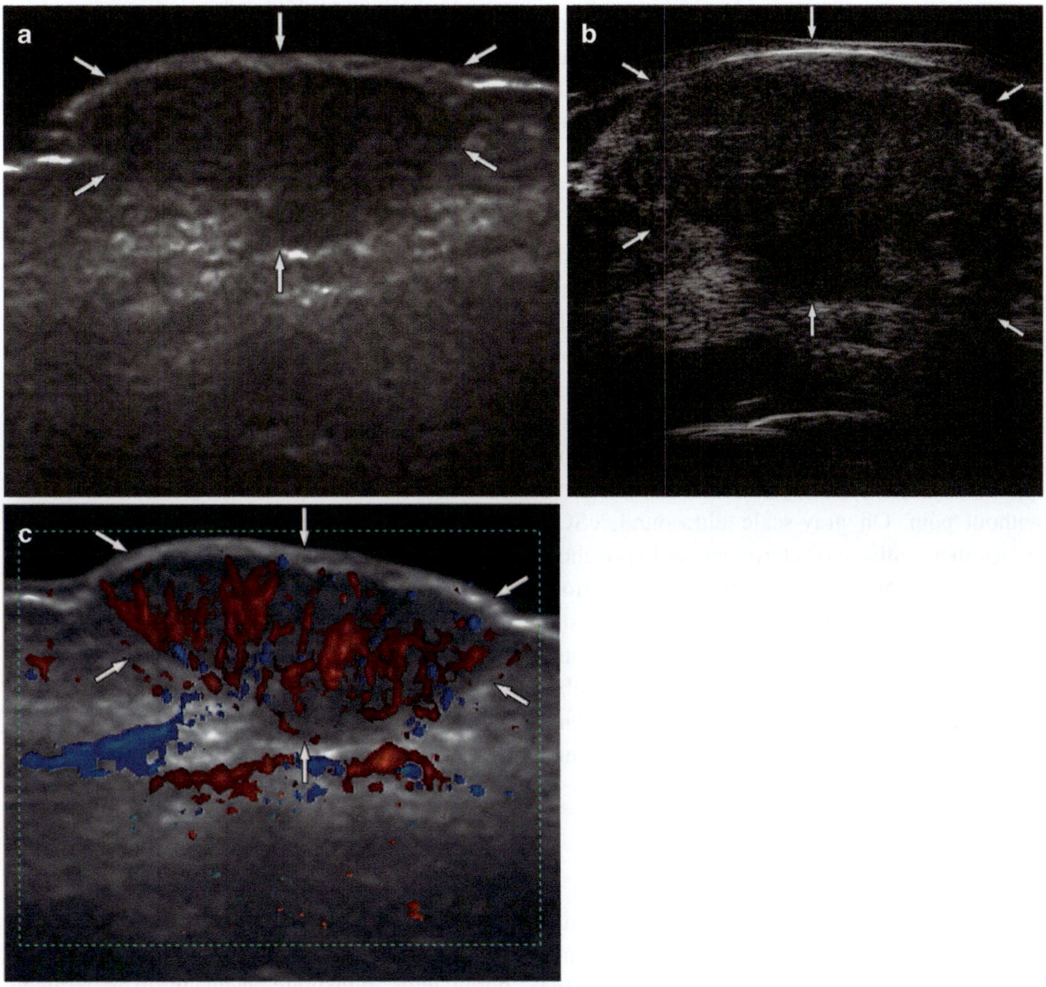

Fig. 5.72 Sebaceous gland carcinoma. Female, 78 years of age. (**a**) Gray-scale ultrasound shows an irregular, well-defined, and homogeneous hypoechoic lesion (arrows) in the dermis and subcutaneous tissue (size: 9.4 mm × 7.9 mm; thickness: 4.7 mm). The surface is elevated without abnormal keratinization (Frequency: 22 MHz). (**b**) Gray-scale ultrasound shows the lesion located in the dermis and subcutaneous tissue (arrows), and the ultrasound features are the same as above (Frequency: 50 MHz). (**c**) Color Doppler ultrasound shows rich blood flow signals inside the lesion (arrows) (Frequency: 22 MHz)

5.3.8.3 Differential Diagnosis

Nodular BCC

Nodular BCC often occurs in the face and appears as a painless papule or nodule. Some of lesions with ulcers on the surface are in the late stage. Sebaceous gland carcinoma, on the other hand, is mostly located around the eye and often presents as diffuse thicken and stiff eyelid, or a single, yellow, and firm nodule without pain. Characteristic anechoic areas and hyperechoic spots are visualized in typical BCC, and there is generally no abnormal keratinization on the surface. However, sebaceous gland carcinoma is homogeneous, some with abnormal keratinization on the surface. When nodular BCC has no characteristic features, it is difficult to differentiate the two entities by ultrasound.

cSCC

cSCC often occurs in the head and face. In the early stage, it is mainly characterized by infiltrative morphea in the early stage, and gradually develops into plaque and nodule. Some lesions appear as cauliflower-like bumps, and some lesions have central ulcers. While sebaceous gland carcinoma is common around the eye and typically presents as a yellow and firm nodule without pain. On gray-scale ultrasound, cSCC shows an irregular and heterogeneous hypoechoic lesion in the epidermis and dermis, with various degrees of abnormal keratinization on the surface. The demarcation between the lesion and surrounding tissue is unclear. However, sebaceous gland carcinoma is relatively regular and homogeneous with mild or no abnormal keratinization.

Nevus Sebaceus

Nevus sebaceus is a benign skin hamartoma of congenital onset and composed of epidermis, dermis, and epidermal appendages, predominantly of sebaceous glands. It often occurs in the scalp and face, and is common in infants and children. The lesions often show yellow hairless plaques with verrucous and papillomatous or nodular convex. Most patients are asymptomatic. Nevus sebaceus is mainly located in the epidermis and dermis and does not involve subcutaneous tissues. While sebaceous gland carcinoma is often around the eye, and typically presents as a yellow and firm nodule without pain. The lesion can infiltrate deeply in depth, involving the whole layers of the skin. The location and the layers of involvement are helpful to differentiate the two entities.

5.3.8.4 Diagnosis Clues

The diagnosis of sebaceous gland carcinoma should be considered if there is a single, yellow, painless, and firm nodule around the eye or a diffuse thick and stiff eyelid. Timely biopsy of the lesion is helpful for early diagnosis. Ultrasound features are non-specific, mainly showing a solid hypoechoic lesion involving the whole layers of the skin, which can be helpful to evaluate the extent and depth of the lesion.

5.3.8.5 Clinical Significance

At present, there are few studies reporting the diagnostic value of ultrasound in sebaceous gland carcinoma. Shen et al. summarized the ultrasound features of 11 cases of sebaceous gland carcinoma in the eyelid. They concluded that sebaceous gland carcinoma appeared as a regular, ill-defined, heterogeneous, or homogeneous hypoechoic lesion on ultrasound. Mandeep et al. summarized the features of 16 cases of sebaceous gland carcinoma on ultrasound biomicroscopy as solid lesions, involving the whole layers of the eyelid, without normal appearance. The lipid aggregation area shows hyperechogenicity on ultrasound, the liquefactive necrosis shows hypoechogenicity, and the fibrovascular component shows linear or round hyperechogenicity.

Although many studies have described the ultrasound features of sebaceous gland carcinoma initially, the number of cases is relatively small. The diagnosis of sebaceous gland carcinoma with ultrasound needs more experience. Ultrasound evaluates the layers of involvement, depth of invasion, and other information of the lesion, providing a reference for preoperative diagnosis.

Key Points

- Sebaceous gland carcinoma is rare, with 3/4 periocular sebaceous gland carcinoma and 1/4 extraocular sebaceous gland carcinoma. It often occurs in middle-aged and elderly people, and is prone to metastasize with a poor prognosis.
- Ultrasound features of sebaceous gland carcinoma are non-specific and resemble BCC. It is mainly characterized by an irregular and ill-defined hypoechoic lesion involving the whole layers of the skin, with rich blood flow signals inside.
- The diagnosis of sebaceous gland carcinoma should be considered if there is a single, yellow, painless, and firm nodule around the eye or a diffuse thick and stiff eyelid. It should be mainly differentiated from nodular BCC, cSCC, and nevus sebaceus.

5.3.9 Trichilemmal Carcinoma

5.3.9.1 Clinical Manifestation and Pathology

Trichilemmal carcinoma (TLC) is a low-grade malignant tumor derived from skin appendage differentiated from the outer root sheath of hair follicles. Although the histological characteristics suggest that the disease may be invasive, it grows slowly. This disease is uncommon clinically, mostly occurs in scalp, ears, neck, and other ultraviolet exposed areas. It is rare in trunk and extremities, and it is often single. The disease is more common in the elderly females.

The visual appearance of TLC is diverse, and some of the lesions are polypoid, cauliflower-like bumps, and some appear as papules or plaques. The surface can rupture or scab. Sometimes it appears as a subcutaneous nodule without obvious appearance changes.

Pathologically, TLC is mainly formed by the variation of transparent cells in the outer root sheath, and keratinization of the outer root sheath is common.

5.3.9.2 Ultrasound Manifestation

Gray-Scale Ultrasound

Gray-scale ultrasound of TLC shows no obvious specific findings. It mostly appears as a solid hypoechoic lesion in the epidermis and dermis. It shows aggressive behavior with invasion, which could deeply invade the subcutaneous tissue and even the bone cortex. The lesion is oval or irregular, heterogeneous, well-defined or ill-defined.

Color Doppler Ultrasound

Color Doppler ultrasound shows rich blood flow signals in most lesions (Figs. 5.73 and 5.74).

5.3.9.3 Differential Diagnosis

cSCC

cSCC can occur all over the body, while TLC mostly occurs in scalp, ears, and neck. The visual appearance of the two entities is similar.

On gray-scale ultrasound, cSCC appears as an irregular and ill-defined hypoechoic lesion in the epidermis and dermis. The surface of cSCC is uneven and appears as thick linear hyperechogenicity resulted from hyperkeratosis, with various degrees of posterior acoustic shadowing, which leads to insufficient visualization of the lesion. However, TLC is regular or irregular without abnormal keratinization and it is heterogenous.

KA

KA often occurs in the face of elderly males. It is a reddish, elevated, and hemispherical nodule. The center of the lesion is filled with keratin plugs, and appears "volcano-like". The disease grows rapidly and tends to regress spontaneously. TLC often occurs in scalp, ears, and neck in the elderly female. It grows slowly and sometimes the surface ruptures or scabs.

On gray-scale ultrasound, KA has a characteristic central hyperkeratotic area, forming an "inverted triangle" posterior acoustic shadowing, while TLC often does not have abnormal keratinization and posterior acoustic shadowing.

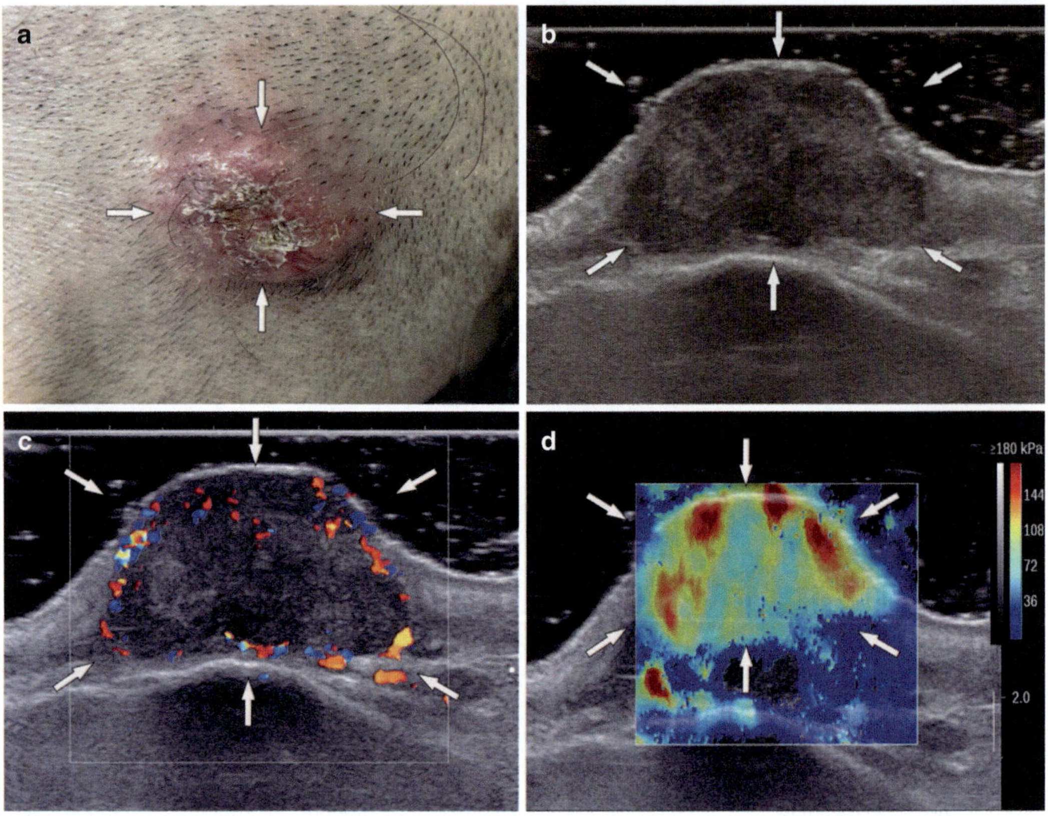

Fig. 5.73 Trichilemmal carcinoma. Female, 84 years of age. (**a**) Visual observation shows a dark red, well-defined bump in the left occiput (arrows), the size of which is about 35.0 mm × 25.0 mm, with ulceration, scab, and no exudates on the surface. (**b**) Gray-scale ultrasound shows a regular, ill-defined hypoechoic nodule (arrows) (size: 30 mm × 22 mm; thickness: 16.6 mm). The surface is elevated without abnormal keratinization. The bottom of the lesion deeply invades to the surface of the bone. The lesion is heterogeneous (Frequency: 15 MHz). (**c**) Color Doppler ultrasound shows rich blood flow signals in the periphery of the lesion (arrows) (Frequency: 15 MHz) (**d**) The lesion is covered by uneven and mixed colors on two-dimensional SWE image (arrows), with maximum elastic modulus of 191.6 kPa and mean elastic modulus of 74.5 kPa

5.3.9.4 Diagnosis Clues

1. Visual appearance of TLC is similar to that of cSCC. Some of the lesions appear as polypoid, cauliflower-like bumps, and some appear as papules or plaques. Sometimes the surface ruptures or scabs.
2. TLC is rare clinically, and there are few studies on its ultrasound features at present. Li et al. reported the ultrasound features of a case of TLC, but the diagnosis was difficult because of lacking specificity. According to our experience, the ultrasound features of TLC are ill-defined, hypoechoic areas in the epidermis and dermis, with rich blood flow signals in the lesion.

More experience is needed in the ultrasound diagnosis of TLC. Ultrasound can evaluate the involved layers and the invasion depth, providing reference for surgeons.

Key Points

- TLC originates from the outer hair root sheath of the hair follicle, and it mostly occurs in the scalp, ears, and neck. It is more common in elderly females.
- Gray-scale ultrasound of TLC shows a solid hypoechoic lesion in the epidermis and dermis. TLC appears aggressive behavior with invasion, which could deeply invade the subcutaneous tissue and even the bone cortex.

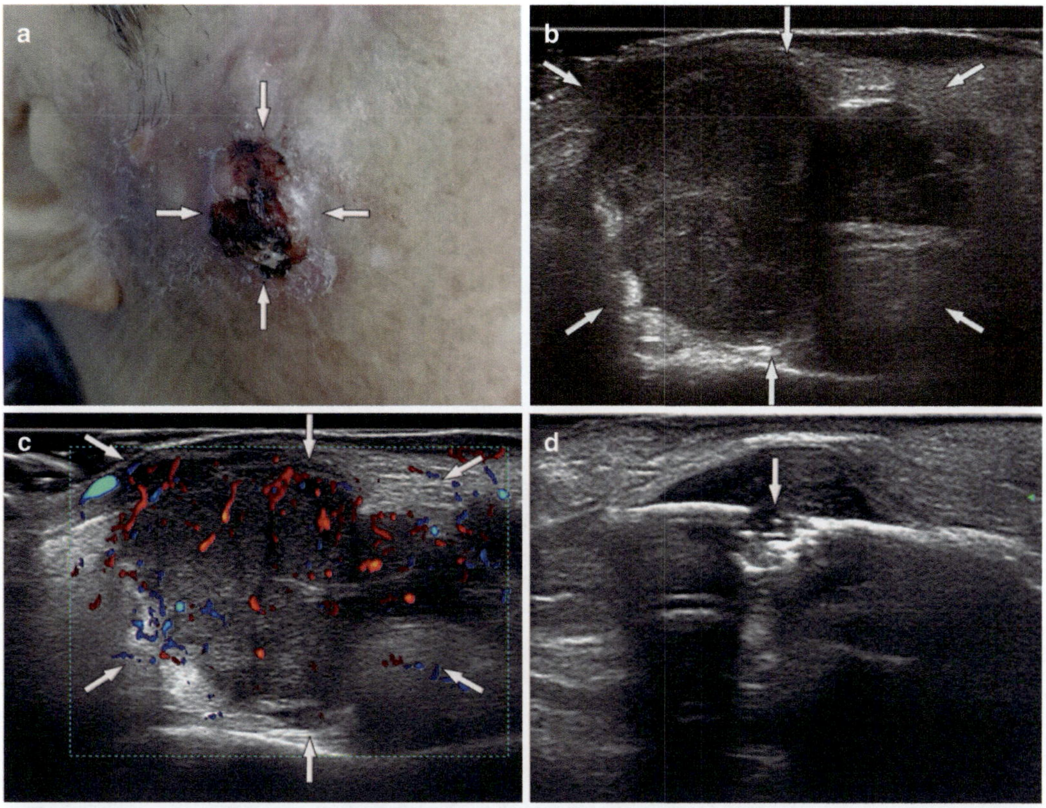

Fig. 5.74 Trichilemmal carcinoma. Female, 92 years of age. (**a**) Visual observation shows a dark red, irregular, and ill-defined bump in the right cheek, with ulceration, scab, and exudates on the surface (arrows). (**b**) Gray-scale ultrasound shows an irregular, ill-defined hypoechoic nodule (arrows) (thickness: 13 ~ 28.1 mm). The lesion is heterogeneous (Frequency: 15 MHz). (**c**) Color Doppler ultrasound shows rich blood flow signals in the lesion (arrows) (Frequency: 15 MHz). (**d**) The lesion invades to the bone convex, appearing as discontinuity of local cortical bone (arrow)

Color Doppler ultrasound shows rich blood flow signals in most lesions.

- TLC should be differentiated from cSCC, KA, and so on.

5.3.10 Mycosis Fungoides

5.3.10.1 Clinical Manifestation and Pathology

Mycosis fungoides (MF) is the most common subtype of primary cutaneous T cell lymphoma (CTCL), accounting for approximately 60% of CTCL. MF originates from peripheral CD4+ effector memory T cells and is a T cell lymphoma with mainly small and medium cell proliferation. The onset of MF is insidious, and it develops slowly and progressively. It usually occurs in non-exposed parts such as trunk and perineum.

In the early stage, the lesion appears as a scaly, infiltrative erythema or plaque. As the disease progresses, the lesion becomes thickened gradually. In the late stage, the lesion appears as an exophytic mass. MF is a low-grade malignancy with a good prognosis in the early stage and a mean survival time of 10 ~ 20 years. In the late stage, lymph nodes and internal organs are involved and the prognosis is poor.

5.3.10.2 Ultrasound Manifestation

Gray-Scale Ultrasound

In the early stage, gray-scale ultrasound shows a homogeneous subepidermal low echoic band (SLEB). The surface is slightly elevated or flat, with abnormal keratinization sometimes. The lesion is crawling, and the bottom is mostly flat. With the progress of the disease, the lesion invades the deep tissue with a funnel-like shape. It is nodular or irregular, ill-defined and heterogeneous.

Color Doppler Ultrasound

Color Doppler ultrasound shows rich blood flow signals in most of lesions (Fig. 5.75).

5.3.10.3 Differential Diagnosis

Eczema

MF needs to be differentiated from eczema in the early stage. The appearance of both lesions is similar, and both of them are scaly erythema. The epidermal hyperplasia and hyperkeratinization of chronic eczema are more obvious than those of

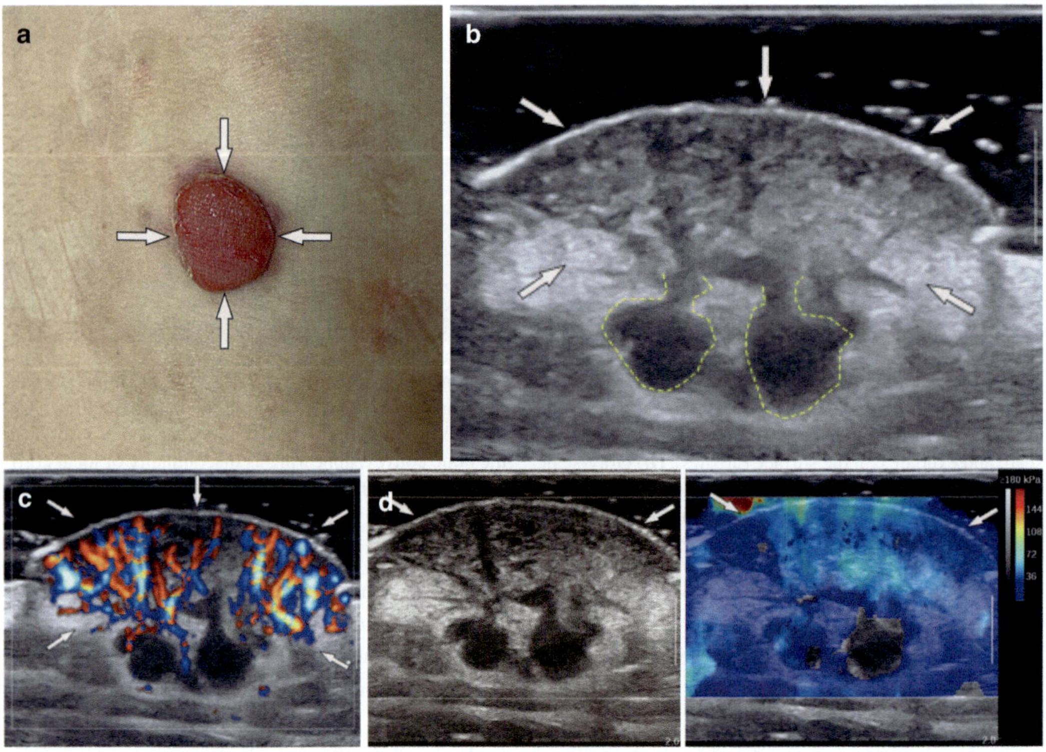

Fig. 5.75 Mycosis fungoides. Female, 30 years of age. (**a**) Visual observation shows a red, irregular, and well-defined nodule about 20.0 × 20.0 mm with exudates in the back (arrows). (**b**) Gray-scale ultrasound shows an irregular, ill-defined hypoechoic lesion in the whole layers of the skin (size: 21.3 mm × 22.7 mm; thickness: 13.2 mm). The surface is elevated without abnormal keratinization. The bottom of the lesion is funnel-like. The lesion is heterogeneous with branch-like hypoechogenicity (Frequency: 15 MHz) (dotted line). (**c**) Power Doppler ultrasound shows rich blood flow signals inside the lesion (Frequency: 15 MHz). (**d**) The lesion is covered by uneven and mixed colors including green, yellow, and blue on two-dimensional SWE image, with maximum elastic modulus of 64.6 kPa and mean elastic modulus of 41.8 kPa. Arrows piont to lesions

early MF. Both of them appear as SLEB on gray-scale ultrasound, but the epidermal thickness and SLEB width of MF are less than those of chronic eczema (Fig. 5.76).

Psoriasis

In the early stage, MF was similar to psoriasis vulgaris in visual appearance and ultrasound, so it is difficult to distinguish the two diseases.

However, the epidermis of psoriasis is thicker, and the number of hypoechoic shadowing behind the epidermis is more, which is related to the complete reflection of ultrasound caused by the local thick scales of the psoriasis.

5.3.10.4 Diagnosis Clues

1. In the early stage, the lesion appears as a scaly, infiltrative erythema or plaque. As the disease progresses, the lesion becomes thickened gradually. In the late stage, the lesion appears as a exophytic mass.
2. Gray-scale ultrasound appears as a SLEB in the early stage. The lesion invades the deep tissue with a funnel-like shape in the late stage. It is nodular or irregular and ill-defined.
3. Color Doppler ultrasound shows rich blood flow signals in most lesions.

5.3.10.5 Clinical Significance

High-frequency ultrasound can be used to differentiate early MF from inflammatory skin diseases such as eczema and psoriasis. Liu et al. found that epidermal thickness, SLEB width, and the number of hypoechoic shadowing behind the epidermis can be used to differentiate the above diseases. At present, there are few studies on the high-frequency ultrasound of late MF, and we found that the funnel-like invasion pattern may

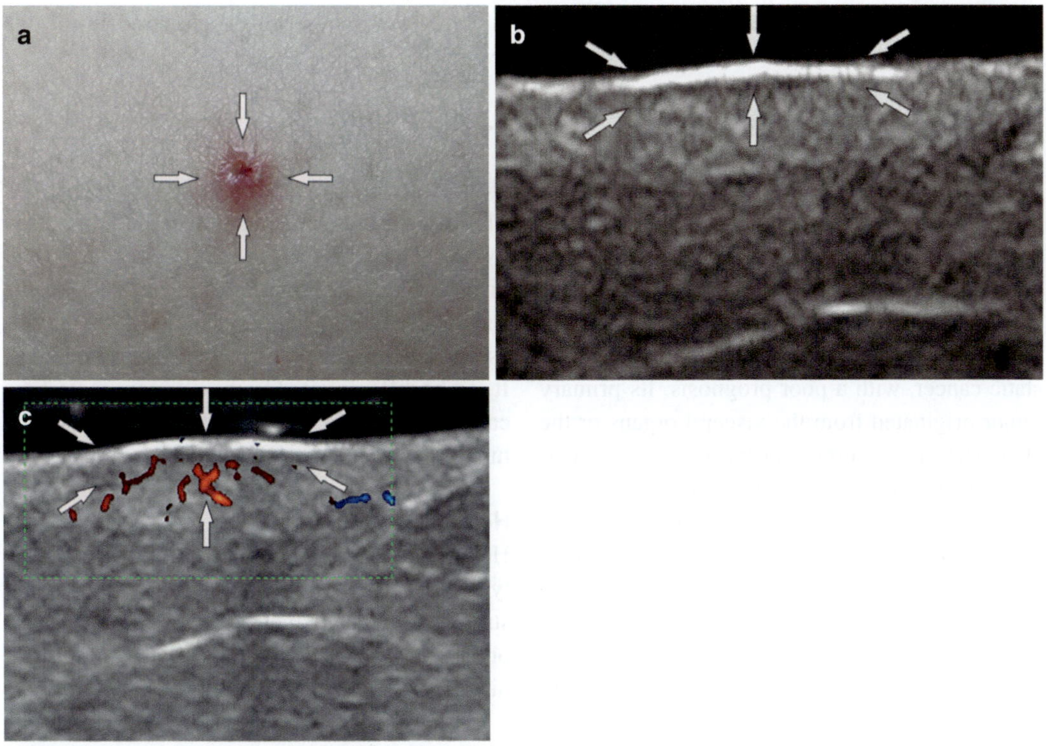

Fig. 5.76 Eczema. Female, 69 years of age. (**a**) Visual observation shows a red patch with scab in the abdominal wall (arrows). (**b**) Gray-scale ultrasound shows an SLEB in the skin (size: 5.2 mm × 3.8 mm; thickness: 0.8 mm). The surface is slightly elevated with abnormal keratinization (arrows) (Frequency: 22 MHz). (**c**) Color Doppler ultrasound shows rare blood flow signals inside the lesion (arrows) (Frequency: 22 MHz)

be its characteristic finding, but further validation is needed. High-frequency ultrasound can also provide depth and morphological characteristics of MF, providing reference for treatment.

Key Points

- MF is the most common subtype of primary CTCL. The onset of MF is insidious, and it develops slowly and progressively.
- Gray-scale ultrasound appears as a subepidermal low echoic band in the early stage. The lesion invades the deep tissue with a funnel-like shape in the late stage. It is nodular or irregular and ill-defined. Color Doppler ultrasound shows rich blood flow signals in most lesions.
- MF should be differentiated from inflammatory skin diseases such as eczema and psoriasis.

5.3.11 Cutaneous Metastatic Carcinoma

5.3.11.1 Clinical Manifestation and Pathology

Cutaneous metastatic carcinoma is a skin metastasis in patients with malignant tumors through vascular, lymphatic vessel, direct invasion, or surgical implantation. Cutaneous metastatic carcinoma is less common than metastatic cancer of other organs, accounting for 2% to 9% of metastatic cancer, with a poor prognosis. Its primary tumor originated from the visceral organs or the skin. The most common primary tumor of cutaneous metastatic carcinoma in females is breast cancer, and about 23.9% of patients with breast cancer suffered from cutaneous metastatic carcinoma. The most common primary tumor of cutaneous metastatic carcinoma in males is lung cancer.

The lesions are often multiple, arranged in clusters, and connected to each other. It is commonly found around the surgical incision, drainage vessel, or puncture site. The appearance of cutaneous metastatic carcinoma is diverse. The surface of the lesion is flat or elevated, and when the epidermis is involved, papules, erythema, ulcerations, and nodules may occur. Therefore, it is often misdiagnosed as herpes zoster, skin infection, or hemangioma clinically. The most common histopathological type of cutaneous metastatic carcinoma is adenocarcinoma.

5.3.11.2 Ultrasound Manifestation

Gray-Scale Ultrasound

Gray-scale ultrasound shows multiple, irregular, and ill-defined hypoechoic lesions in the subcutaneous tissue, often without capsule. The lesions are heterogeneous, and may be accompanied by posterior acoustic shadowing. The disease can involve the whole layers of the skin or even the muscles.

Color Doppler Ultrasound

Blood flow signals can be observed inside the lesion (Fig. 5.77).

5.3.11.3 Differential Diagnosis

Herpes Zoster

This disease is an inflammation of the skin caused by varicella-zoster virus. The lesions are often distributed on one side of the body in bands, showing painful patchy erythema, which may be associated with ulcerations without firm nodules. It can be differentiated from cutaneous metastatic carcinoma based on clinical symptoms and history.

Hemangioma

Hemangiomas are mostly present at birth, and typically present as red-blue patches on the skin surface. Cutaneous metastatic carcinoma is secondary to tumor history and related to surgical history.

Ultrasound findings are useful to differentiate the two entities. On gray-scale ultrasound, most hemangiomas appear as hypoechoic lesions in

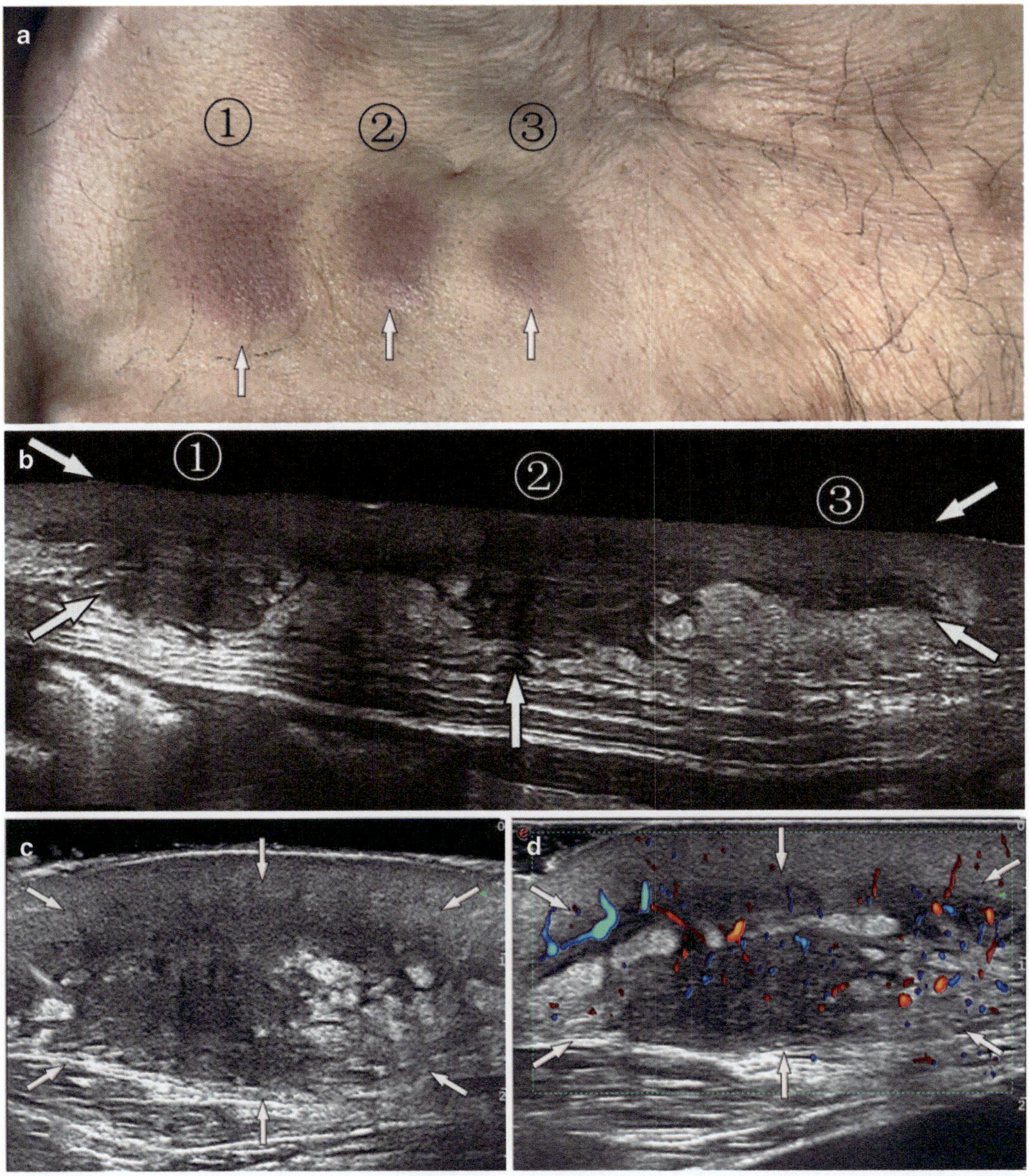

Fig. 5.77 Cutaneous metastatic carcinoma (from gastric cancer). Male, 67 years of age. (**a**) Visual observation shows three adjacent elevated and ill-defined dark red nodules (①, ②, ③) in the abdominal wall, with diameters of 30 mm, 20 mm, and 10 mm, respectively, without rupture on the surface (arrows). (**b**) Gray-scale ultrasound shows the overall morphology of the three lesions (①, ②, and ③ in Fig. A, respectively) by extended field of view, appearing as multiple, irregular, ill-defined, and heterogeneous hypoechoic lesions (arrows) involving the dermis and subcutaneous tissues (size: 31.2 mm × 28.3 mm; 22.0 mm × 18.6 mm, and 13.7 mm × 12.9 mm, respectively; thicknesses: 28.8 mm, 27.9 mm, and 6.3 mm, respectively). The lesions are connected to each other. Peripheral subcutaneous tissue is swollen with increased echogenicity (Frequency: 22 MHz). (**c**) Gray-scale ultrasound shows locally magnified lesion ②, appearing as a hypoechoic lesion (arrows) in the dermis and subcutaneous tissue. The lesion is heterogeneous with patchy hyperechogenicity inside (Frequency: 22 MHz). (**d**) Color Doppler ultrasound shows rare blood flow signals inside the lesion (arrows) (Frequency: 22 MHz)

the subcutaneous tissues, and some lesions appear spongiform or honeycombed, with posterior acoustic enhancement. The diagnosis can be identified by the "compression test" on color Doppler ultrasound. However, cutaneous metastatic carcinoma shows an irregular, ill-defined, and heterogeneous hypoechoic lesion in the subcutaneous tissue, which involves the whole layers of the skin.

5.3.11.4 Diagnosis Clues

1. Patients have a history of malignant tumors.
2. Papules, erythemas, ulcerations, or nodules appear in the skin without obvious inducement.
3. Ultrasound shows an irregular and ill-defined hypoechoic lesion in the subcutaneous tissue. The lesion is heterogeneous, with patchy hyperechogenicity inside. The lesion may involve the whole layers of skin.

The ultrasound features of cutaneous metastatic carcinoma are non-specific and easily misdiagnosed in clinical practice. For lesions with unexplained reasons, the diagnosis of cutaneous metastatic carcinoma should be considered in patients with a history of malignancy. Ultrasound can be helpful to assess benign and malignant tumors by visualizing the extent and the layers of involvement of the lesions. Biopsy is required for qualitative diagnosis.

Key Points

- Cutaneous metastatic carcinoma is rare with a poor prognosis. Breast cancer is the most common primary tumor in women with cutaneous metastatic carcinoma, and lung cancer is most common in men.
- Ultrasound shows multiple, irregular, and ill-defined hypoechoic lesions in the subcutaneous tissues, often without capsule. This disease can involve the whole layers of skin, even muscle.
- The history of malignant tumors is the most important basis for diagnosing cutaneous metastatic carcinoma. It should be mainly differentiated from herpes zoster and hemangioma.

5.3.12 Lymph Node Metastasis

5.3.12.1 Clinical Manifestation and Pathology

Lymph node is an important immune organ of the human body, producing lymphocytes, plasma cells, and other immune cells to participate in the immune process of the body, and it is also the most common metastasis site of malignant tumors. Lymph node metastasis occurs in cutaneous malignancies, and the possibility of metastasis varies among different malignancies. The clinical stage will change as a result of lymph node metastasis, with a worse prognosis of the disease.

BCC has a possibility of lymph node metastasis <0.5% and is considered rarely fatal; primary SCC has a possibility of lymph node metastasis of 4% with a better prognosis; while the possibility of lymph node metastasis in recurrent SCC rapidly increases to 45% with a very poor prognosis. The lymph node metastasis rate of EMPD is high, up to 37.2%, and the 5-year survival rate after lymph node metastasis is only 7%. Domestic studies reported that the overall lymph node metastasis rate of melanoma was more than 30%, with a poor prognosis.

In general, lymph node metastasis follows a trend of "from the near to the distant," "from the superficial to the deep" and "ipsilateral high risk."

1. Cutaneous malignancies of the head and neck involve the neck firstly and subsequently the supraclavicular fossa, followed by the mediastinum and further afield.
2. Cutaneous malignancies of the upper extremity may metastasize to the ipsilateral trochlea and subsequently to the axilla.
3. Cutaneous malignancies of the lower extremity may metastasize to the ipsilateral popliteal fossa and subsequently to the inguinal region.
4. Cutaneous malignancies of the trunk have the potential to metastasize both ipsilaterally upward (supraclavicular fossa) and downward (inguinal region).
5. It should be noted that inguinal lymph node metastasis is more common in the perineal cutaneous malignancies, which often involve

both sides and is more likely to be accompanied by abdominal lymph node metastasis.

Clinically, the typical lymph node metastasis appears as a palpable, painless, and firm nodule, and occasionally arranged in clusters. However, most lymph node metastasis does not have typical clinical symptoms and is difficult to diagnose in clinic. At this time, ultrasound can be used to assist in further clinical diagnosis and treatment.

5.3.12.2 Ultrasound Manifestation (Fig. 5.78)

1. Volume: The affected side is usually significantly larger than the contralateral side or the previous lesion (usually more than doubled compared with the unaffected side).
2. Shape: The shape is oval or round (longest diameter/shortest diameter < 2). Or it appears irregular shape due to the tumor breaking through the capsule. Metastatic lymph nodes are often multiple and appear beaded, and sometimes fuse with each other. Single lymph node metastasis is rare.
3. Internal echogenicity: The cortex can be thickened locally or diffusely. Even the entire lymph node appears as a diffuse hypoechoic lesion, with the thinning, deformation, or disappearance of the medulla, or the indistinct demarcation between the cortex and medulla.
4. Lymphatic hilum: It is unclear or completely disappears.
5. Types of blood flow distribution: Abnormal lymph nodes may show rich blood flow signals, usually in the periphery or with an irregular distribution pattern, and the "portal type" blood supply pattern disappears completely.

5.3.12.3 Differential Diagnosis

Normal Lymph Nodes (Fig. 5.79)

1. Clinical manifestation: Normal lymph nodes have no obvious clinical symptoms, most of them are non-palpable. A few thin people have palpable superficial normal lymph nodes.
2. Volume: In general, the volume of normal lymph nodes is smaller than that of abnormal lymph nodes, but there is no uniform reference value for the volume of lymph node. Whether its volume is abnormal or not, it is judged by comparing with the lymph nodes on the unaffected side and the previous volume.
3. Morphology: Normal lymph nodes generally show an oblate shape (longest diameter/shortest diameter > 2), sometimes the longest diameter is even more than 30.0 mm. The morphology cannot be considered abnormal if the longest diameter is not significantly increased.
4. Internal echogenicity: The normal lymph node is "kidney-shaped", that is, the outside is a hypoechoic cortex, which is thin and homogeneous; the inside is a hyperechoic medulla, which is zonal or oval. The cortex rings around the medulla, which generally does not exceed the medulla in thickness.

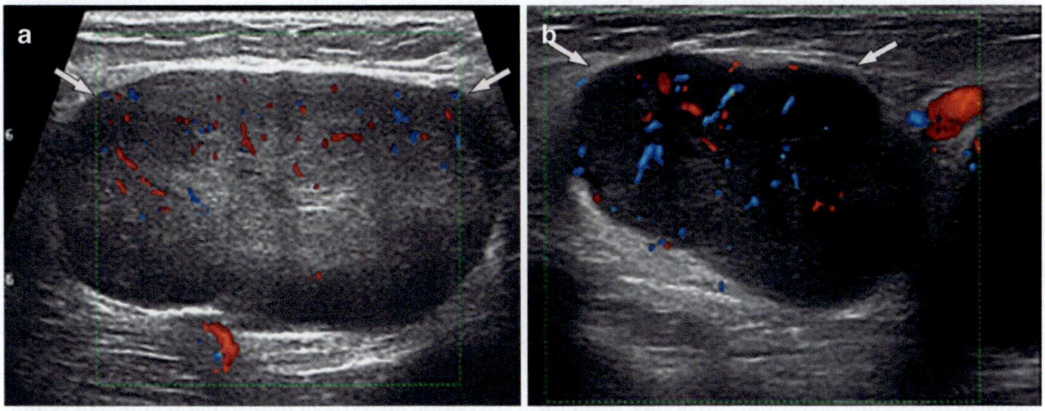

Fig. 5.78 Abnormal lymph nodes. (**a**) Inguinal lymph node metastasis of Paget's disease (arrows) (Frequency: 6–15 MHz). (**b**) Popliteal lymph node metastasis of malignant melanoma (arrows) (Frequency: 6–15 MHz)

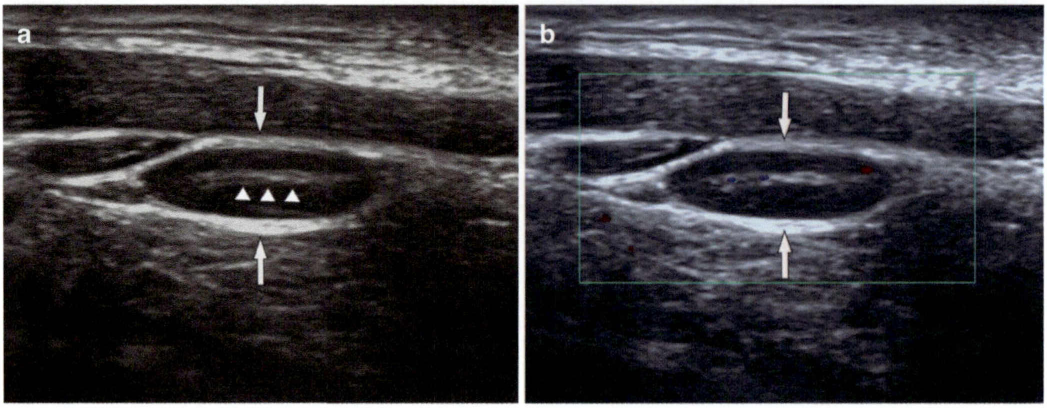

Fig. 5.79 Ultrasound features of normal cervical lymph nodes. (**a**) Gray-scale ultrasound shows a hypoechoic lesion (arrows), with a well-defined lymphatic hilum (△) and corticomedullary demarcation (longest diameter/shortest diameter > 2) (Frequency: 15 MHz). (**b**) Color Doppler ultrasound shows rare "portal type" blood flow distribution in the normal lymph node (arrows) (Frequency: 18 MHz)

5. Lymphatic hilum: The lymphatic hilum is the hub site for lymphatic vessels and blood vessels to enter and exit the lymph nodes. It often locates in the depression side of the lymph node and connects to the medulla, which is important for differentiating benign and malignant lymph nodes.
6. Types of blood flow distribution: The blood flow distribution of normal lymph node is "portal type" i.e., blood vessels pass through the lymphatic hilum in bundles and spread out in a branch-like manner in the lymph nodes.

Malignant Lymphoma

The disease is common in children and young adults and clinically appears as painless, progressive proliferation of lymph node tissue. On ultrasound, it appears a heterogeneous hypoechoic area with thickened cortex and disorganized blood flow signals. It is difficult to differentiate lymphoma from lymph node metastases by relying independently on ultrasound features. But they can be differentiated based on clinical symptoms and history.

Reactive Lymph Node Hyperplasia

Reactive lymph node hyperplasia is a common benign lesion, which can present as an enlarged and firm mass clinically, often involving bilateral lymph nodes. Patients often have a history of inflammation and symptoms such as pain and discomfort; some patients may not. On ultrasound, it shows a hypoechoic lesion in full shape (longest diameter/shortest diameter < 2), thickened cortex, well-defined corticomedullary demarcation, and lymphatic hilum. Occasionally, owing to being squeezed by the significantly thickened cortex, the medulla and lymphatic hilum cannot be visualized. Rich blood flow signals are observed on color Doppler ultrasound, with "portal type" blood flow distribution (Fig. 5.80).

It should be noted that cutaneous malignancies and their treatment can cause inflammation, resulting in reactive lymph nodes hyperplasia. It may be difficult to diagnose at this time and require biopsy to confirm the diagnosis. Table 5.8 summarizes the key points in differentiating lymph node metastasis from normal lymph nodes and reactive lymph nodes hyperplasia.

5.3.12.4 Diagnosis Clues

1. If patients have a history of skin malignancies, with abnormal ultrasound findings of adjacent regional lymph nodes, the diagnosis of metastasis needs to be considered.
2. Diffuse decreased echogenicity, absence of corticomedullary demarcation and lymphatic hilum, and non-portal type blood flow distribution are typical ultrasound features of lymph node metastasis of cutaneous malignancies.

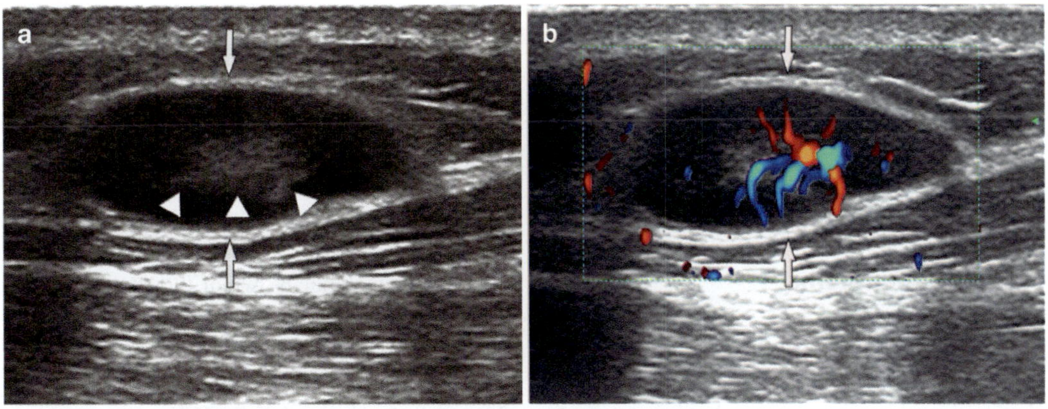

Fig. 5.80 Ultrasound features of reactive lymph node hyperplasia. (**a**) Gray-scale ultrasound shows a hypoechoic lesion (arrows), appearing full in shape (maximum longest diameter/shortest diameter < 2), and thickened cortex, with well-defined corticomedullary demarcation and lymphatic hilum (△) (Frequency: 15 MHz). (**b**) Color Doppler ultrasound shows rich blood flow signals in the lymph nodes, with "portal type" blood flow distribution (arrows) (Frequency: 15 MHz)

Table 5.8 Differentiation of lymph node metastasis, normal lymph nodes, and reactive lymph node hyperplasia

Clinical and ultrasound features	Normal lymph nodes	Lymph node metastasis of cutaneous malignancy	Reactive lymph node hyperplasia
Clinical symptoms	Asymptomatic	Asymptomatic/palpable painless mass	Asymptomatic/palpable painful mass
Clinical history	No clinical history	History of malignancy	Inflammation history/no clinical history
Clinical outcome	No change	Enlarged, increased, capsular invasion	No change/reduction
Volume	Small	Swollen	Swollen
Shape	Oblate	Full/irregular	Full
Longest diameter/shortest diameter	> 2	< 2	< 2
Corticomedullary demarcation	Well-defined	Ill-defined	Well-defined/ill-defined
Lymphatic hilum	Well-defined	Absent	Well-defined
Cortex	Thin	Thick	Thick
Medulla	Banded	Absent	Thin/linear
Extent of involvement	/	Unilateral mostly	Bilateral mostly
Types of blood flow distribution	Portal	Irregular or peripheral	Portal

3. Acral lentiginous melanoma commonly metastasize to popliteal and trochlear lymph nodes, so attention should be paid during examination.

Key Points

- Cutaneous malignancies have the possibility of lymph node metastasis, and the superficial lymph nodes on the same side should be examined.
- Ultrasound examinations of lymph node should follow the order of "from the near to the distant, from the superficial to the deep," and attention should be paid to comparison with the unaffected side.
- Lymph node metastasis and reactive lymph node hyperplasia cannot be differentiated by size. It is necessary to combine the history and ultrasound features such as internal echogenicity and blood flow signals of lymph

nodes. If necessary, biopsy and other methods can be used for further diagnosis.

5.4 Hemangioma and Congenital Vascular Malformation

5.4.1 Hemangioma

5.4.1.1 Clinical Manifestation and Pathology

Hemangioma is a congenital benign tumor or vascular malformation formed by the proliferation of angioblasts during the embryonic period. And it is commonly located in the skin and soft tissues. It typically appears as a red-blue patch on the skin surface at birth. Hemangioma occurs throughout the body, and the most common locations of hemangioma are oral and maxillofacial region (60%), followed by the trunk (25%) and extremities (15%). It is more common in females, with a male to female ratio of (1:3) to (1:4).

5.4.1.2 Ultrasound Manifestation

Gray-Scale Ultrasound

The ultrasound findings of hemangioma are diverse and mainly divided into two types.

1. Nodular type: The lesion appears as a hypoechoic lesion in the subcutaneous tissue. It is oval or round-shaped and well-defined. Slit-like anechogenicity is observed in some lesions, so that some lesions appear spongiform or honeycombed. Sometimes, dot-like or patchy hyperechogenicity formed by thrombus is observed inside the lesion. The lesion is non-encapsulated.
2. Diffuse type: It shows a slightly hyperechoic lesion in the subcutaneous tissue without capsule and space-occupying effect. Contrast to the nodular type, the diffuse type is irregular and ill-defined, but the internal echogenicity is similar to the nodular type. The lesion often shows the posterior acoustic enhancement.

Color Doppler Ultrasound

Color Doppler ultrasound plays an important role in the diagnosis of hemangioma. Due to the thin lumen of the internal vessels of the hemangioma and the slow blood flow velocity, blood flow signals on color Doppler ultrasound are often rare, and even absent. Given this circumstance, it can be further identified by the "compression test." That is, when the pressure from the transducer rapidly squeezes the lesion, the blood flow signals increased transiently, followed by rare or even disappearance of blood flow signals in the lesion. When the pressure from the transducer is quickly relieved, the transient increase of blood flow signals is observed, then returns to the status before compression. This phenomenon is a characteristic feature of hemangioma, caused by blood flowing in and out the hemangioma rapidly (Fig. 5.81 and 5.82).

5.4.1.3 Differential Diagnosis

Giant Cell Tumor of Tendon Sheath

The disease is common on the tendon sheath of the fingers, wrists, and appears as a hard and painless nodule. There is no tendency for spontaneous regression. On gray-scale ultrasound, it shows a well-defined, regular, or irregular hypoechoic lesion in the tendon or para-articular region. The lesion may wrap the joint and invade the adjacent bone. While, most of hemangiomas show the feature of spongiform or honeycombed. The "compression test" on color Doppler ultrasound is the important feature to differentiate the two entities.

Schwannoma

Visual appearance of the two entities is different. Hemangioma typically appear as a red-blue patch, while schwannoma appears as a skin-colored bump.

On gray-scale ultrasound, schwannoma appears as an oval or spindle-shaped hypoechoic lesion. Cystic change, necrosis, and hemorrhage are visualized in some lesions. If cystic areas appear, the lesion is heterogeneous, and it needs to be differentiated from hemangioma. The rat tail sign on gray-scale ultrasound and "squeeze

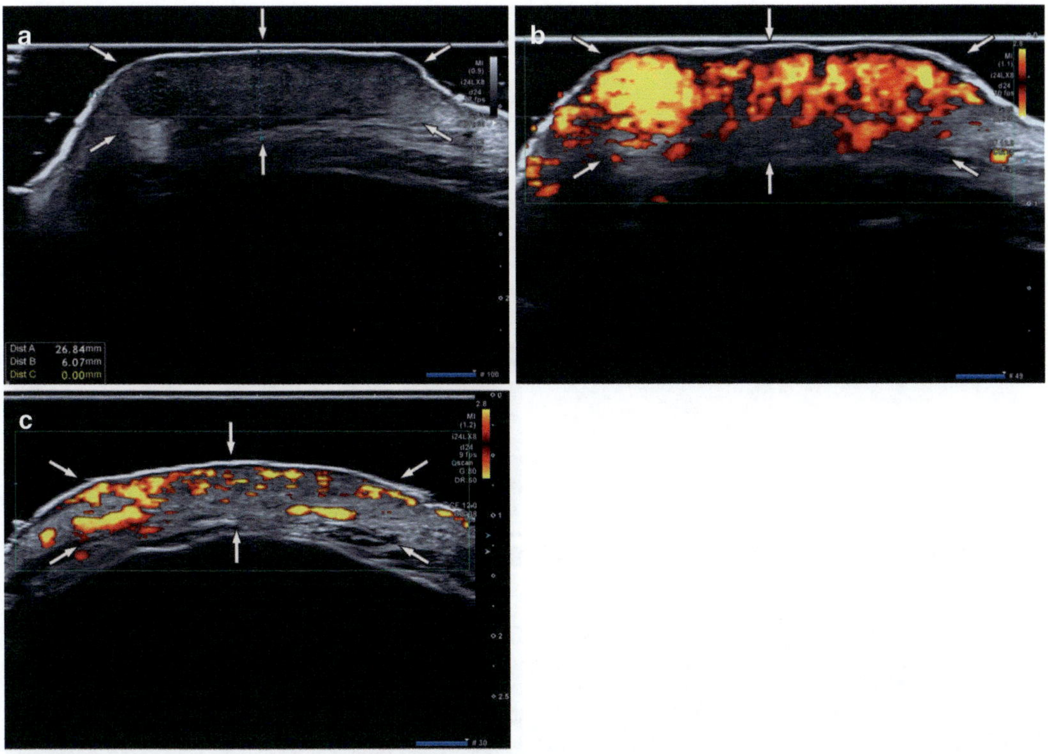

Fig. 5.81 Hemangioma. Male, 72 years of age. (**a**) Gray-scale ultrasound shows an irregular, well-defined hypoechoic lesion (arrows) in the subcutaneous tissue (size: 26.0 mm × 19.0 mm; thickness: 1.9 mm). The surface is slightly elevated. The lesion is heterogeneous, and slit-like hypoechogenicity is observed inside the lesion (Frequency: 24 MHz). (**b**) Power Doppler ultrasound shows the blood flow signals increased transiently once the transducer is pressed onto the surface of the lesion (arrows) (Frequency: 24 MHz). (**c**) Power Doppler ultrasound shows the blood flow signals inside the lesion decreased significantly under continuous compression from the transducer (arrows) (Frequency: 24 MHz)

test" on color Doppler ultrasound are valuable in differentiating the two entities.

Epidermoid Cyst

Epidermoid cyst is similar to nodular hemangioma in terms of visual appearance and ultrasound features. Both diseases appear as round or oval mixed echogenic lesions. Epidermoid cyst shows slit-like hypoechogenicity, with capsule and no blood flow signals. However, hemangioma is encapsulated, spongiform, or honeycombed. It is characterized by "compression test" on color Doppler ultrasound.

5.4.1.4 Diagnosis Clues

1. Hemangioma typically appears as a red-blue patch on the skin surface at birth, and clinical history is helpful in the diagnosis of the disease.
2. Gray-scale ultrasound shows a hypoechoic lesion in the subcutaneous tissue. And some lesions show spongiform or honeycombed change, with posterior acoustic enhancement.
3. Color Doppler ultrasound is important for the diagnosis of hemangioma. The diagnosis can be validated by the "compression test." That is, when the transducer rapidly squeezes the lesion, the blood flow signals increased transiently, followed by sparse or even disappearance of blood flow signal in the lesion. When the pressure from the transducer is quickly relieved, the transient increase of blood flow signal can be observed, then returns to the status before compression.

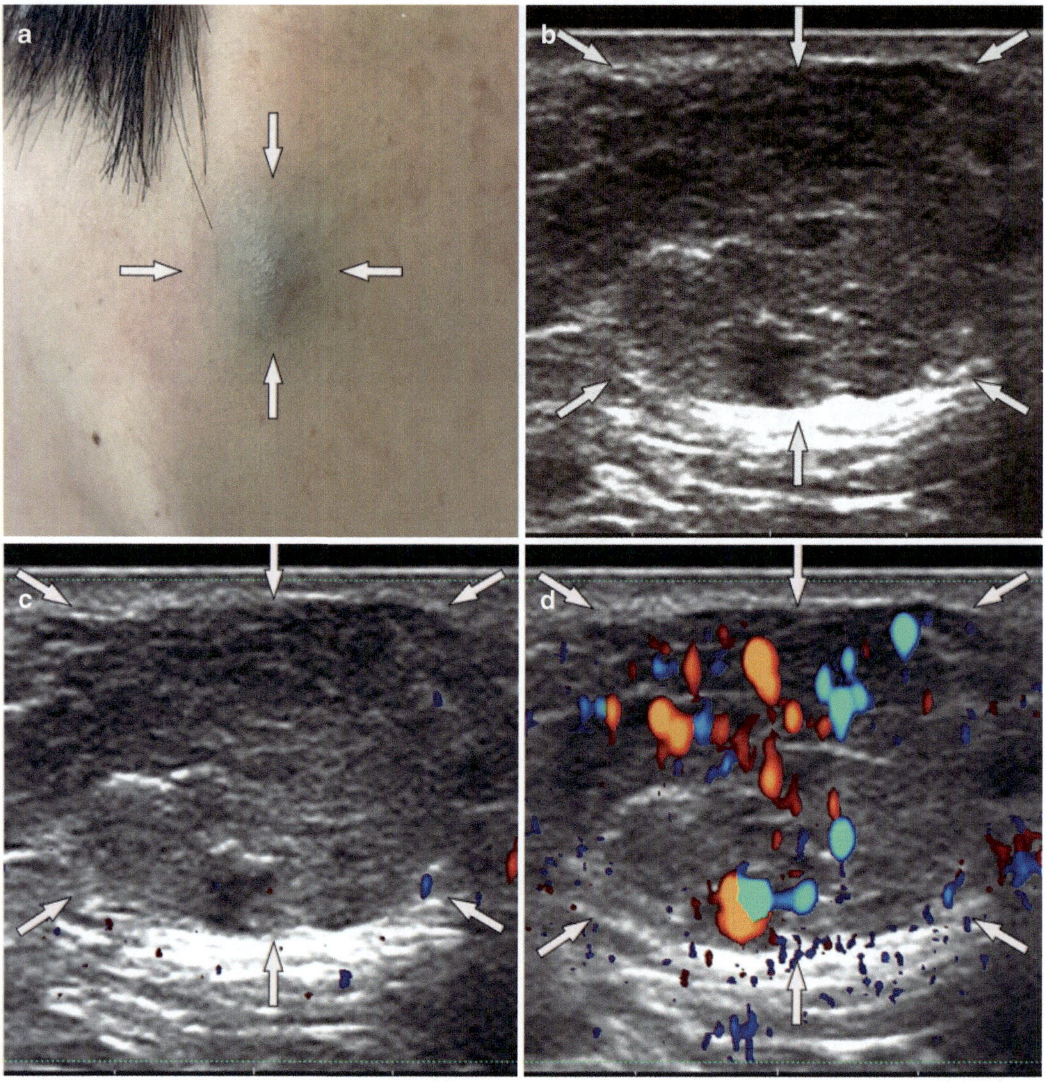

Fig. 5.82 Hemangioma. Male, 43 years of age. (**a**) Visual observation shows a blue bump in the right side of the face. The surface is smooth (arrows). (**b**) Gray-scale ultrasound shows a regular, well-defined hypoechoic lesion (arrows) in the subcutaneous tissue (size: 22.0 mm × 19.0 mm; thickness: 9.4 mm). The lesion is heterogeneous, and banded hyperechogenicity is observed inside the lesion (Frequency: 22 MHz). (**c**) Color Doppler ultrasound shows no blood flow signals inside the lesion under the transducer compression (arrows) (Frequency: 22 MHz). (**d**) Color Doppler ultrasound shows rich blood flow signals inside the lesion once the compression relieved (arrows) (Frequency: 22 MHz)

Key Points

- Hemangioma is a common congenital benign tumor.
- On gray-scale ultrasound, it is mainly divided into nodular and diffuse types.
- Most of the nodular types show subcutaneous hypoechoic lesions. Some of lesions show spongiform or honeycombed appearance, with posterior acoustic enhancement.
- The diffuse types show hyperechoic, irregular, and ill-defined lesions without space-occupying effect.
- The diagnosis can be identified by the "compression test" on color Doppler ultrasound.

5.4.2 Port Wine Stains

5.4.2.1 Clinical Manifestation and Pathology

Port wine stain (PWS) is the most common capillary malformations. PWS is a congenital disease with an incidence of 0.3% ~ 0.5%. PWS occurs most frequently in the head, face, and neck, followed by the extremities, chest, and back. Visual appearance of the lesion shows erythema at birth, and the color of erythema will change with influencing factors such as temperature and mood, fading or partially fading on compression. The lesion is irregular and well-defined. It is difficult to resolve spontaneously, and with age, the area of erythema increases correspondingly and the color gradually deepens. As the disease progresses, PWS tends to form nodules, known as thickened nodular PWS, which is rare.

Clinically, PWS can be divided into three types:

1. Pink type: The lesion is flat, light pink to red, and totally fading with compression.
2. Purple-red type: The lesion is flat, light to deep purple-red, and not totally fading with compression.
3. Thickened type: The lesion is thickened or nodular hyperplasia, not fading or slightly fading with compression.

The pathogenesis of PWS is still unclear, and it has been shown that the nerve distribution in PWS is significantly reduced compared with normal skin. A decrease in the neurovascular ratio may lead to vasodilator malformations, which may be an important factor in its pathogenesis.

The pathological changes of PWS are dilatation of capillaries and venules in the dermal papillary layer and reticular layer. Histology shows that it is mainly a superficial dermal telangiectasia malformation caused by congenital weakness of the capillary wall. The wall of the malformed vessels is composed of a single layer of endothelial cells without proliferation, which is different from hemangiomas characterized by vascular endothelial cell proliferation.

5.4.2.2 Ultrasound Manifestation

Gray-Scale Ultrasound

The dermis of the erythematous area is usually thicker than that in the normal side. Without compression, ultrasound biomicroscopy can show hypoechoic "reticular formation" in a hyperechoic dermis, which corresponds to telangiectasia and venular dilatation of the dermal papillary layer and reticular layer. However, high frequency ultrasound cannot show the above structures (Fig. 5.83). It should be noted that "reticulation" is common in adult patients and can be used for assessment after treatment. The "reticular formation" of the lesion in adolescents and children is not clear, which may be related to the fact that the lesion is too tiny to be visualized by ultrasound.

Color Doppler Ultrasound

Theoretically, the blood flow signals in the erythematous area should be rich. However, due to the thin lumen of the dilated vessels and the slow blood flow velocity, blood flow signals on color Doppler are often rare, and even absent. At present, for most patients with PWS, color Doppler ultrasound cannot reflect the changes of blood flow. Only in some adult patients with PWS, increased blood flow signals is visualized on color Doppler ultrasound.

5.4.2.3 Differential Diagnosis

Infantile Hemangioma

PWS in children less than 6 months needs to be differentiated from infantile hemangioma. Both diseases appear as erythema in the face early. PWS shows a flat erythema, while infantile hemangioma has a proliferative process and appears as gradually elevated bright red granular erythema. Color Doppler ultrasound shows richer blood flow signals in infantile hemangioma than in PWS.

5.4.2.4 Diagnosis Clues

1. The diagnosis of PWS is mainly based on clinical history and manifestations. The erythema appears at birth, and the color will

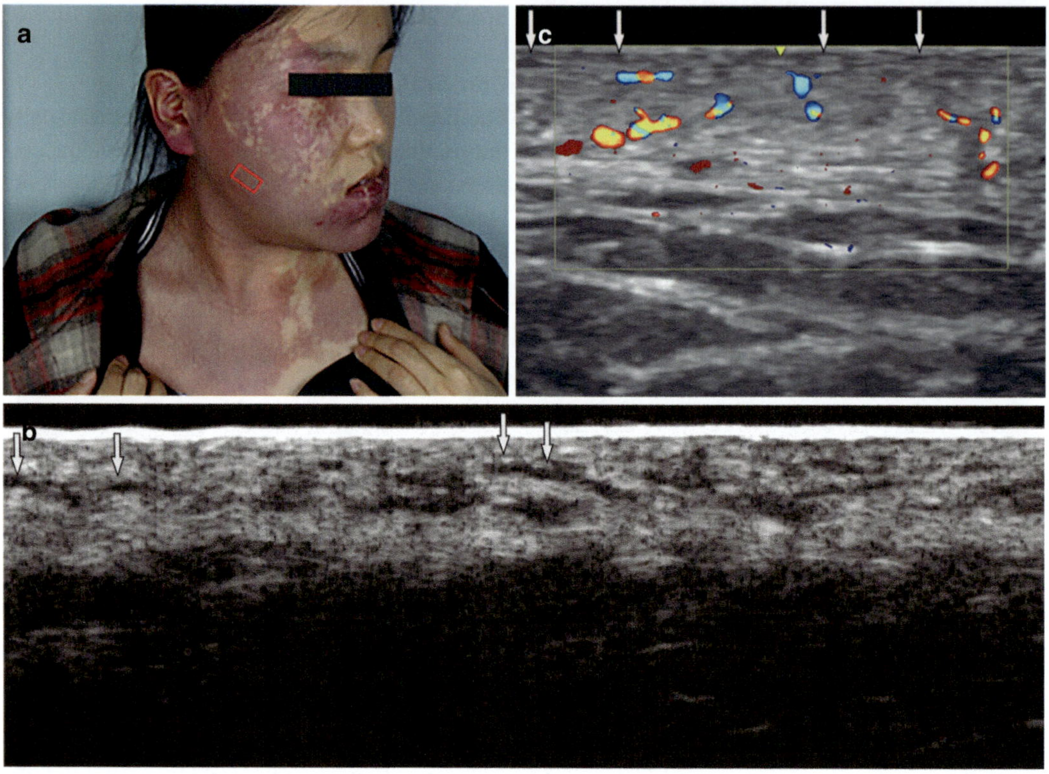

Fig. 5.83 Port wine stains. Female, 29 years of age. (**a**) Visual observation shows a large area of erythema in the right side of the face and neck. The surface is smooth. (**b**) Gray-scale ultrasound biomicroscopy shows that the dermis layer is thicker than the normal side, with several transverse tubular hypoechoic structures, parallel to the body surface (arrows) (Frequency: 50 MHz). (**c**) Color Doppler ultrasound shows that the tubular hypoechoic structure in the dermis is not clearly visualized with blood flow signals (arrows) (Frequency: 22 MHz)

change with temperature, mood, and other factors, fading or partially fading by compression. When necessary, histological examination is needed to establish the diagnosis.

2. Gray-scale ultrasound shows that the dermis in the erythematous area is thicker than that of normal side. Without compression, ultrasound biomicroscopy shows the "reticular formation" in the dermis of the erythematous area parallel to the body surface.

Key Points

- PWS is the most common congenital malformation of capillaries.
- Gray-scale ultrasound shows that the dermis in the erythematous area is thicker than that of normal side. Ultrasound biomicroscopy will show the "reticular formation" in the dermis.
- Blood flow signals in PWS is difficult to visualize on high-frequency ultrasound.

5.5 Summary

5.5.1 Summary of Benign Skin Tumors

Benign skin tumors have a high incidence and often cause unnecessary concerns for patients, and some benign tumors are easily identified by high-frequency ultrasound. Kuwano et al. conducted a retrospective study of 183 patients with lipoma, epidermal cyst, and ganglion cyst. The results indicated that compared with palpation, high-frequency ultrasound improved the accuracy of preoperative diagnosis of the above soft tumor significantly (29% vs. 46%). However, it should be noted that the high-frequency ultrasound features of benign skin tumors are more diverse compared with malignant tumors, and there are often different ultrasound features with the same disease.

For example, according to the patient's age, lesion location and depth, human intervention, vascularization degree, and the formation of thrombosis, the high-frequency ultrasound features of hemangioma are especially various as hyperechogenicity, isoechogenicity, hypoechogenicity, and mixed echogenicity. Spongiform structure and the changes of blood flow signals with compression are diagnostic clues for hemangioma.

In addition, there are a wide variety of benign diseases originated from skin appendages such as sweat glands. High-frequency ultrasound features of this category of tumor need to be summarized to improve the diagnostic accuracy.

Previous studies confirmed that high-frequency ultrasound played an active role in the preoperative planning of benign skin tumors. Among them, Takemura et al. found that high-frequency ultrasound helped to assess the wall of epidermoid cysts, facilitating the surgeon to handle the cyst wall more accurately. In some cases, hemangioma appears as an ill-defined heterogeneous area, but the boundary on ultrasound can still provide some hints to dermatologists, especially the relationship with deep blood vessels.

5.5.2 Summary of Malignant Skin Tumors

In general, most cutaneous malignancies, such as MM, BCC, and SCC, all present as solid and irregular hypoechoic lesions on ultrasound. Various diseases also have characteristic features, such as the presence of scattered or clustered hyperechogenic spots in BCC, the tendency of deep invasion of MM, the special crawling growth pattern of EMPD or BD, and the "whirlpool sign" of fat infiltration in dermatofibrosarcoma protuberans.

In addition, high-frequency ultrasound also provides information on the margins of malignant tumors. Previous studies have confirmed that high-frequency ultrasound can accurately delineate the contour of BCC before surgery, and the preoperative tumor volume on high-frequency ultrasound has a good correlation with the result on histopathology.

One previous study indicated that high-frequency ultrasound of 20 MHz was more sensitive to subclinical invasion of bulky tumors (> 17.4 mm in diameter). With the development of high-frequency ultrasound, some studies have confirmed that in MM with an average thickness of 0.4 mm, the value of high-frequency ultrasound of 75 MHz is correlated with Breslow thickness (the distance from the granular layer to the bottom of the tumor). Our study found that high-frequency ultrasound of 50 MHz could clearly show the layers of involvement and skin appendageal invasion of EMPD, providing the information for the staging of tumors.

In addition, there are some special cases of skin malignancies, such as bulky tumors, including tumors with large surface area, which is much larger than the transducer field. At this time, the splicing of multiple images or EFOV imaging is needed. However, none of the above methods can overcome the distortion and deformation of the images. On the other hand, for tumors that extend in depth, the focus of clinicians is whether there is involvement of deep muscles, bones, and lymph nodes. At this time, lower frequency ultrasound (< 15 MHz) is recommended.

5.5.3 Diagnostic Clues of Common Skin Tumors

Skin tumors are complex and diverse, and dermatologists often make an initial diagnosis based on the visual appearance of the lesion previously. The diagnosis of skin tumors are mainly based on skin biopsy. High-frequency ultrasound is used to preoperatively assess the size, layers of involvement, and boundary of skin tumors. Therefore, it is favored by dermatologists due to its non-radiation, convenience, and real-time. Although skin tumors are complex, most of them have their characteristic features on ultrasound. The authors have analyzed a large number of cases in Shanghai Skin Disease Hospital and summarized the diagnostic points of common skin tumors (Table 5.9).

Table 5.9 Diagnostic clues of common skin tumors on high-frequency ultrasound

Diagnostic clues	Basal cell carcinoma	Squamous cell carcinoma	Bowen's disease	Actinic keratosis	Seborrheic keratosis
Layers of involvement	Epidermis and/or dermis	Epidermis and dermis, or the whole layers of the skin	Epidermis	Epidermis	Epidermis
Echogenicity	Heterogeneous, lesions often with hyperechoic spots and/or anechoic areas	Homogeneous or heterogeneous, some lesions with anechoic areas	Homogeneous, hypoechogenicity	Homogeneous, hypoechogenicity	Homogeneous, hypoechogenicity
Growth pattern	Regular, nodular or crawling	Nodular, irregular	Crawling	Nodular or crawling	Nodular or crawling
Boundary of bottom	Well-defined	Ill-defined	Clear demarcation between bottom and dermis	Unclear demarcation between bottom and dermis	Clear demarcation between bottom and dermis
Keratinization	No abnormal keratinization	Various degrees of abnormal keratinization with posterior acoustic shadowing	Severe hyperkeratosis with posterior acoustic shadowing	Mild abnormal keratinization with pale acoustic shadowing	Severe hyperkeratosis with posterior acoustic shadowing
Color Doppler ultrasound	Rich, visible nutrient vessels	Rich, visible nutrient vessels/ vessels cannot be visualized due to abnormal keratinization	Rare/vessels cannot be visualized due to abnormal keratinization	Rare/vessels cannot be visualized due to abnormal keratinization	Rich/rare /vessels cannot be visualized due to abnormal keratinization

Key Points

- Ultrasound is valuable in preoperatively assessing the size, layers of involvement, and boundary of skin tumors.
- Although skin diseases are complex, most of them have their characteristic features on ultrasound.

Suggested Reading

1. Yu CW. Ultrasonographic observation of superficial epidermoid cyst by high frequency ultrasonography [J] (in Chinese). J Clinical Ultrasound Med. 2015;17(12):860–1.
2. Liu PP, Zhang CP, He P, et al. Value of high frequency ultrasound in diagnosis of external hair root sheath cyst [J] (in Chinese). Chinese J Ultrasound Med. 2019;35(3):266–8.
3. Guo WX. Ultrasound medicine [M] (in Chinese). 6th ed. Beijing: People's Military Medical Press; 2011.
4. Zeng HC, Guo L, Han W, et al. Value of high frequency ultrasonography in differential diagnosis of pilomatrixoma and epidermoid cyst [J] (in Chinese). J Clinical Ultrasound Med. 2016;18(5):326–9.
5. Wang LH, Chen FM, Zhao B, et al. Clinical and ultrasound diagnosis of pilomatrixoma [J] (in Chinese). Chinese J Ultrasound Med. 2017;33(9):806–8.
6. W CY, Zhao XM, Xia YH et al., Analysis of ultrasonic misdiagnosis of surface angioleiomyoma [J] (in Chinese). J Clinical Ultrasound Med. 2015;17(10):702–4.
7. Wang SQ, Liu J, Liu ZR, et al. Analysis of skin high-frequency ultrasonography and dermoscopy characteristics of lipid keratosis [J] (in Chinese). Chinese J Dermatol. 2018;51(11):815–9.
8. Li YF, Liu XQ, Yu M, et al. Clinicopathological analysis of 25 cases of poroma [J] (in Chinese). J Diagnostic Pathol. 2017;24(3):170–3.
9. Wang Y, Xu HX, Xie XY. High-frequency ultrasonographic findings of rare focal lesions of sialic gland [J] (in Chinese). Chinese J Med Ultrasound. 2011;8(6):70–3.
10. Liu LN, Xu HX, Xie XY, et al. Discussion on high-frequency ultrasonographic diagnosis of superficial

soft tissue [J] (in Chinese). Chinese J Ultrasound Med. 2010;26(6):558–62.
11. Chinese expert consensus on standardized pathological diagnosis of melanoma (2017 Edition) [J] (in Chinese). Chinese J Pathol. 2018:1.
12. Zhu XL, Qiu L. Clinical and ultrasonographic characteristics of cutaneous basal cell carcinoma and squamous cell carcinoma [J] (in Chinese). Chinese J Ultrasound Med. 2018;34(11):1045–8.
13. Wang J, Zhao L, Li HH, et al. Clinical characteristics of 62 cases of cutaneous metastatic carcinoma [J] (in Chinese). J Clin Oncol. 2016;21(4):336–9.
14. Chen XC, Lu XM, Zhou GZ, et al. Clinical and histopathological analysis of 47 cases of Paget's disease [J] (in Chinese). Chinese J Leprosy Dermatol. 2017;33(2):103–5.
15. Yue LX. Practical ultrasonic diagnostics of superficial organs and soft tissues [M] (in Chinese). Version 2. Beijing: People's Medical Publishing House; 2017.
16. Wang ML, Liu HX. Progress in pathogenesis and treatment of nevus flammeus [J] (in Chinese). Chinese J Leprosy Dermatol. 2019;35(9):564–7.
17. Yuan WH, Hsu HC, Lai YC, et al. Differences in sonographic features of ruptured and unruptured epidermal cysts [J]. J Ultrasound Med. 2012;31(2):265–72.
18. Huang CC, Ko SF, Huang HY, et al. Epidermal cysts in the superficial soft tissue: sonographic features with an emphasis on the pseudotestis pattern [J]. J Ultrasound Med. 2011;30(1):11–7.
19. Kuwano Y, Ishizaki K, Watanabe R, et al. Efficacy of diagnostic ultrasonography of lipomas, epidermal cysts, and ganglions [J]. Arch Dermatol. 2009;145(7):761–4.
20. He P, Cui LG, Wang JR, et al. Trichilemmal cyst: clinical and sonographic features [J]. J Ultrasound Med. 2019;38(1):91–6.
21. Ramaswamy AS, Manjunatha HK, Sunilkumar B, et al. Morphological spectrum of Pilar cysts [J]. N Am J Med Sci. 2013;5(2):124–8.
22. Sadath HN, Ramachandra S, Kumar MA, et al. Multicentric calcified trichilemmal cysts with alopecia universalis affecting siblings [J]. Indian J Dermatol Venereol Leprol. 2013;79(1):88–91.
23. Wagner JM, Rebik K, Spicer PJ. Ultrasound of soft tissue masses and fluid collections [J]. Radiol Clin N Am. 2019;57(3):657–69.
24. Buehler A, Diot G, Volz T, et al. Imaging of fatty tumors: appearance of subcutaneous lipomas in optoacoustic images [J]. J Biophotonics. 2017;10(8):983–9.
25. Tsuruta D, Nakagawa K, Taniguchi S, et al. Combined cutaneous hamartoma encompassing benign melanocytic naevus, vellus hair cyst and epidermoid cyst [J]. Clin Exp Dermatol. 2000;25(1):38–40.
26. de Giorgi V, Massi D, Sestini S, et al. Cutaneous collision tumour (melanocytic, naevus, basal cell carcinoma, seborrhoeic keratosis): a clinical, dermoscopic and pathological case report [J]. Br J Dermatol. 2005;152(4):787–90.
27. Kittler H. Dermatoscopic-pathological correlation of melanocytic skin lesions [J]. Hautarzt. 2018;69(7):528–35.
28. Malvehy J, Pellacani G. Dermoscopy, confocal microscopy and other non-invasive tools for the diagnosis of non-melanoma skin cancers and other skin conditions [J]. Acta Derm Venereol. 2017;Suppl 218:22–30.
29. Askari SK, Schram SE, Wenner RA, et al. Evaluation of prospectively collected presenting signs/symptoms of biopsy-proven melanoma, basal cell carcinoma, squamous cell carcinoma, and seborrheic keratosis in an elderly male population [J]. J Am Acad Dermatol. 2007;56(5):739–47.
30. Wollina U. Seborrheic keratoses-the most common benign skin tumor of humans. Clinical presentation and an update on pathogenesis and treatment options [J]. Open access Maced. J Med Sci. 2018;6(11):2270–5.
31. Hawkes JE, Woodcock J, Christensen LC, et al. Giant pilomatricoma with angiomyxoid stroma: unusual presentation of a benign tumor [J]. JAAD Case Rep. 2015;1(4):169–71.
32. Solivetti FM, Elia F, Drusco A, et al. Epithelioma of malherbe: new ultrasound patterns [J]. J Clin Exp Cancer Research. 2010;29(1):42–8.
33. Ogawa R. Keloid and hypertrophic scars are the result of chronic inflammation in the reticular dermis [J]. Int J Mol Sci. 2017;18(3):606.
34. Reinholz M, Schwaiger H, Poetschke, et al. Objective and subjective treatment evaluation of scars using optical coherence tomography, sonography, photography, and standardised questionnaires [J]. Eur J Dermatol. 2016;26(6):599–608.
35. Kwiek B, Schwartz RA. Keratoacanthoma (KA): an update and review [J]. J Am Acad Dermatol. 2016;74(6):1220–33.
36. Ra SH, Su A, Li X, et al. Keratoacanthoma and squamous cell carcinoma are distinct from a molecular perspective [J]. Mod Pathol. 2015;28(6):799–806.
37. Watchorn RE, Thomas S, Miller C, et al. Keratoacanthoma management: results of a survey of U.K. dermatologists and surgeons [J]. Br J Dermatol. 2018;178(1):e49–50.
38. Won KY, Park SY, Jin W, et al. Dermatofibroma: sonographic findings and pathologic correlation [J]. Acta Radiol. 2018;59(4):454–9.
39. Zarchi K, Kromann CB, Wortsman X, et al. Usefulness of ultrasound for the diagnosis of dermatofibroma [J]. Med Ultrason. 2016;18(1):132–3.
40. Ryu JA, Lee SH, Cha EY, et al. Sonographic differentiation between schwannomas and neurofibromas in the musculoskeletal system [J]. J Ultrasound Med. 2015;34(12):2253–60.
41. Raffin D, Zaragoza J, Georgescou G. High-frequency ultrasound imaging for cutaneous neurofibroma in patients with neurofibromatosis type I [J]. Eur J Dermatol. 2017;27(3):260–5.

42. Lin AL, Gutmann DH. Advances in the treatment of neurofibromatosis-associated tumours [J]. Nat Rev Clin Oncol. 2013;10(11):616–24.
43. Zarchi K, Wortsman X, Jemec GB. Ultrasound as a diagnostic aid in identifying neurofibromas [J]. Pediatr Dermatol. 2014;31:535–7.
44. Yang JW, Kim JS, Lee DC, et a1. The radial artery superficial palmar branch flap: a modified free thenar flap with constant innervation [J]. J Reconstr Microsurg, 2010, 26(8): 529–38.
45. Li MX, Guo LH, Wang Q, et al. Imaging findings of Bowen's disease: a comparison between ultrasound biomicroscopy (UBM) and conventional high-frequency ultrasound (HFUS) [J]. Skin Res Technol. 2020;26(5):654–63.
46. Zhang JZ, Zhou J, Zhang ZC. Subcutaneous angioleiomyoma: clinical and sonographic features with histopathologic correlation [J]. J Ultrasound Med. 2016;35(8):1669–73.
47. Bosic M, Kirchner M, Volckmar AL, et al. Targeted molecular profiling reveals genetic heterogeneity of poromas and porocarcinomas [J]. Pathology. 2018;50(3):327–32.
48. Col C, Yilmaz EE. Caesarean scar endometrioma: case series [J]. World J Clin Cases. 2014;2(5):133–6.
49. Lumbiganon P, Laopaiboon M, Gulmezoglu AM, et al. Method of delivery and pregnancy outcomes in Asia: the WHO global survey on maternal and perinatal health 2007-2008 [J]. Lancet. 2010;375(9713):490–9.
50. Djaković I, Vuković A, Bolanča I, et al. Abdominal wall endometriosis eleven years after cesarean section: case report [J]. Acta Clin Croat. 2017;56(1):162–5.
51. Rindos NB, Mansuria S. Diagnosis and management of abdominal wall endometriosis: a systematic review and clinical recommendations [J]. Obstet Gynecol Surv. 2017;72(2):116–22.
52. Morton CA, Birnie AJ, Eedy DJ. British Association of Dermatologists' guidelines for the management of squamous cell carcinoma in situ (Bowen's disease) 2014 [J]. Br J Dermatol. 2014;170(2):245–60.
53. Neagu TP, Tiglis M, Botezatu D, et al. Clinical, histological and therapeutic features of Bowen's disease [J]. Romanian J Morphol Embryol. 2017;58(1):33–40.
54. Petrella LI, Pereira WC, Valle HA, et al. Study of superficial basal cell carcinomas and Bowen disease by qualitative and quantitative ultrasound biomicroscopy approach [J]. Conf Proc IEEE Eng Med Biol Soc. 2010;2010:5999–6002.
55. Cameron MC, Lee E, Hibler BP, et al. Basal cell carcinoma: epidemiology; pathophysiology; clinical and histological subtypes; and disease associations [J]. J Am Acad Dermatol. 2019;80(2):303–17.
56. Vega N, Wortsman X, Navarrete N, et al. Color Doppler ultrasound supports early diagnosis of mixed high and low risk of recurrence subtypes in the same basal cell carcinoma lesion [J]. Dermatol Surg. 2018;44(5):741–3.
57. Wang SQ, Liu J, Zhu QL, et al. High-frequency ultrasound features of basal cell carcinoma and its association with histological recurrence risk [J]. Chin Med J. 2019;132(17):2021–6.
58. Wortsman X, Vergara P, Castro A, et al. Ultrasound as predictor of histologic subtypes linked to recurrence in basal cell carcinoma of the skin [J]. J Eur Acad Dermatol Venereol. 2015;29(4):702–7.
59. Hernández-Ibáñez C, Blazquez-Sánchez N, Aguilar-Bernier M, et al. Usefulness of high-frequency ultrasound in the classification of histologic subtypes of primary basal cell carcinoma [J]. Actas Dermosifiliogr. 2017;108(1):42–51.
60. Desai TD, Desai AD, Horowitz DC, et al. The use of high-frequency ultrasound in the evaluation of superficial and nodular basal cell carcinomas [J]. Dermatol Surg. 2007;33(10):1220–7.
61. Hogue L, Harvey VM. Basal cell carcinoma, squamous cell carcinoma, and cutaneous melanoma in skin of color patients [J]. Dermatol Clin. 2019;37(4):519–26.
62. Korhonen N, Ylitalo L, Luukkaala T, et al. Characteristics and trends of cutaneous squamous cell carcinoma in a patient cohort in Finland 2006-2015 [J]. Acta Derm Venereol. 2019;99(4): 412–6.
63. Que SKT, Zwald FO, Schmults CD. Cutaneous squamous cell carcinoma: incidence, risk factors, diagnosis, and staging [J]. J Am Acad Dermatol. 2018;78(2):237–47.
64. Hernández Ibáñez C, Aguilar Bernier M, de Troya Martín M. Ultrasound in the management of non-melanoma skin cancer [J]. Actas Dermosifiliogr. 2015;106(Suppl 1):21–8.
65. Kozovska Z, Gabrisova V, Kucerova L. Malignant melanoma: diagnosis, treatment and cancer stem cells [J]. Neoplasma. 2016;63(4):510–7.
66. Wong SL, Faries MB, Kennedy EB, et al. Sentinel lymph node biopsy and management of regional lymph nodes in melanoma: American society of clinical oncology and society of surgical oncology clinical practice guideline update [J]. J Clin Oncol. 2018;36(4):399–413.
67. Niebling MG, Haydu LE, Karim RZ, et al. Reproducibility of AJCC staging parameters in primary cutaneous melanoma: an analysis of 4924 cases [J]. Ann Surg Oncol. 2013;20(12):3969–75.
68. Uematsu T, Kasami M, Kiyohara Y. B-mode ultrasound imaging, Doppler imaging, and real-time elastography in cutaneous malignant melanoma and lymph node metastases [J]. Healthcare (Basel). 2013;1(1):84–95.
69. Blum A, Schmid-Wendtner MH, Mauss-Kiefer V, et al. Ultrasound mapping of lymph node and subcutaneous metastases in patients with cutaneous melanoma: results of a prospective multicenter study [J]. Dermatology. 2006;212(1):47–52.
70. Cohen JM, Granter SR, Werchniak AE. Risk stratification in extramammary Paget disease [J]. Clin Exp Dermatol. 2015;40(5):473–8.

71. Keung EZ, Gershenwald JE. The eighth edition American joint committee on cancer (AJCC) melanoma staging system: implications for melanoma treatment and care [J]. Expert Rev Anticancer Ther. 2018;18(8):775–84.
72. Hata M, Koike I, Wada H, et al. Radiation therapy for extramammary Paget's disease: treatment outcomes and prognostic factors [J]. Ann Oncol. 2014;25(1):291–7.
73. Llombart B, Serra C, Requena C, et al. Guidelines for diagnosis and treatment of cutaneous sarcomas: dermatofibrosarcoma protuberans [J]. Actas Dermosifiliogr. 2018;109(10):868–77.
74. Ma C, Sun Y, Yang X, et al. Improving precision of resection by pre-surgery inspections with contrast-enhanced ultrasound for dermatofibrosarcoma protuberans [J]. Dermatol Ther. 2016;29(6):473–5.
75. Criscito MC, Martires KJ, Stein JA. Prognostic factors, treatment, and survival in dermatofibrosarcoma protuberans [J]. JAMA Dermatol. 2016;152(12):1365–71.
76. Cardoso JC, Calonje E. Malignant sweat gland tumours: an update [J]. Histopathology. 2015;67(5):589–606.
77. Tolkachjov SN, Hocker TL, Baum CL, et al. Treatment of porocarcinoma with mohs micrographic surgery: the Mayo clinic experience [J]. Dermatol Surg. 2016;42(6):745–50.
78. Worley B, Owen JL, Bolotin D, et al. Evidence-based clinical practice guidelines for microcystic adnexal carcinoma: informed by a systematic review [J]. JAMA Dermatol. 2019;155(9):1059–68.
79. Hadravsky L, Kazakov DV, Stehlik J, et al. Aggressive extraocular sebaceous carcinoma of the scalp involving the brain in a patient with Muir-Torre syndrome [J]. Am J Dermatopathol. 2016;38(8):618–22.
80. Cicinelli MV, Kaliki S. Ocular sebaceous gland carcinoma: an update of the literature [J]. Int Ophthalmol. 2019;39(5):1187–97.
81. Kaliki S, Gupta A, Ali MH, et al. Prognosis of eyelid sebaceous gland carcinoma based on the tumor category of the American joint committee on cancer (AJCC) classification [J]. Int Ophthalmol. 2016;36(5):681–90.
82. Baum SH, Mohr C. Metastases from distant primary tumours on the head and neck: clinical manifestation and diagnostics of 91 cases [J]. Oral Maxillofac Surg. 2018;22(2):119–28.
83. Wong CY, Helm MA, Helm TN, et al. Patterns of skin metastases: a review of 25 years' experience at a single cancer center [J]. Int J Dermatol. 2014;53(1):56–60.
84. Thompson JF, Haydu LE, Uren RF, et al. Preoperative ultrasound assessment of regional lymph nodes in melanoma patients does not provide reliable nodal staging: results from a large multicenter trial [J]. Ann Surg. 2021;273(4):814–20.
85. He L, Huang G. Spectral Doppler ultrasound for predicting long-term response to topical timolol in children with infantile hemangioma [J]. J Clin Ultrasound. 2017;45(8):480–7.
86. Requena L, Santonja C, Martinez-Amo JL, et al. Cutaneous epithelioid sarcomalike (pseudomyogenic) hemangioendothelioma: a little-known low-grade cutaneous vascular neoplasm [J]. JAMA Dermatol. 2013;149(4):459–65.
87. Latrive A, Teixeira LR, Gomes AS, et al. Characterization of skin port-wine stain and hemangioma vascular lesions using Doppler OCT [J]. Skin Res Technol. 2016;22(2):223–9.
88. Johnson CM, Navarro OM. Clinical and sonographic features of pediatric soft-tissue vascular anomalies part 2: vascular malformations [J]. Pediatr Radiol. 2017;47(9):1196–208.
89. Gong X, Yu W, Li J, et al. High-frequency ultrasound investigation of port-wine stains: hemodynamic features revealed by 10- and 22- MHz transducers [J]. J Ultrasound Med. 2019;38(3):641–8.
90. Troilius A, Svendsen G, Ljunggren B. Ultrasound investigation of port wine stains [J]. Acta Derm Venereol. 2000;80(3):196–9.
91. Chen ST, Guo LH, Yan JN, et al. Ultrasound biomicroscopy and high-frequency ultrasound for evaluating extramammary Paget disease with pathologic correlation [J]. J Ultrasound Med. 2019;38(12):3229–37.
92. Jambusaria-Pahlajani A, Schmults CD, Miller CJ, et al. Test characteristics of high-resolution ultrasound in the preoperative assessment of margins of basal cell and squamous cell carcinoma in patients undergoing Mohs micrographic surgery [J]. Dermatol Surg. 2009;35(1):9–15.
93. Marmur ES, Berkowitz EZ, Fuchs BS, et al. Use of high-frequency, high-resolution ultrasound before Mohs surgery [J]. Dermatol Surg. 2010;36(6):841–7.
94. Wortsman X, Castro A, Figueroa A. Color Doppler ultrasound assessment of morphology and types of fistulous tracts in hidradenitis suppurativa (HS) [J]. J Am Acad Dermatol. 2016;75(4):760–7.
95. Takemura N, Fujii N, Tanaka T. Epidermal cysts: the best surgical method can be determined by ultrasonographic imaging [J]. Clin Exp Dermatol. 2007;32(4):445–7.
96. Huang SY, Xiang X, Guo RQ, et al. Quantitative assessment of treatment efficacy in keloids using high-frequency ultrasound and shear wave elastography: a preliminary study [J]. Sci Rep. 2020;10(1):1375.
97. Ohara K, Fujisawa Y, Murata Y, et al. A proposal for a TNM staging system for extramammary Paget disease: retrospective analysis of 301 patients with invasive primary tumors [J]. J Dermatol Sci. 2016;83(3):234–9.
98. Bichakjian CK, Olencki T, Aasi SZ, et al. Basal cell skin cancer, version 1.2016, NCCN clinical practice guidelines in oncology [J]. J Natl Compr Cancer Netw. 2016;14(5):574–97.
99. Brantsch KD, Meisner C, Schonfisch B, et al. Analysis of risk factors determining prognosis of

cutaneous squamous-cell carcinoma: a prospective study [J]. Lancet Oncol. 2008;9(8):713–20.
100. Jambusaria-Pahlajani A, Kanetsky PA, Karia PS, et al. Evaluation of AJCC tumor staging for cutaneous squamous cell carcinoma and a proposed alternative tumor staging system [J]. JAMA Dermatol. 2013;149(4):402–10.
101. Work Group, Invited Reviewers, Kim JYS, et al. Guidelines of care for the management of cutaneous squamous cell carcinoma [J]. J Am Acad Dermatol. 2018;78(3):560–78.
102. Tripodi SA, Rocca BJ, Mourmouras V, et al. Benign glomus tumor of the urinary bladder [J]. Arch Pathol Lab Med. 2013;137(7):1005–8.
103. Park HJ, Jeon YH, Kim SS, et al. Gray-scale and color Doppler sonographic appearances of nonsubungual soft-tissue glomus tumors [J]. J Clin Ultrasound. 2011;39(6):305–9.
104. Kaya TI, Ikizoglu G, Kokturk A, et al. A simple surgical technique for the treatment of steatocystoma multiplex [J]. Int J Dermatol. 2001;40(12):785–8.
105. Feng YG, Xiao SX, Ren XR, et al. Keratin 17 mutation in pachyonychia congenita type 2 with early onset sebaceous cysts [J]. Br J Dermatol. 2003;148(3):452–5.
106. Alotaibi L, Alsaif M, Alhumidi A, et al. Steatocystoma multiplex suppurativa: a case with unusual giant cysts over the scalp and neck [J]. Case Rep Dermatol. 2019;11(1):71–6.
107. Headington JT. Tumors of the hair follicle. A review [J]. Am J Pathol. 1976;85:480–502.
108. Headington JT. Tricholemmal carcinoma [J]. J Cutan Pathol. 1992;19(2):83–4.
109. Boscaino A, Terracciano LM, Donofrio V, et al. Tricholemmal carcinoma: a study of seven cases [J]. J Cutan Pathol. 1992;19(2):94–9.
110. Niu Z, Wang Y, Zhu Q, et al. The value of high-frequency ultrasonography in the differential diagnosis of early mycosis fungoides and inflammatory skin diseases: a case-control study. Skin Res Technol. 2021;27(3):453–60.
111. Daniel LA, Fernando G, Luis C, et al. Diagnostic value of genotypic analysis in primary cutaneous lymphomas using standardized BIOMED-2 polymerase chain reaction protocols: experience in daily clinical practice. Acta Derm Venereol. 2021;
112. Dippel E, Assaf C, Becker JC, et al. S2k Guidelines – Cutaneous Lymphomas Update 2016 – Part 1: Classification and Diagnosis (ICD10 C82 - C86). John Wiley & Sons, Ltd (101111) 2017; 15(12).
113. Wang Y, Niu Z, Liu J, et al. Value of high-frequency ultrasound in accurate staging of mycosis fungoides/Sézary syndrome. J Ultrasound Med. 2020;39(10):1927–37.

6 Non-tumorous Skin Lesions

Qiao Wang, Xiao-Long Li, Le-Hang Guo, Hui Shi, and Hong-Yan Chen

6.1 Inflammatory Skin Diseases

6.1.1 Cutaneous Edema

6.1.1.1 Clinical Manifestation and Pathology

Cutaneous edema is defined as the retention of excessive fluid in the skin layers and is classified as local or generalized edema. Many diseases can cause cutaneous edema. Generalized edema is mainly caused by cardiogenic, nephrogenic, hepatogenic, and metabolic diseases. Local edema is mainly caused by local trauma, burns, venous thrombosis, and so on.

Clinical manifestations of cutaneous edema include varying degrees of swelling, which are more common in the lower extremities. When pressing the area of edema, there may be depression or not.

6.1.1.2 Ultrasound Manifestation

Gray-Scale Ultrasound

Edema is often characterized by thickened subcutaneous tissue, increased echogenicity, with banded or slit-like hypoechoic structures. There may be manifestations of fluid retention (Fig. 6.1).

6.1.1.3 Differential Diagnosis

Lymphangitis and Erysipelas

These diseases are manifested as swelling of the skin and soft tissues. However, lymphangitis and erysipelas show the increased tension of soft tissue, with redness, swelling, heat, and pain. Color Doppler ultrasound shows rich blood flow signals.

Etiological Identification

Gray-scale ultrasound can detect skin edema without clinical signs, which can prompt clinicians for further examination. Ultrasound can rule out edema caused by thrombosis, but there

Q. Wang (✉)
Department of Medical Ultrasound, Shanghai Skin Disease Hospital, Ultrasound Research and Education Institute, School of Medicine, Tongji University, Shanghai, China

Department of Medical Ultrasound, Shanghai Tenth People's Hospital, Ultrasound Research and Education Institute, School of Medicine, Tongji University, Shanghai, China

X.-L. Li · H. Shi
Department of Medical Ultrasound, Shanghai Tenth People's Hospital, Ultrasound Research and Education Institute, School of Medicine, Tongji University, Shanghai, China

L.-H. Guo
Department of Medical Ultrasound, Shanghai Skin Disease Hospital, Ultrasound Research and Education Institute, School of Medicine, Tongji University, Shanghai, China

H.-Y. Chen
Department of Ultrasound, Shanghai Minhang District Central Hospital, Fudan University, Shanghai, China

H. Xu et al. (eds.), *Diagnostic Ultrasound in Dermatology*,
https://doi.org/10.1007/978-981-16-7345-0_6

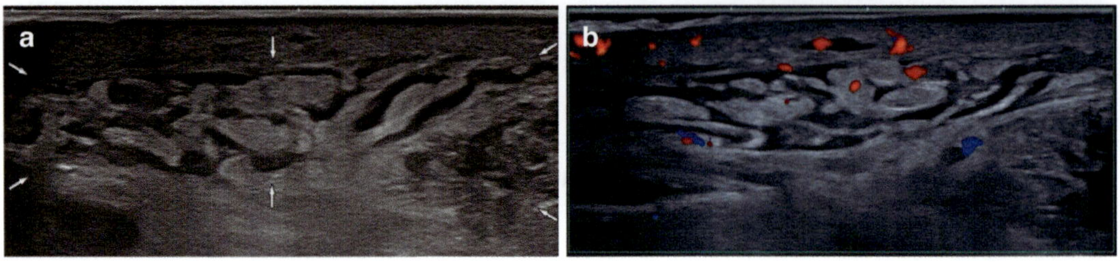

Fig. 6.1 Subcutaneous edema. (**a**) Gray-scale ultrasound shows thickened subcutaneous tissue, increased echogenicity, and slit-like changes (arrows) (Frequency: 24 MHz). (**b**) Color Doppler ultrasound shows rare blood flow signals in the thickened subcutaneous tissue (Frequency: 24 MHz)

are many causes of skin edema, which often need to be combined with clinical history.

6.1.1.4 Diagnosis Clues

1. Cutaneous edema can be diagnosed based on clinical manifestations.
2. Gray-scale ultrasound shows thickened subcutaneous tissue, increased echogenicity, with banded or slit-like hypoechoic structures.

Key Points

- Cutaneous edema is classified as local or generalized edema.
- Gray-scale ultrasound shows thickened subcutaneous tissue, increased echogenicity, with banded or slit-like hypoechoic structures.
- It should be mainly differentiated from lymphangitis and erysipelas.

6.1.2 Panniculitis

6.1.2.1 Clinical Manifestation and Pathology

Panniculitis is an inflammation that occurs in the subcutaneous fat layer. Systemic adipose tissue can be involved, and it is more common in the subcutaneous superficial fat layer. The disease can be a non-suppurative inflammation originated from fat lobule, that is, nodular panniculitis, also known as Weber—Christian disease. It can also be caused by trauma and other causes. The disease often occurs in women. Clinically, the lesions appear as small firm nodules that are red, purplish, or skin-colored, and most of lesions are accompanied by pain.

Histopathologically, it can be divided into lobular panniculitis and septal panniculitis. Pathological findings in the early stage are mainly intralobular adipocytes degeneration and necrosis, with varying degrees of vasculitis changes. The subcutaneous adipose tissue atrophies and fibrosis occur during the later stage, and some lesions have internal calcification. With the progression of the disease, fat liquefaction occurs in some lesions, which called liquefying panniculitis. According to different stages of its pathological process, panniculitis can be divided into nodular panniculitis, liquefying panniculitis, and calcific panniculitis.

6.1.2.2 Ultrasound Manifestation

Gray-Scale Ultrasound

The ultrasound findings of panniculitis are related to the stages of disease pathological process.

1. Nodular panniculitis: It is characterized by increased echogenicity and thickened subcutaneous adipose tissue, with patchy hyperechoic and irregular hypoechoic areas in the lesion. The lesion is irregular and ill-defined without space-occupying effect.
2. Calcific panniculitis: Along with the progression of the disease, hyperechogenicity is visualized in the lesion, with regular or irregular shape and posterior acoustic shadowing.
3. Liquefying panniculitis: Hypoechoic or anechoic areas are visualized in the lesions, which are manifestations of liquefaction necrosis of adipose tissue.

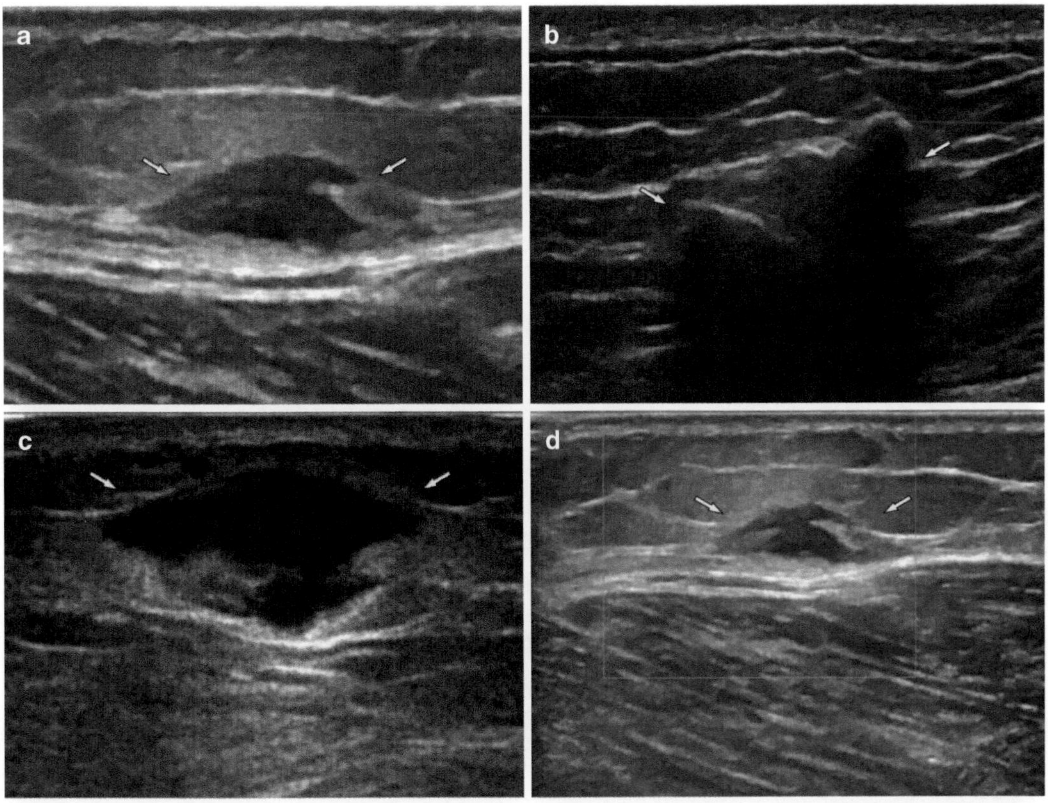

Fig. 6.2 Panniculitis of different stages. (**a**) Nodular panniculitis: Gray-scale ultrasound shows thickened subcutaneous adipose layer with increased echogenicity. The lesion is heterogeneous, with a patchy hypoechoic area inside the hyperechoic area (arrows). The lesion has no space-occupying effect (size: 8.3 mm × 6.9 mm; thickness: 5.1 mm) (Frequency: 15 MHz). (**b**) Calcific panniculitis: Gray-scale ultrasound shows a patchy hyperechoic lesion (arrows) in the subcutaneous adipose layer (size: 10.8 mm × 9.6 mm; thickness: 3.7 mm). The lesion is irregular with a wide posterior acoustic shadowing (Frequency: 15 MHz). (**c**) Liquefying panniculitis: Gray-scale ultrasound shows a mixed echogenic lesion (arrows) in the subcutaneous adipose layer, which is mainly anechoic (size: 11.9 mm × 10.4 mm; thickness: 10.7 mm). The lesion is irregular and well-defined, with the posterior acoustic enhancement (Frequency: 15 MHz). (**d**) Color Doppler ultrasound shows no blood flow signals in the lesion (arrows) (Frequency: 15 MHz)

Color Doppler Ultrasound

Color Doppler ultrasound shows no or rare blood flow signals in the lesion (Fig. 6.2).

6.1.2.3 Differential Diagnosis

Superficial Lipoma

Superficial lipoma is located in subcutaneous tissue, partially appearing as a skin-colored lump. The lesion is soft and most of patients are asymptomatic. Panniculitis, on the other hand, appears as a red or skin-colored hard nodule, and most patients have pain.

On gray-scale ultrasound, lipomas appear as regular, well-defined hyperechoic, isoechoic, or hypoechoic lesions in the subcutaneous tissue. Most of lesions show banded hyperechoic septa. Panniculitis are also heterogeneous, often with liquefaction and calcification. The lesion has no space-occupying effect.

Nodular Fasciitis

Nodular fasciitis originates from fascial tissue and is a benign fibroproliferative lesion. Patients often present with palpable subcutaneous nodules with pain, and the clinical duration is short.

The lesion is usually small in size and grows rapidly. Clinical manifestation of panniculitis is similar to nodular fasciitis.

On gray-scale ultrasound, the location of panniculitis is superficial without space-occupying effect. The lesion is heterogeneous, often with liquefaction and calcification. Nodular fasciitis is deep and closely related to the fascia tissue, appearing as solid hypoechogenicity with rare liquefaction and calcification.

6.1.2.4 Diagnosis Clues

1. Clinical manifestations are helpful in the diagnosis of panniculitis. The lesion appears as a red or skin-colored firm nodule. Most patients have pain.
2. On ultrasound, nodular panniculitis is characterized by thickened subcutaneous adipose tissue, with patchy hyperechoic and irregular hypoechoic areas. Calcific panniculitis appears as a hyperechogenicity in subcutaneous adipose tissue with posterior acoustic shadowing. Liquefying panniculitis is characterized by hypoechoic or anechoic areas in the lesion.

Although ultrasound findings are various at different pathological stages, the lesions are located in the subcutaneous fat layer.

3. On Color Doppler ultrasound, most of lesions have no blood flow signals.

Key Points

- Panniculitis can be divided into nodular panniculitis, liquefying panniculitis, and calcific panniculitis according to disease progression. The disease often occurs in women.
- Ultrasound findings are various at different pathological stages, but the lesions are located in the subcutaneous fat layer. It should be mainly differentiated from superficial lipoma and nodular fasciitis.

6.1.3 Folliculitis

6.1.3.1 Clinical Manifestation and Pathology

Folliculitis is an inflammatory reaction in the superficial aspect of the hair follicle and can involve the follicular opening or the perifollicular hair follicles. The main pathogen is *Staphylococcus aureus*. Weakened body immunity, unclean skin, and sweating are easy to induce the disease.

Folliculitis is common in adult males, and often occurs on scalp, neck, chest, and back. The initial appearance of the lesion is a small papule at follicle opening, with hair passing through the center, and a blush around it. A few days later, small pustules are formed, and yellow scabs will be formed after the pustules rupture or dry up. The disease can heal after the crust falls off and generally leave no scar.

6.1.3.2 Ultrasound Manifestation

Gray-Scale Ultrasound

The dermis where the lesion located is thickened with oblique hypoechoic and ill-defined bands passing through the lesion.

Color Doppler Ultrasound

Color Doppler ultrasound shows blood flow signals in the lesion.

6.1.3.3 Differential Diagnosis

Cellulitis

Clinical manifestations can be used to differentiate the two entities. Cellulitis often occurs on calves and feet. Visual appearance of cellulitis is erythematous, and the surface area is extensive. It involves the deep dermis and subcutaneous tissues. Folliculitis typically appears as a red papule at follicle opening, with hair passing through the center.

Ultrasound also can be used to differentiate the two entities. Characteristic ultrasound features are oblique hypoechoic and ill-defined bands passing through the lesion in folliculitis. Cellulitis is a heterogeneous and hypoechoic lesion in the subcutaneous tissue, with hyperechoic septa. And soft tissues arround the lesion become thickening and hyperechoic.

6.1.3.4 Diagnosis Clues

1. Diagnosis can be based on clinical manifestations. The clinical manifestations of folliculitis are red papules at follicle opening, with hair passing through the center.

2. Ultrasound shows thickened dermis with oblique hypoechoic bands, which is the follicle.

Key Points
Folliculitis is a suppurative inflammation of the follicle opening, and often occurs on scalp, neck, chest, and back. The main pathogenic bacteria are *Staphylococcus aureus*.

Ultrasound shows thickened dermis, with hypoechoic and ill-defined bands passing through the lesion.

6.1.4 Cellulitis

6.1.4.1 Clinical Manifestation and Pathology

Cellulitis is a group of diffuse suppurative infections involving the dermis and lymphatic vessels. The disease is induced by tinea pedis and local infection. Most lesions are caused by Streptococci, and a few lesions are caused by *Staphylococcus aureus*. Cellulitis involves the deep dermis and subcutaneous tissues.

The lesion appears as an extensive and poorly circumscribed red macule. It often occurs on calves and feet. The clinical manifestations are redness, swelling, heat, and pain of the local skin. Patients always have high fever. In severe cases, the lesions will develop into local abscesses, and gangrene will occur. Laboratory tests show increased leukocyte, erythrocyte sedimentation rate, and C-reactive protein.

6.1.4.2 Ultrasound Manifestation

Gray-Scale Ultrasound

Gray-scale ultrasound shows a heterogeneous and hypoechoic lesion located in the subcutaneous tissue, with hyperechoic septa. The lesion has no capsule and space-occupying effect. At the same time, soft tissues around the lesion become thickening and hyperechoic significantly. Anechoic areas with poor acoustic transmission will appear in the lesion, that is, abscess.

Color Doppler Ultrasound

Color Doppler ultrasound shows increased blood flow signals predominantly in the periphery of the lesion (Fig. 6.3).

6.1.4.3 Differential Diagnosis

The ultrasound findings of cellulitis are similar to lymphangitis and erysipelas. However, lesion involvement in depth is deeper than that of lymphangitis and erysipelas, and the area of lesion's

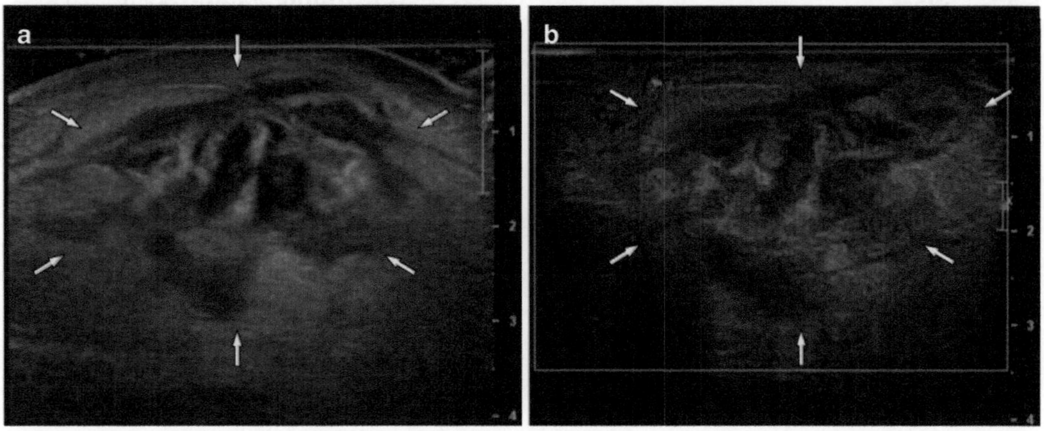

Fig. 6.3 Cellulitis. Male, 32 years of age. (**a**) Gray-scale ultrasound shows a mixed echogenic lesion (arrows) in the subcutaneous tissue. It is heterogeneous with hyperechoic septa (size: 62.6 mm × 58.7 mm; thickness: 55.6 mm). The lesion is irregular and ill-defined (Frequency: 15 MHz). (**b**) Color Doppler ultrasound shows rare blood flow signals in the periphery, and no blood flow signals inside the lesion (arrows) (Frequency: 15 MHz)

visual appearance is not as large as the both entities. Further, abscesses are more likely to occur in cellulitis. It is difficult to differentiate the three entities by ultrasound. The diagnosis needs to combine with clinical manifestations.

6.1.4.4 Diagnosis Clues

The diagnosis of cellulitis is mainly based on clinical manifestations and laboratory tests. Ultrasound examination can provide important information such as the depth of lesion involvement, presence of abscess, foreign body, or vascular injury. Besides, ultrasound is used for follow-up after treatment.

Key Points

- Cellulitis is a group of diffuse suppurative infections involving the dermis and lymphatic vessels.
- Ultrasound shows a heterogeneous and hypoechoic lesion located in the subcutaneous tissue, with hyperechoic septa. Peripheral tissues are thickened and hyperechoic significantly. The lesion has no space-occupying effect.
- Diagnosis of cellulitis is mainly based on clinical manifestations and laboratory tests. It should be mainly differentiated from lymphangitis and erysipelas.

6.1.5 Wart

6.1.5.1 Clinical Manifestation and Pathology

Warts are common entities that form when keratinocytes are infected with human papilloma virus (HPV). With the infection and clonal proliferation of the basal layer, the epidermis is thickened and hyperkeratotic. After a few weeks or months, warts will be detected by the naked eye. Visual appearance is largely determined by the location. In the areas of hands, feet, or trunk, warts initially appear as tiny papules. Gradually, the lesions increase in size, and become round or polygonal in shape. The lesions are skin-colored or yellowish-gray with papillomatous and keratotic ("verruciform") surface (Fig. 6.4). In the areas of plantar foot, warts often grow in an endophytic manner due to pressure they are exposed to. Therefore, only the surface part of the lesion can be clinically visible, while the bulk of the lesion extends into deeper layers and is invisible.

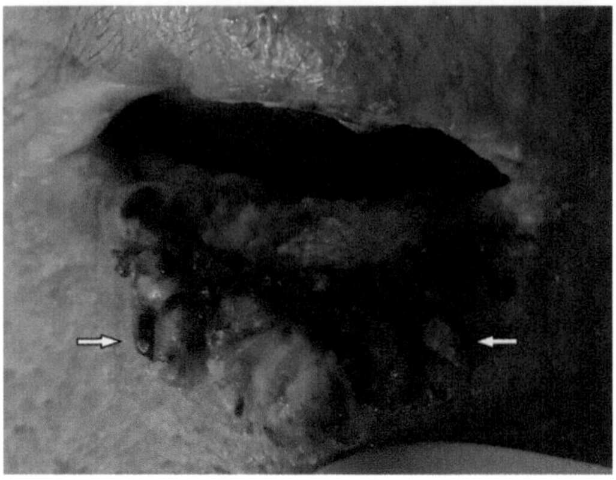

Fig. 6.4 Visual appearance of wart. A yellowish-gray rough plaque in the lower lip (arrows)

Warts are common skin diseases that can occur at any age, especially in childhood. Studies have showed that 5% to 30% of children and young adults suffer from warts. Warts can persist for many years without inflammation, and it is self-limited. The spontaneous remission rates of warts are significantly higher in children than in adults.

The main pathology of warts is vacuolar cell and papillomatous hyperplasia in the upper part of the spinous layer and granular layer, hyperkeratosis and parakeratosis in the stratum corneum. Warts can be subdivided into common warts, plantar warts, flat warts, and genital warts (condyloma acuminatum) on an anatomical or morphological basis.

6.1.5.2 Ultrasound Manifestation

Gray-Scale Ultrasound

Warts usually appear as irregular and ill-defined hypoechoic lesions located in the epidermis and dermis. The surface is rough caused by abnormal keratinization, with thick posterior acoustic shadowing, which affects the visualization of the interior and bottom of the lesion.

Color Doppler Ultrasound

Color Doppler ultrasound shows blood flow signals in the lesion, but abnormal keratinization will disturb the visualization of blood flow signals (Figs. 6.5 and 6.6).

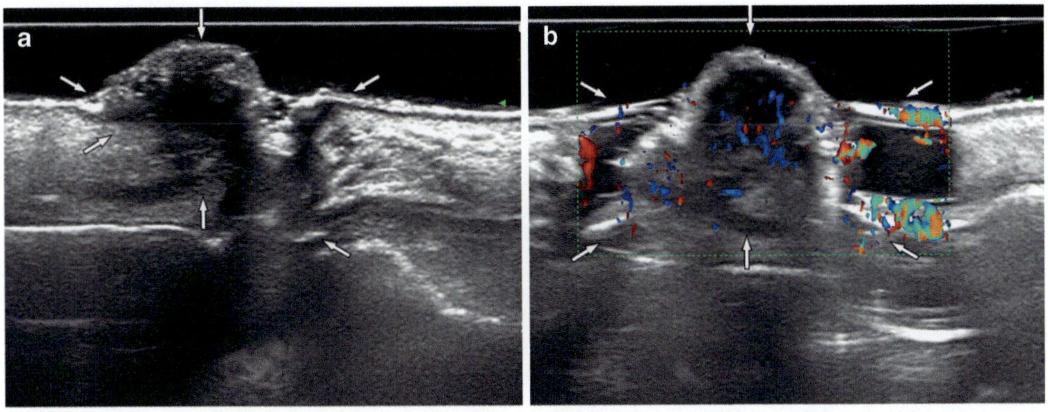

Fig. 6.5 Viral wart. Female, 89 years of age. (**a**) Gray-scale ultrasound shows an irregular, ill-defined, and nodular hypoechoic lesion (arrows) in the epidermal layer (size: 26.0 mm × 10.8 mm; thickness: 5.3 mm). Thick linear hyperechogenicity is observed on the surface, accompanied by posterior acoustic shadowing. The lesion is heterogeneous (Frequency: 22 MHz). (**b**) Color Doppler ultrasound shows blood flow signals in the lesion (arrows) (Frequency: 22 MHz)

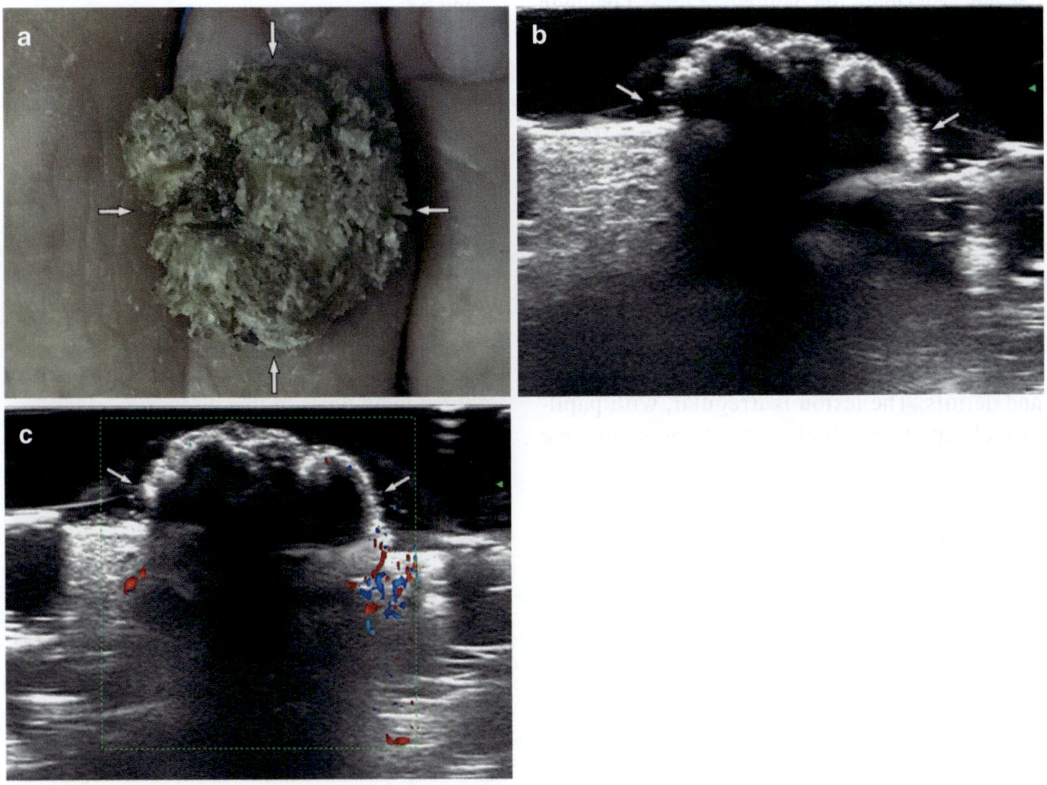

Fig. 6.6 Common wart. Female, 76 years of age. (**a**) Visual observation shows a brown papule about 20.0 mm in diameter on the third toe of the left foot with a rough cauliflower-like surface (arrows). The lesion is hard as cartilage. (**b**) Gray-scale ultrasound shows an irregular hypoechoic lesion (arrows) in the epidermal layer (size: 23.2 mm × 21.9 mm; thickness: 13.0 mm). The surface is convex, and appears as thick linear hyperechogenicity. Posterior acoustic shadowing affects the visualization of the interior and bottom of the lesion (Frequency: 22 MHz). (**c**) Color Doppler ultrasound shows no blood flow signals in the lesion (arrows) (Frequency: 22 MHz)

6.1.5.3 Differential Diagnosis

AK

AK often occurs in the head and face of middle-aged and elderly people. On ultrasound, AK is located in the epidermis. The surface appears as linear hyperechogenicity with posterior acoustic shadowing, but the interior and bottom of the lesion are still be visualized.

Wart often occurs on the feet, lips, and external genitals. On ultrasound, the thick linear hyperechogenicity on the surface is more severe than that of AK, in addition, the interior and bottom are often not visualized.

SK

SK often occurs in middle-aged and elderly people, while wart often occurs in adolescents. SK appears as a small, flat, yellow, or brown patch in the early stage, and characteristics of "cerebriform-like" change in the later stage. Most of warts initially appear as tiny papules, and later appear as round or polygonal bumps. Wart is skin-colored or yellowish-gray with a papillomatous and keratotic ("verruciform") surface.

On gray-scale ultrasound, SK is confined to the epidermis, showing a typical morphology of arcuate elevation with hyperechogenic surface. The lesion is regular in overall morphology. In contrast, wart is located in epidermis and dermis. The lesion is irregular, with papillary elevated and thick linear hyperechogenic surface.

6.1.5.4 Diagnosis Clues

1. Wart is common in adolescents. Most of warts initially appear as tiny papules, and gradually become round or polygonal in shape. The lesion is skin-colored or yellowish-gray with a papillomatous and keratotic ("verruciform") surface.
2. Plantar warts often grow in an endophytic manner, so only the surface part of the lesion can be clinically visible.
3. Ultrasound shows an irregular hypoechoic lesion located in epidermis and dermis. The surface is papillary convex, and shows abnormal keratinization with posterior acoustic shadowing, disturbing the visualization of the interior and bottom of the lesion.
4. Color Doppler ultrasound shows no or rare blood flow signals in the lesion.

Key Points

- Warts are common entities that form when keratinocytes are infected with human papilloma virus (HPV) and common in adolescents.
- Ultrasound shows an irregular hypoechoic lesion in epidermis and dermis. The surface is papillary convex, and shows abnormal keratinization with posterior acoustic shadowing, disturbing the visualization of the interior and bottom of the lesion.
- Wart should mainly be differentiated from AK and SK.

6.1.6 Nodular Fasciitis

6.1.6.1 Clinical Manifestation and Pathology

Fasciitis is a non-specific aseptic inflammation that occurs in the location of muscular fascia attached to the bone. Fasciitis can occur all over the body, mostly in the area of lumbar region, posterior iliac crest, and scapular region. There are three main types of this disease:

1. eosinophilic fasciitis: It is an inflammatory reaction dominated by eosinophils and the skin becomes hard, thickened, and orange-like;
2. necrotizing fasciitis (the most dangerous type): It causes extensive necrosis of the fascia and subcutaneous tissue leading to severe systemic toxicity (usually caused by β-hemolytic streptococci);
3. nodular/pseudosarcomatous/proliferative fasciitis (the most common type): It is characterized by rapid growth of fibroblasts accompanied by mononuclear inflammatory cell infiltration and proliferative capillaries in soft tissues. The disease is benign, but it sometimes mimics a fibrosarcomatous lesion.

Nodular fasciitis (NF) is a benign and rapid proliferation of fibroblasts and myofibroblasts. The etiology of NF is unknown and may be related to trauma, inflammation, and infection. It occurs at all ages, mostly in the 20s ~ 40s. Clinically, it presents as a solitary, palpable, and firm nodule with occasional pain. NF grows rapidly within 2 ~ 4 weeks, and the diameter of most lesions is less than 4 cm. The disease duration is short, often less than 3 months. NF is self-limited.

Histologically, NF can be divided into three subtypes: myxoid or reactive (type I), cellular (type II), and fibrous (type III). The histopathological type can progress with the duration of the disease, from the early active myxoid type to the cellular type, then to the late fibrous type. These subtypes are continuous, so the lesion may contain different histological types.

6.1.6.2 Ultrasound Manifestation

Gray-Scale Ultrasound

Most of NFs appeared as homogeneous hypoechoic or mixed echogenic (predominantly hypoechoic) lesions. The lesion is regular and well-defined, with no capsule. NF can be divided into subcutaneous type, fascial type, and intramuscular type according to anatomical location of the lesion, and different types of NF have characteristic ultrasound findings respectively.

(1) Subcutaneous type (the most common): The lesion is located in the superficial fat layer, which appears as a regular, well-defined, and homogeneous hypoechoic lesion. (2) Fascial type: The lesion is located in the superficial or deep fascia, and this type includes NF in intermuscle. Some lesions extend along the fascia to the fibrous septa of fat lobules, in these cases, lesions show infiltrative growth, ill-defined border, and "string-like" shape. Capsular-like hyperechogenicity is observed around some lesions, and it continues with the fascia around the lesions, showing a "fascial tail sign". (3) Intramuscular type: The lesion is located in the muscle, which is deeply located and bulky. NF of this type appears as a well-defined hypoechoic lesion, with unclear demarcation from muscle bundles and fascia.

The subcutaneous and fascial types belong to the superficial type of NF, that is, lesions located between the dermis and muscle.

Color Doppler Ultrasound

Color Doppler ultrasound shows no or rare blood flow signals in the lesion, mainly in the periphery (Fig. 6.7).

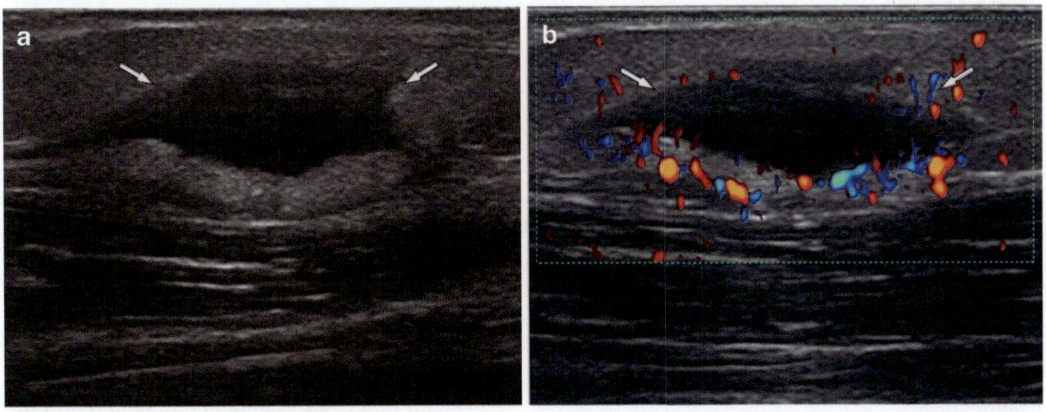

Fig. 6.7 Nodular fasciitis. Female, 25 years of age. (**a**) Gray-scale ultrasound shows an irregular and ill-defined hypoechoic lesion in subcutaneous tissue, with increased echogenicity of the surrounding tissue (arrows). The lesion is closely related to the superficial fascia tissue (size: 15.4 mm × 14.7 mm; thickness: 6.7 mm) (Frequency: 15 MHz). (**b**) Color Doppler ultrasound shows rich blood flow signals in the periphery of the lesion (arrows) (Frequency: 15 MHz)

6.1.6.3 Differential Diagnosis

Superficial Lipoma

Lipomas are soft nodules located in subcutaneous tissue. Some lipomas are elevated with skin-colored surface. Most of patients are asymptomatic. While NFs are usually small in size and grow rapidly, patients often present with a palpable nodule with pain.

On gray-scale ultrasound, lipomas appear as hyperechoic, isoechoic, or hypoechoic lesions in the subcutaneous tissue, with banded hyperechoic septa inside. The lesions are regular and well-defined. While NFs appear as small solid hypoechogenic lesions, closely related to the deep and superficial fascia.

Epidermoid Cyst

Most epidermoid cysts appear as skin-colored hemispherical masses. The cysts are soft and grow slowly, and patients are asymptomatic. While the duration of NF is short, and the lesion often grows rapidly, patients often present with a palpable nodule with pain.

On gray-scale ultrasound, characteristic features of epidermoid cysts are “dot-like” hyperechogenicity, “slit-like” anechogenicity, and/or “onion-like” change. Some lesions show sinus tracts. The location of NFs is closely related to the deep and superficial fascia, appearing as solid hypoechoic small nodules, and there are no sinus tracts.

Panniculitis

Both of the two entities can appear as small firm subcutaneous nodules. Most patients have pain.

On gray-scale ultrasound, the location of panniculitis is superficial without space-occupying effect. The lesion is heterogeneous, often with internal liquefaction and calcification. However, nodular fasciitis is deeply located and closely related to the fascia tissue, showing solid hypoechogenicity and rare liquefaction and calcification.

6.1.6.4 Diagnosis Clues

1. Clinical manifestations are helpful in the diagnosis of NF. The lesion appears as a single rapidly growing nodule, and some patients have pain.
2. On ultrasound, most of NFs appear as regular, well-defined, and homogeneous hypoechoic or mixed echogenic lesions, with no capsule. Different types of NF have different characteristic ultrasound features respectively.
3. Color Doppler ultrasound shows no or rare blood flow signals in the lesion.

Key Points

- NF can be divided into subcutaneous, fascial, and intramuscular types according to the location. It often occurs in young and middle-aged patients. The lesion grows rapidly, and patients will be accompanied by pain.
- Different types of NF show different ultrasound features. The lesion is closely related to the deep and superficial fascia. It should be mainly differentiated from superficial lipoma, epidermoid cyst, and sarcoma.

6.1.7 Scleroderma

6.1.7.1 Clinical Manifestation and Pathology

Scleroderma is a connective tissue disease, including localized scleroderma (LS) and systemic sclerosis (SSc). LS, is also known as morphea, is characterized by inflammation, degeneration, thickening, and fibrosis of the skin and subcutaneous tissues. SSc is characterized by microangiopathy, immune dysregulation, and fibrotic changes affecting the skin and internal organs. SSc can cause multisystem damage, including the digestive tract, lungs, heart, and kidneys, and is one of the connective tissue diseases with the highest mortality rate. Although LS and SSc have some pathophysiologic pathways, they represent different diseases rather than a single disease continuum. The etiology is uncertain, but people who are often exposed to silica have an increased risk of this disease.

The disease often occurs in young and middle-aged women. Clinically, typical skin lesions go through three stages in turn: edema stage, sclerosis stage, and atrophy stage.

1. Edema stage: Skin is non-pitting and hard swelling. Generally, it starts from the hands

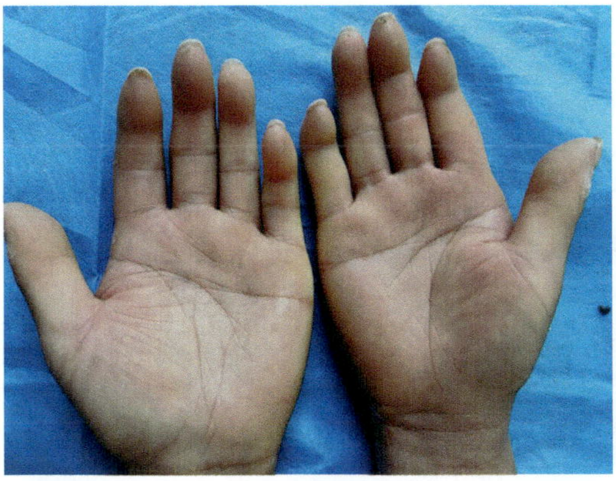

Fig. 6.8 Visual appearance of LC. The skin is smooth and shows waxy yellow leathery changes in hands

and face, and fingers may appear as "sausage-like".

2. Sclerosis stage: The skin gradually becomes thickened and hardened, and the skin surface is smooth and shows waxy yellow leathery changes (Fig. 6.8). And at this stage, skin adheres to deeper tissues, cannot be moved and pinched up, with less hairs. The lesions may involve the face, extremities, and trunk. When the face is involved, "mask face" will be present.
3. Atrophy stage: The lesions may involve subcutaneous tissues and muscles. The whole layers of the skin becomes atrophic and thinned. In some patients, the skin is directly attached to the bone surface, appearing "skinny-like" changes. The skin involved by the lesion is hypohidrotic and hair loss. The degree of skin involvement is related to the severity of organs involvement, adverse reactions, increased disability, and decreased life expectancy.

Pathologically, it can be divided into early (inflammatory and edematous phase) and late (sclerotic and atrophic phase) stages. In the early stage, it is characterized by swelling of dermal collagen fibers, infiltration of inflammatory cells dominated by lymphocytes between dermal collagen and around blood vessels, edema of the vessel wall, and break of elastic fibers. In the late stage, the collagen fiber bundles are hypertrophic and sclerotic, and closely arranged, with inflammatory cell infiltration in perivascular area, wall thickening and sclerosis, narrow or even obstruction of the lumen, atrophy of sebaceous and sweat glands, thinning of the fat layer, and calcium deposition. Anti-Scl-70 antibodies are specific for SSc.

6.1.7.2 Ultrasound Manifestation

Gray-Scale Ultrasound

The ultrasound features of scleroderma are related to the pathological process. In the early stage, scleroderma is characterized by diffuse thickening of the dermis with normal or slightly increased echogenicity. As the disease progresses, the thickness of skin becomes thinner and the echogenicity gradually increases. In the late stage, atrophy of the dermis, subcutaneous soft tissue, and even muscle may occur (Fig. 6.9).

Color Doppler Ultrasound

Color Doppler ultrasound shows no or rare blood flow signals inside the lesion.

SWE

SWE features of scleroderma are related to the degree of skin involvement.

The mean elastic modulus of normal skin is usually less than 100 kPa, and the color is uniform blue or blue-green on two-dimensional SWE image. The mean elastic modulus in scleroderma is usually greater than 200 kPa, and it increases accordingly as the lesion progresses.

6.1.7.3 Differential Diagnosis

Eosinophilic Fasciitis

Eosinophilic fasciitis is a connective tissue disease involving the deep fascia of the skin with scleroderma-like manifestations. The lesion is common on lower extremities. Clinical manifestations of eosinophilic fasciitis range from edema to sclerosis of the skin, also known as orange peel or cobblestone. Groove sign resulting from venous furrowing along the veins in the infiltrated areas is observed in some patients, which is highly suggestive of fasciitis or deep fibrosis. In the early stage of scleroderma, Raynaud's phe-

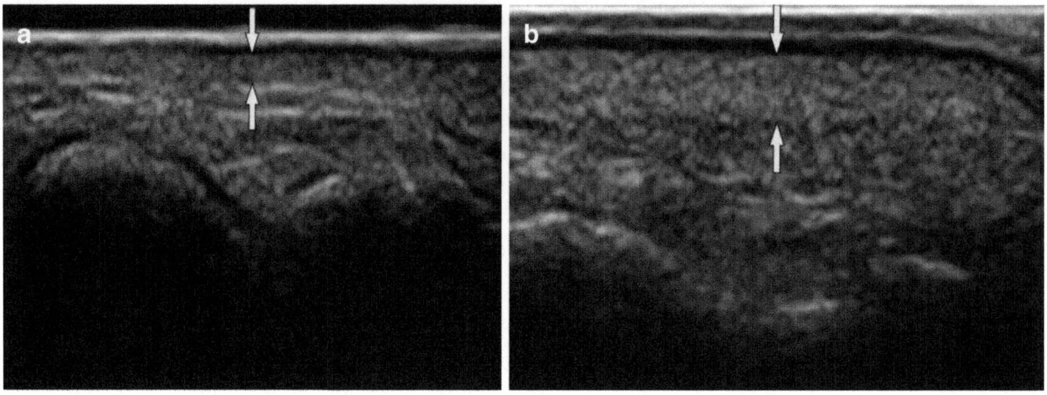

Fig. 6.9 Comparison of skin thickness in healthy individuals and patients with LC. (**a**) Thickness of normal skin is 0.8 mm (arrows). The echogenicity is normal and homogeneous (Frequency: 18 MHz). (**b**) In the early stage of LC, the dermis is thickened to 1.9 mm (arrows). The echogenicity of dermis is homogeneous and slightly increased (Frequency: 18 MHz)

nomenon is more common, and the skin surface will not appear depression.

On ultrasound, scleroderma is mainly located in dermis without space-occupying effect. While, eosinophilic fasciitis is mainly located in the deep subcutaneous tissue, which is closely related to the deep and superficial fascia, and solid hypoechoic lesions are visible sometimes.

Scleredema Adultorum of Buschke

Scleredema adultorum of Buschke is a rare connective tissue disease characterized by fibromucinous thickening of the dermis. It is common in the nape of the neck, the upper back, and shoulders. The lesion progresses symmetrically with diffuse skin hardening, and without skin atrophy and hair loss. The skin of patients with scleredema adultorum of Buschke is wrinkled by pinching and pressing. In contrast, the skin of patients with scleroderma is tight and does not wrinkle. In the advanced stage of scleroderma, skin atrophy and hair loss will occur. The above clinical manifestations can be used to differentiate the two entities.

On gray-scale ultrasound, the dermis of scleredema adultorum of Buschke is thickened, with the thickness about three times that of normal skin. The echogenicity of skin is normal or slightly increased, with hyperechogenic spots sometimes. It is difficult to differentiate from scleroderma.

6.1.7.4 Diagnosis Clues

1. Clinical manifestations are helpful for the diagnosis of scleroderma. The disease is commonly found on the face and lower extremities. The skin becomes hard and not wrinkled, with sweat gland and sebaceous gland dysfunction, hair loss. Raynaud's phenomenon is common.
2. Positive antinuclear antibody and anti-Scl-70 antibody are used to assist the diagnosis.
3. Ultrasound can evaluate changes of skin thickness, reflecting the stage of the disease.
4. SWE can quantitatively assess the degree of skin involvement and the clinical stage of scleroderma.

Key Points

- On gray-scale ultrasound, scleroderma in the early stage shows thickened dermis. With the progression of the disease, the thickness of the skin becomes thinner and the echogenicity increases. Atrophy of dermis, subcutaneous soft tissue, and even muscle will occur in the late stage.
- SWE is used to assess the severity of scleroderma.
- It should be mainly differentiated from eosinophilic fasciitis and scleredema adultorum of Buschke.

6.1.8 Cutaneous Lupus Erythematosus

6.1.8.1 Clinical Manifestation and Pathology

Cutaneous lupus erythematosus (CLE) is a chronic relapsing autoimmune disease. CLE is the cutaneous manifestation of lupus erythematosus and may precede systemic involvement. The etiology of the disease is uncertain, of which genetic factors, environmental factors (sun exposure and smoking), and drugs play an important role. The disease is most common in women, and may be accompanied by pruritus. Most lesions appear as psoriasis-like or pityriasis-like erythema covered with scales.

CLE can be divided into the following subtypes according to clinical manifestations:

1. acute CLE, including localized and generalized CLE;
2. subacute CLE, including annular erythematous and papulosquamous CLE;
3. chronic CLE, including localized and disseminated discoid lupus erythematosus, verrucous lupus erythematosus, swollen lupus erythematosus, deep lupus erythematosus, chilblain lupus erythematosus, and Blaschko linear lupus erythematosus.

Histopathologically, CLE is characterized by dermatitis with liquefaction degeneration of basal cells, accompanied by lymphocytic infiltration of dermal vessels and around appendages. Abnormal keratinization is seen in the epidermis. Materials positively expressed by periodic acid-Schiff reaction (PAS) are deposited at the epidermal/dermal junction, resulting in the formation of atrophic scar. The treatment of CLE aims to prevent recurrence and the formation of scar. Local therapy mainly uses steroids and calcineurin inhibitors, while hydroxychloroquine is used for systemic therapy.

6.1.8.2 Ultrasound Manifestation

Gray-Scale Ultrasound

The lesion appears as thickened dermis and a hypoechoic area within it. The lesion is heterogeneous and well-defined. Meanwhile, the echogenicity of the subcutaneous tissue is increased.

Color Doppler Ultrasound

Color Doppler ultrasound shows blood flow signals inside the lesion (Fig. 6.10).

6.1.8.3 Differential Diagnosis

Psoriasis Vulgaris

Visual appearance of CLE is similar to psoriasis vulgaris, and both diseases can present with scaly erythema. Psoriasis vulgaris is common on the scalp and extremities; while CLE is common on the face.

On gray-scale ultrasound, psoriasis vulgaris is located in the epidermis. The lesion shows thickened spinosum with abnormal keratinization. CLE is mainly located in the dermis and shows thickened dermis with hypoechoic area within it, and the echogenicity of the subcutaneous tissue is increased.

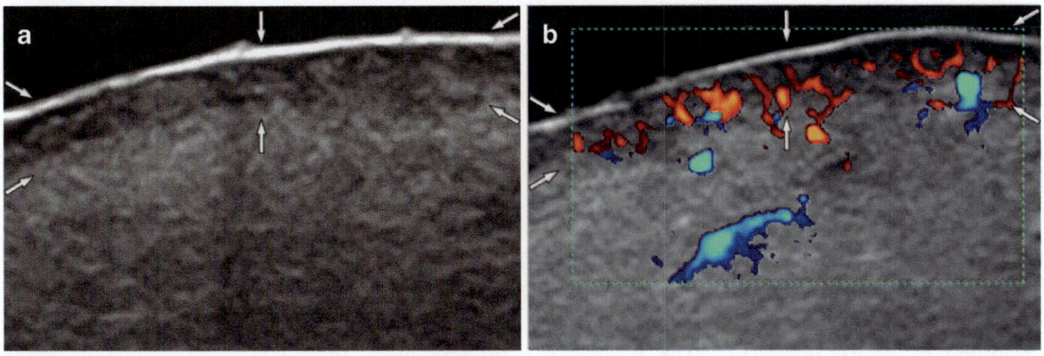

Fig. 6.10 CLE. (**a**) Gray-scale ultrasound shows dermal thickening, with a heterogeneous hypoechoic area under the epidermis (arrows), and the echogenicity of subcutaneous tissue is increased (Frequency: 22 MHz). (**b**) Color Doppler ultrasound shows rich blood flow signals inside the lesion (arrows) (Frequency: 22 MHz)

Dermatomyositis

Both diseases appear as skin erythema. CLE is clinically characterized by butterfly-like erythema on both cheeks. CLE and dermatomyositis can occur at the same time.

On gray-scale ultrasound, CLE shows dermal thickening with a hypoechoic area within it, and increased echogenicity of subcutaneous tissue. However, dermatomyositis shows increased echogenicity of the muscle and subcutaneous soft tissue. Calcification is detected in some lesions. Ultrasound findings are useful to differentiate the two entities.

6.1.8.4 Diagnosis Clues

1. CLE often appears as a round, psoriasis-like or pityriasis-like lesion with squamous erythema, and some patients have pruritus.
2. Gray-scale ultrasound shows thickened dermis and a hypoechoic area within it. The echogenicity of the subcutaneous tissue is increased.
3. Color Doppler ultrasound shows blood flow signals in the lesion.

Key Points

- CLE is divided into acute, subacute, and chronic types based on clinical manifestations. This disease often occurs in women.
- Lesions often show dermal thickening with hypoechoic area within it and increased echogenicity of subcutaneous tissues.
- It should be mainly differentiated from psoriasis vulgaris and dermatomyositis.

6.1.9 Dermatomyositis

6.1.9.1 Clinical Manifestation and Pathology

Dermatomyositis (DM) is an autoimmune connective tissue disease that occurs in the skin, small blood vessels, and skeletal muscle. Clinically, it is characterized by Gottron's papules, Gottron's sign, or muscle weakness, often involving a variety of organs. The disease is accompanied with tumors and other connective tissue diseases sometimes. The etiology is uncertain and is generally considered to be related to gene alterations and virus infections. There are significant ethnic differences in this disease, with African-Americans having the highest incidence. Clinically, 55% of patients present with erythema before myositis, 25% present with erythema during myositis, and 15% present with erythema after myositis.

The skin lesions of DM are mainly manifested as:

1. Gottron papules, that is, facial violaceous eruption on the upper eyelids. These violaceous papules appear on the forehead, zygoma, nose, nasolabial folds, and anterior neck, upper chest (V-shaped distribution), and posterior neck, upper back, shoulders, and lateral upper arm (shawl-shaped distribution).
2. Gottron's sign: Atrophic papules with a few scales on the dorsal of the metacarpophalangeal and proximal interphalangeal joints. The skin of fingerpad is keratinized, thickened, and chapped. Dark black transverse striae can appear on the palmar and lateral surfaces of the fingers.
3. Other mucocutaneous changes: Red atrophic plaques will appear at the scalp, covered with scales, and it is often misdiagnosed as psoriasis or seborrheic dermatitis. Photosensitivity, pruritus, panniculitis, mucin deposition, leukoplakia, lipoatrophy, and Raynaud's phenomenon will also occur.

Pathologically, the skin changes of DM are not specific. In the early stage, erythematous area shows liquefaction and degeneration of basal cells, and atrophy of the spinosum layer. Dermal collagen fibers are edematous, and blood vessels are dilated surrounded by lymphocyte infiltration. In the late stage, the lesion shows atrophy of the epidermis and skin appendages, sclerosis of collagen fibers, and calcification in a few cases. Immunofluorescence examination sometimes shows deposition of IgG, IgM, and C3 at the junction of the epidermis and dermis. The muscle changes of DM are myofibrosis and perivascular inflammatory. In the late stage, lesions show muscular fiber atrophy, sclerosis, and calcification.

6.1.9.2 Ultrasound Manifestation

Gray-Scale Ultrasound

Gray-scale ultrasound shows increased echogenicity of the muscle resulted from edema. Increased echogenicity of the subcutaneous tissue resulted from panniculitis is detected sometimes. Calcification is detected in some lesions and appears as hyperechogenicity with posterior acoustic shadowing.

Color Doppler Ultrasound

There is no blood flow signals inside the lesion (Fig. 6.11).

6.1.9.3 Differential Diagnosis

CLE

CLE is clinically characterized by butterfly erythema on both cheeks. The erythema is psoriasis-like or pityriasis-like and covered with scales, and most lesions are round in shape. CLE and DM will occur at the same time.

On gray-scale ultrasound, CLE shows dermal thickening with a hypoechoic area within it, and increased echogenicity of subcutaneous tissue. However, DM shows increased echogenicity of the muscle and subcutaneous tissue. Calcification would be detected in the lesion sometimes.

Solar Dermatitis

Solar dermatitis is an acute phototoxic reaction that occurs after excessive exposure of normal skin to ultraviolet irradiation, and often involves epidermis. The disease duration is short and the disease usually heals within 1 week. Ultrasound shows increased echogenicity of epidermis.

On the other hand, DM usually lasts for months to years and will be worsen after sun exposure. The two diseases can be differentiated with the assistance of ultrasound findings and patients' clinical history.

6.1.9.4 Diagnosis Clues

1. Clinical manifestations are helpful in the diagnosis of DM: Gottron's papule, Gottron's sign, or muscle weakness.
2. Ultrasound shows increased echogenicity of the muscle and subcutaneous tissue. Calcification with posterior acoustic shadowing is detected sometimes.
3. Most lesions show no blood flow signals on color Doppler ultrasound.

Key Points

- DM shows increased echogenicity of the muscle and subcutaneous tissue. Calcification with posterior acoustic shadowing is detected sometimes.

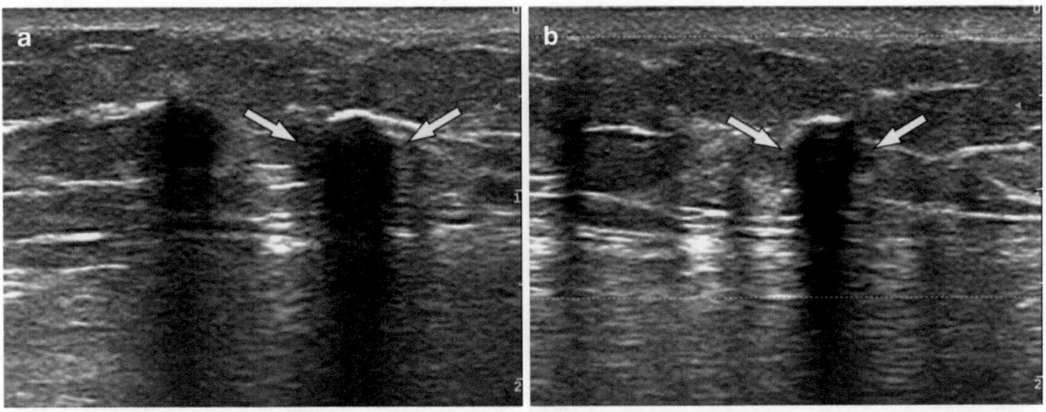

Fig. 6.11 DM. (**a**) Gray-scale ultrasound shows several hyperechoic lesions in the subcutaneous tissue, the size of which is about 13.2 mm × 10.1 mm (arrows). The lesions are curved with posterior acoustic shadowing (Frequency: 15 MHz). (**b**) Color Doppler ultrasound shows no blood flow signals inside the lesion (arrows) (Frequency: 15 MHz)

- It should be mainly differentiated from CLE and solar dermatitis, and ultrasound is used as an adjunct modality in the differential diagnosis of DM.

6.1.10 Radiodermatitis

6.1.10.1 Clinical Manifestation and Pathology

Radiodermatitis is called cutaneous radiation injury, which is an inflammatory change of the skin caused by radiation exposure (mainly X-ray, β ray, or γ ray). The pathogenesis of the disease is that DNA in the nucleus absorbs radiation energy, affecting DNA synthesis and cell differentiation and further resulting in changes in genes.

Radiodermatitis is a very common side effect in radiotherapy of cancer. Radiation has an incubation period for skin damage. Generally, symptoms of skin will appear a few days later when the skin is exposed to high-dose radiation for a short time. Low-dose radiation in skin for a long time has a cumulative effect. After several years or decades, radiodermatitis and even cancer can occur. Clinical manifestations include dermatitis, pigmentation, and irreversible skin atrophy, destruction of sebaceous glands and sweat glands, and permanent hair loss, resulting in ulcer and necrosis of the skin. According to clinical history of radiation exposure, the skin damage occurs at the radiation site and the features are similar to thermal burn, and this disease is easy to diagnose. Once radiodermatitis occurs, radiation exposure should be stopped in time, and attention should be paid to avoid external stimulation.

Pathologically, acute radiodermatitis shows spinosum edema and vacuolar degeneration, mitotic cell differentiation and nuclear pyknosis, liquefaction and necrosis of basal layer, and increased melanin in dermal, and so on. Chronic radiodermatitis shows fibrous thickening of vascular wall, with various degrees of obstruction, hyperkeratosis, granulosum thickened or epidermal atrophy, and various degrees of damage to sebaceous glands, hair follicles, sweat glands, and so on.

6.1.10.2 Ultrasound Manifestation

Gray-Scale Ultrasound

Gray-scale ultrasound shows that the dermis is thickened with decreased echogenicity. It is heterogenous with posterior acoustic shadowing. However, there is no space-occupying effect. The acute radiodermatitis may be accompanied by subcutaneous edema.

Color Doppler Ultrasound

Color Doppler ultrasound shows no or rare blood flow signals in the dermis (Fig. 6.12).

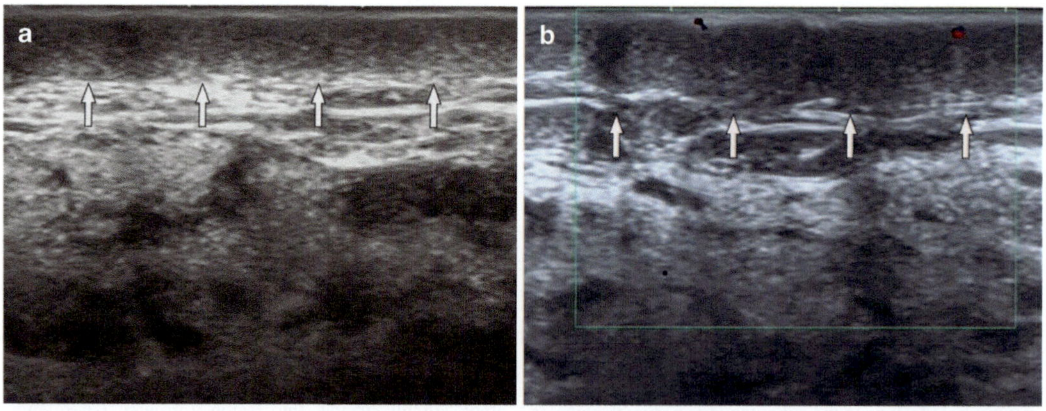

Fig. 6.12 Radiodermatitis after radiotherapy for breast cancer. Female, 30 years of age. (**a**) Gray-scale ultrasound shows the dermis in left breast is thickened (arrows), and the echogenicity is decreased. It is heterogenous with posterior acoustic shadowing (Frequency: 18 MHz). (**b**) Color Doppler ultrasound shows rare blood flow signals in the dermis (arrows) (Frequency: 18 MHz)

6.1.10.3 Differential Diagnosis

Paget's Disease of the Breast

Paget's disease of the breast is a rare disorder of the nipple-areola complex, which is often associated with an underlying in situ or invasive carcinoma.

Eczematoid changes of the nipple-areola complex and soreness or itching should raise suspicion of this disease. Ultrasound shows that the hypoechogenic lesion can involve epidermis, dermis, and even breast glands. Color Doppler ultrasound shows rich blood flow signals. When it is accompanied by ductal carcinoma, an irregular and hypoechoic mass is seen below the nipple.

Radiodermatitis shows that dermis is thickened with decreased echogenicity. Color Doppler ultrasound shows no or rare blood flow signals. Patients with radiodermatitis often have a history of exposure to radiation.

6.1.10.4 Diagnosis Clues

1. Patients often have a history of exposure to radiation.
2. Gray-scale ultrasound shows that the dermis is thickened with decreased echogenicity. Sometimes it is heterogenous with posterior acoustic shadowing. The acute radiodermatitis may be accompanied by subcutaneous edema. Color Doppler ultrasound shows no or rare blood flow signals in the dermis.

Key Points

- Radiodermatitis is an inflammatory change of the skin caused by radiation exposure.
- Radiodermatitis is a very common side effect in radiotherapy of cancer.
- Gray-scale ultrasound shows that the dermis is thickened with decreased echogenicity. Sometimes it is heterogenous with posterior acoustic shadowing. Color Doppler ultrasound shows no or rare blood flow signals in the dermis.

6.1.11 Odontogenic Cutaneous Fistula

6.1.11.1 Clinical Manifestation and Pathology

Fistula is the pathological channel connecting the hollow organ with the body surface or another hollow organ. Odontogenic cutaneous fistula is an abnormal channel between facial skin and oral cavity. Studies showed that 80% of fistulas in maxilloface and neck are odontogenic. When the teeth are not treated in time due to caries, trauma, or developmental deformity, bacteria can invade the pulp directly and cause pulp infection, which further leads to infection of periapical tissue. With the lesion developing, it will extend to the skin through the path with the least resistance and cause skin ulceration, thus forming facial skin fistula.

Odontogenic cutaneous fistula is uncommon in clinic. It appears as a red, smooth nodule with purulent discharge or not (Fig. 6.13). Studies showed that 80% of lesions arised from chronic periradicular abscess of a mandibular tooth. Therefore, most fistulas occur in the area of chin and mandible, and some in the neck. In the patients with odontogenic cutaneous fistula, only

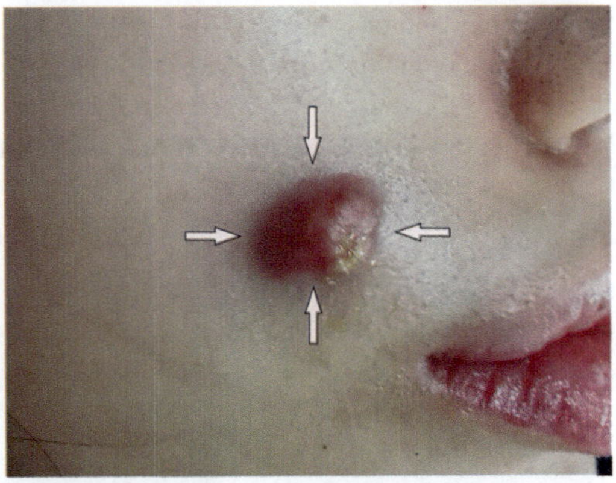

Fig. 6.13 Visual appearance of odontogenic cutaneous fistula. Visual observation shows a dark red nodule in the right cheek with purulent discharge (arrows)

about 50% of the patients had ever presented with toothache. Most of patients have no discomfort.

6.1.11.2 Ultrasound Manifestation

Gray-Scale Ultrasound

Gray-scale ultrasound shows a tubular hypoechoic lesion extending deeply to the maxillary and mandibular edge throughout the epidermis, dermis, and subcutaneous tissue. The surface is elevated without abnormal keratinization. The lesion is irregular, ill-defined, and heterogeneous.

Color Doppler Ultrasound

Color Doppler ultrasound shows rich blood flow signals in the lesion (Fig. 6.14).

6.1.11.3 Differential Diagnosis

Epidermoid Cyst

Epidermoid cyst often occurs in trunk, the lesion is hemispherical, soft, skin-colored and grows slowly. Some lesions have black spots in the center. However, odontogenic cutaneous fistula often occurs in the area of chin and mandible, it appears as a red nodule, sometimes with purulent discharge.

On gray-scale ultrasound, "dot-like" hyperechogenicity and/or irregular "slit-like" anechogenicity are often visualized in epidermoid cyst. Sometimes the lesion is connected to the surface of skin through a hypoechoic sinus tract. Odontogenic cutaneous fistula extends deeply from the skin to the edge of the maxilla or mandible. On color Doppler ultrasound, there are often no blood flow signals in the epidermoid cyst. If the cyst wall ruptures with granulomatous inflammation, blood flow signals will be detected in and around the lesion. However, the skin lesion and fistula of odontogenic cutaneous fistula often show rich blood flow signals.

Skin Abscess

The two diseases are similar in visual appearance as red nodules, and some of lesions show purulent discharge on the surface. On gray-scale ultrasound, most of skin abscesses are located in the subcutaneous tissue, and some lesions with fluctuations. But skin abscess usually has no fistula-like structure.

6.1.11.4 Diagnosis Clues

1. Odontogenic cutaneous fistula appears as a red and smooth nodule with purulent discharge or not, usually without tenderness.
2. Gray-scale ultrasound shows hypoechoic lesion in the epidermis, dermis, and subcutaneous tissue. The lesion extends deeply to the maxillary and mandibular edge through a fistula.

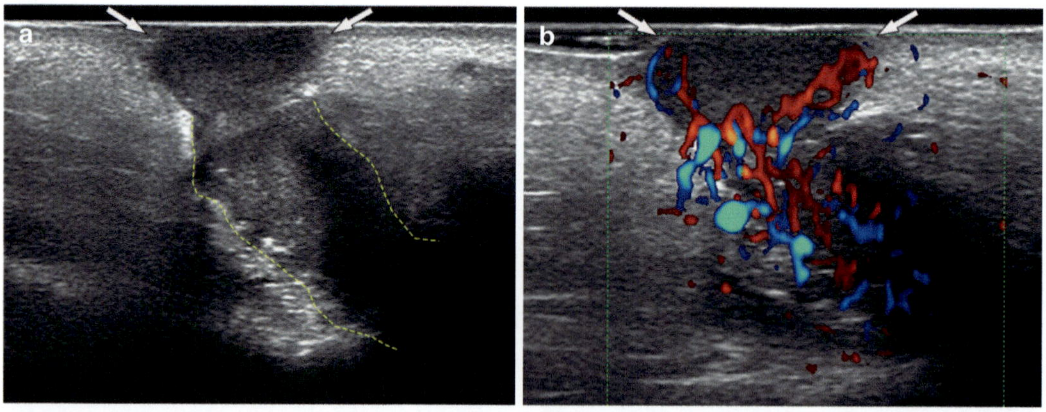

Fig. 6.14 Odontogenic cutaneous fistula. Female, 26 years of age. (**a**) Gray-scale ultrasound shows a hypoechoic lesion (arrows) in the epidermis, dermis, and subcutaneous tissue (size: 12.0 mm × 11.0 mm; thickness: 10.0 mm). The lesion extends deeply to the posterior maxillary edge through a fistula (dotted line) (length: 14.2 mm; width: 8.3 mm). The lesion is irregular, ill-defined, and heterogeneous (Frequency: 15 MHz). (**b**) Color Doppler ultrasound shows rich blood flow signals in the lesion (arrows) (Frequency: 15 MHz)

3. Color Doppler ultrasound shows rich blood flow signals in the lesion.

6.1.11.5 Clinical Significance

Odontogenic cutaneous fistula is rare in clinical practice. Its appearance is similar to skin abscess, furuncle and carbuncle, foreign body injury, and so on. Since the affected teeth often have no obvious clinical symptoms, patients often focus on the negative impacts of fistula on cosmetology, so they often visit the department of surgery, dermatology, or cosmetology.

Ultrasound is a safe and effective method to detect odontogenic cutaneous fistula. Patients with suspected odontogenic cutaneous fistula can be examined by ultrasound firstly. Once diagnosed, the patient should be referred to the department of stomatology in time to avoid delay in treatment.

Key Points

- Odontogenic cutaneous fistula often occurs in the area of chin and mandible, and some of lesions occur in the neck. It appears as a red and smooth nodule with purulent discharge or not.
- Gray-scale ultrasound shows hypoechoic lesion in the epidermis, dermis, and subcutaneous tissue. The lesion extends deeply to the maxillary and mandibular edge through a fistula. Color Doppler ultrasound shows rich blood flow signals in the lesion.
- Odontogenic cutaneous fistula should be differentiated from skin abscess.

6.1.12 Pseudocyst of the Auricle

6.1.12.1 Clinical Manifestation and Pathology

Pseudocyst of the auricle, also known as serous perichondritis of auricle, intracartilage effusion of auricle, is a cystoid swelling containing viscous fluid on the lateral or anterior surface of the cartilage of the auricle. Because there is no epithelial tissue in its cyst wall, it is called pseudocyst. The etiology of pseudocyst of the auricle is uncertain, it may be related to mechanical trauma, compression, immune, congenital dysplasia, and so on. This disease is common in young people between 30 and 50 years old, and is found more in males than females. Pseudocyst of the auricle often occurs in the scaphoid or triangular fossa of the auricle without the back of the auricle involved. It appears as a skin-colored and painless swelling (Fig. 6.15).

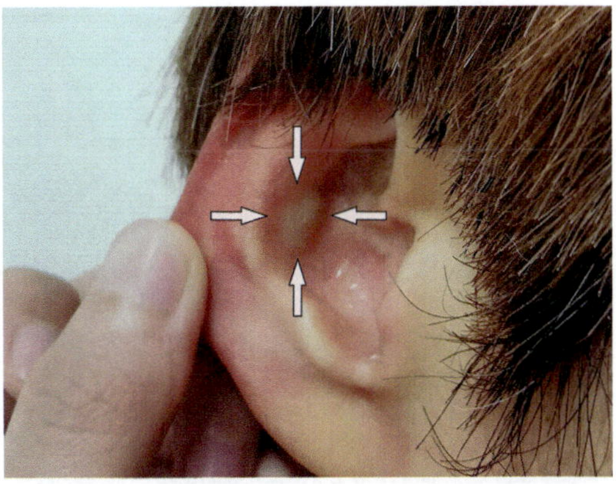

Fig. 6.15 Visual appearance of pseudocyst of the auricle. Visual observation shows a skin-colored lesion with local swelling in the right auricle (size: 18.0 mm × 10.2 mm) (arrows)

6.1.12.2 Ultrasound Manifestation

Gray-Scale Ultrasound

Gray-scale ultrasound often shows local thickening of the auricular cartilage. The lesion is irregular, ill-defined, and heterogenous, with hypoechoic and isoechoic areas found in the lesion.

Color Doppler Ultrasound

Color Doppler ultrasound shows blood flow signals around the lesion (Fig. 6.16).

6.1.12.3 Differential Diagnosis

Epidermoid Cyst

Both of the diseases show skin-colored surface. Epidermoid cyst often occurs in trunk, while pseudocyst of the auricle often occurs in the scaphoid or triangular fossa of the auricle.

On gray-scale ultrasound, "dot-like" hyperechogenicity and/or irregular "slit-like" anechogenicity in the lesion are characteristic features

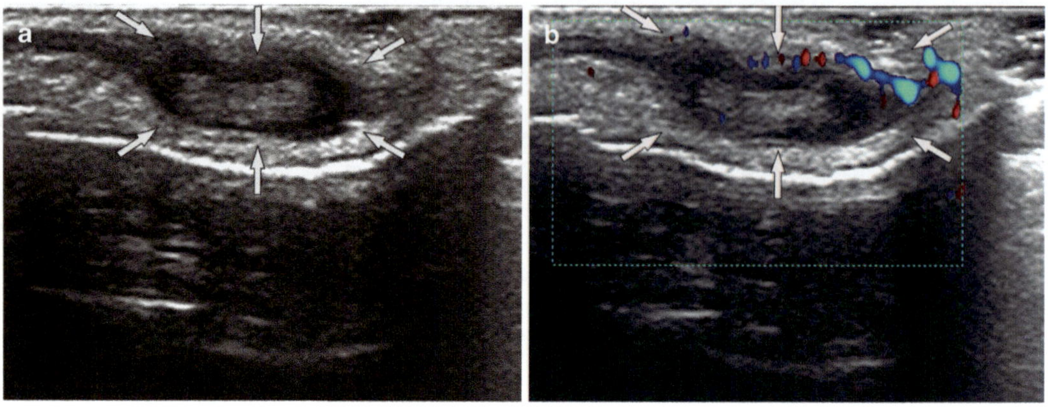

Fig. 6.16 Pseudocyst of the auricle. Male, 39 years of age. (**a**) Gray-scale ultrasound shows local thickening of the auricular cartilage (arrows). It is irregular, ill-defined, and heterogenous with isoechoic areas in the lesion (size: 17.0 mm × 10.2 mm; thickness: 4.5 mm). (**b**) Color Doppler ultrasound shows blood flow signals around the lesion (arrows) (Frequency: 22 MHz)

of epidermoid cyst. Pseudocyst of the auricle is thickening of the auricular cartilage. Gray-scale ultrasound helps to distinguish the two entities.

Gouty Tophi

Gouty tophi appear as draining or chalk-like subcutaneous nodules under transparent skin, often with overlying vascularity. Ears are one of the common sites.

On ultrasound, gouty tophi appear as circumscribed, hypoechoic to hyperechoic, heterogeneous structure with occasional posterior acoustic shadowing, and some lesions show a small anechoic rim. However, pseudocyst of the auricle is local thickening of the auricular cartilage. The ultrasound findings of the two entities are distinct.

6.1.12.4 Diagnosis Clues

1. Pseudocyst of the auricle is more common in young men, mostly in the scaphoid or triangular fossa of the auricle without the back of the auricle involved.
2. Gray-scale ultrasound often shows local thickening of the auricular cartilage with hypoechoic and isoechoic areas in the lesion.
3. Color Doppler ultrasound shows blood flow signals around the lesion.

Key Points

- Pseudocyst of the auricle is common in young men.
- Pseudocyst of the auricle often occurs in the scaphoid or triangular fossa of the auricle without the back of the auricle involved.
- Gray-scale ultrasound shows local thickening of the auricular cartilage with hypoechoic and isoechoic areas in the lesion. Color Doppler ultrasound shows blood flow signals around the lesion.

6.2 Foreign Bodies

6.2.1 Clinical Manifestation and Pathology

Foreign bodies in soft tissues are exogenous objects that enter subcutaneous tissues through the skin. With the rapid development of transportation and construction industry, trauma with subcutaneous tissue foreign bodies is increasingly common. Large foreign bodies are palpable and even visible to the naked eye and are easier to be diagnosed clinically, while tiny foreign bodies embedded in the subcutaneous tissue are difficult to be detected by the naked eye and palpation.

Common foreign bodies are wood chips, glass, metal sheets, and fish bones.

The clinical manifestations are erythema and/or scar on the skin surface of the injured site, or palpable hard mass. Patients have various degrees of pain. Histologically, infiltration of macrophages and inflammatory cells is observed in the lesion.

6.2.2 Ultrasound Manifestation

6.2.2.1 Gray-Scale Ultrasound

Ultrasound can confirm the presence of foreign bodies and provide information about their size and location. However, definite diagnosis of foreign bodies needs to be combined with clinical history. The ultrasound features of foreign bodies of different materials are slightly different, but they have some similarities.

Soft tissue wounds caused by pieces of glass and splinters of wood show punctate, linear, or irregular hyperechoic structures on ultrasound image, with well-defined boundary and no posterior acoustic shadowing (Fig. 6.17A and B).

Broken stone and rubber in soft tissues show punctate or curved hyperechoic structures with posterior acoustic shadowing (Fig. 6.17C, D).

Most fish bones in soft tissues show parallel hyperechoic bands on ultrasound, with well-defined boundary and no posterior acoustic shadowing (Figs. 6.17E and 6.18).

The ultrasound findings of soft tissues around foreign bodies vary according to the presence of infection and bleeding. Sometimes, ultrasound shows hypoechoic areas around foreign body, which are inflammatory or granulomas in the surrounding tissues. If irregular anechoic areas appear in the periphery of the foreign body, there may be abscesses or bleeding.

6.2.2.2 Color Doppler Ultrasound

Color Doppler ultrasound shows blood flow signals around the foreign body. Sometimes, there are no blood flow signals.

6.2.3 Differential Diagnosis

6.2.3.1 Skin Tumor

Some patients do not realize that the foreign body is still left in the tissue at the time of injury, and later present with erythema at the wound site or palpable lumps accompanied by pain. It should be differentiated from skin tumors at this time. Most patients with skin tumors often are asymptomatic, some patients have pruritus and pain. Most of skin tumors show hypoechoic, hyperechoic, or mixed echogenic lesions on gray-scale ultrasound. The foreign bodies show punctate and linear hyperechoic structures. It is easy to differentiate them when ultrasound examination is in combination with clinical history.

6.2.3.2 Erysipelas

The main clinical manifestation of erysipelas is erythema in the lower extremities or face, which is clearly demarcated from the surrounding normal skin. The affected site may be red, swollen, hot, and the patient may feel painful. Gray-scale ultrasound shows thickening of the subcutaneous superficial fat layer. Color Doppler ultrasound shows rich blood flow signals. It is easy to differentiate it from foreign bodies by ultrasound findings and clinical history.

6.2.4 Diagnosis Clues

1. A history of wounds such as glass, wood, or fish bones provide critical information for the diagnosis. Local pain caused by foreign bodies helps to quickly identify the location where foreign bodies may be present.
2. Ultrasound findings of foreign bodies show punctate or linear hyperechoic structures with or without posterior acoustic shadowing. A hypoechoic inflammatory area and/or an anechoic area (abscess or hematoma) may appear around the foreign body in some cases.
3. The location of foreign bodies may migrate, and some of them will be far away from the site of wound. Therefore, it is recommended to expand the scope of ultrasound examination.

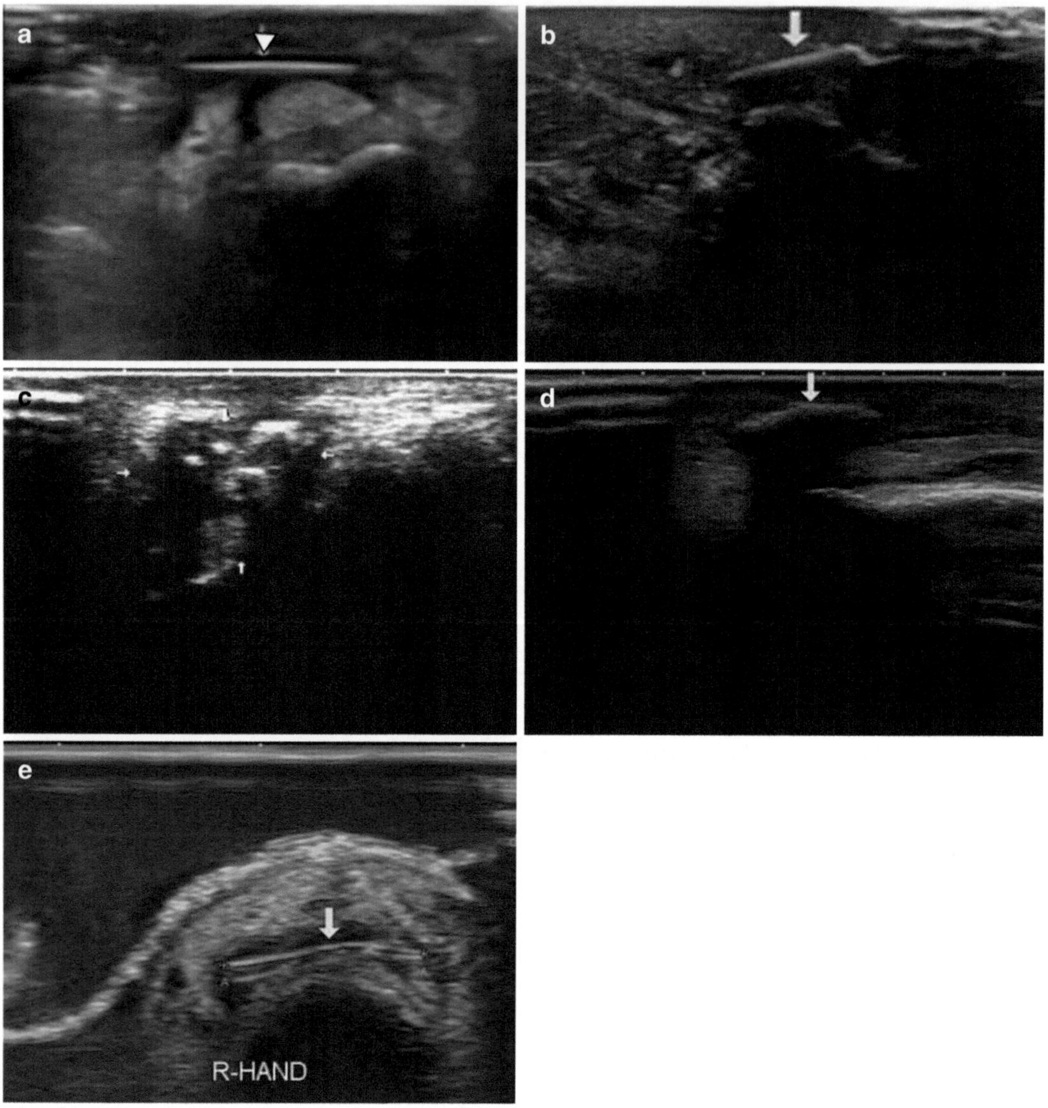

Fig. 6.17 Common foreign bodies in soft tissue. (**a**) Ultrasound image of a piece of glass in subcutaneous tissue of the finger (▽). (**b**) Ultrasound image of a splinter of wood in subcutaneous tissue of the left foot (arrow). (**c**) Ultrasound image of a broken stone in subcutaneous tissue of the face (arrows). (**d**) Ultrasound image of a piece of rubber in subcutaneous tissue of the left arm (arrow). (**e**) Ultrasound image of a fish bone in subcutaneous tissue of the right ring finger (arrow)

Key Points

- Soft tissue foreign bodies are exogenous objects that enter subcutaneous soft tissues through the skin.
- Ultrasound examination usually shows punctate and linear hyperechoic structures.
- Diagnosis of foreign body is mainly based on clinical history. Those with uncertain clinical history should be differentiated from skin tumors and erysipelas.

6.3 Psoriasis and Psoriatic Arthritis

6.3.1 Clinical Manifestation and Pathology

Psoriasis is a chronic inflammatory skin disease. It has a long disease duration, and is prone to recur. The disease often occurs in young adults and

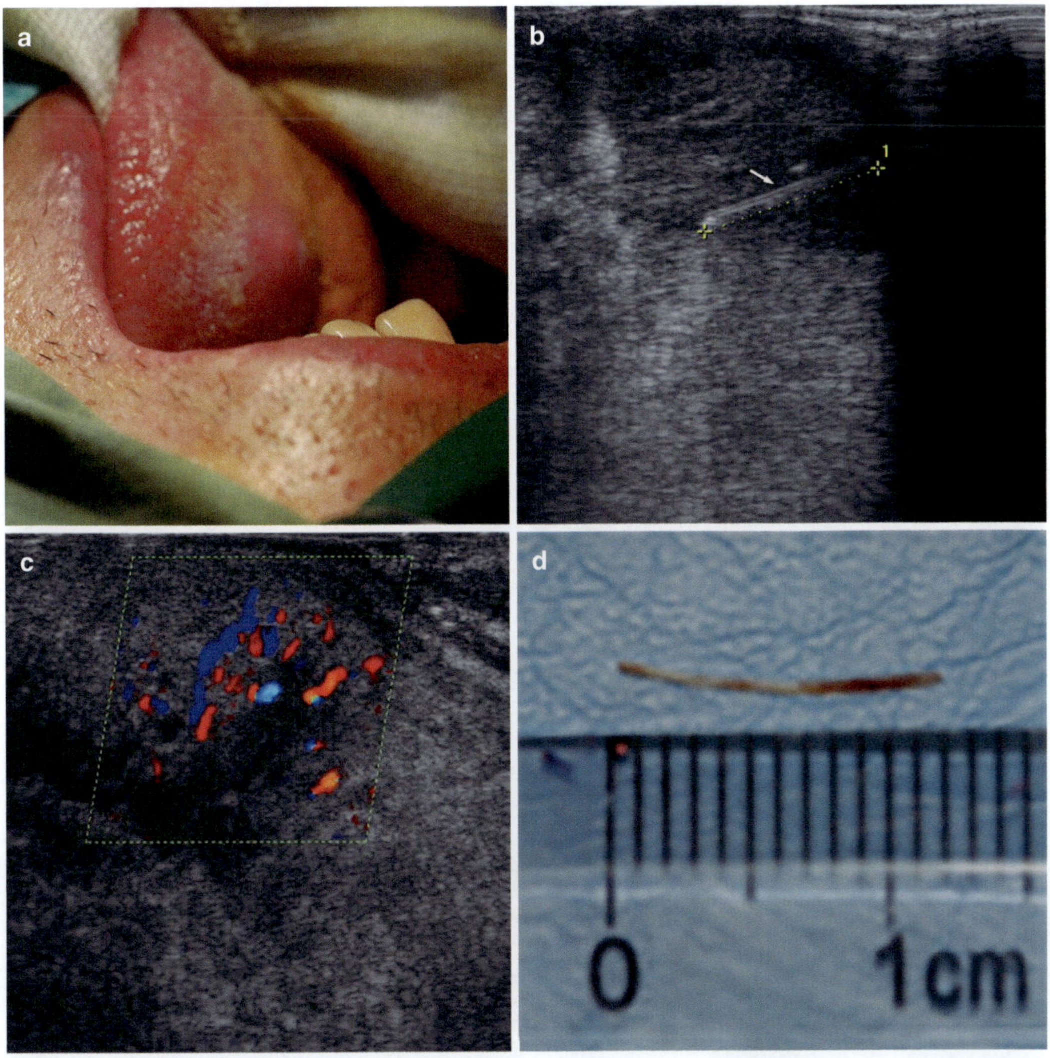

Fig. 6.18 Fish bone in soft tissue. (**a**) Visual observation shows local redness under the tongue. (**b**) Gray-scale ultrasound shows a linear hyperechoic structure (arrow) in the tissue of the tongue, the diameter of which is about 12.0 mm. It is well-defined without posterior acoustic shadowing (Frequency: 15 MHz). (**c**) Color Doppler ultrasound shows rich blood flow signals in hypoechoic areas around the above hyperechoic structure (Frequency: 15 MHz). (**d**) Foreign body of fish bone is removed surgically

mostly affects the skin and joints. The clinical manifestations are mainly erythema and scales. It is common on the scalp and extensor sides of the extremities, and most lesions are aggravated in winter. Genetics, immune, and metabolism have a great impact on its pathogenesis. Besides, infection, drugs, and mental factors also play an important role in its pathogenesis. Psoriasis can be classified into four types based on clinical features: psoriasis vulgaris, pustular psoriasis, erythrodermic psoriasis, and arthropathic psoriasis.

6.3.1.1 Psoriasis Vulgaris

It is the most common type in clinical practice. The lesions are usually multiple with various shape and size. Typical lesion appears as a red papule or maculopapule covered with multiple layers of silvery scales. The scales are easy to be scraped off, and then a light red shiny translucent film was exposed. After scraping off the scales, small bleeding spots, also called "Auspitz sign" are seen. The light red shiny translucent film and the "Auspitz sign" are characteristic features of psoriasis vulgaris. The lesions often occur on the scalp, sacrum, and extensor surfaces of the extremities. Some patients have various degrees of pruritus (Fig. 6.19A).

6.3.1.2 Psoriasis Pustular

It is rare, and often caused by drug irritation, pregnancy, and infection. Clinically, erythema and aseptic pustules are the main features. This disease occurs at any site of the body surface, especially at flexor and ruffled sites of the extremities. Some lesions are confined to the palms. Lesions appear as small pustules on erythema with pruritus or pain. Most of psoriasis pustular have periodic attacks. Psoriatic vulgaris is the type during remission (Fig. 6.19B).

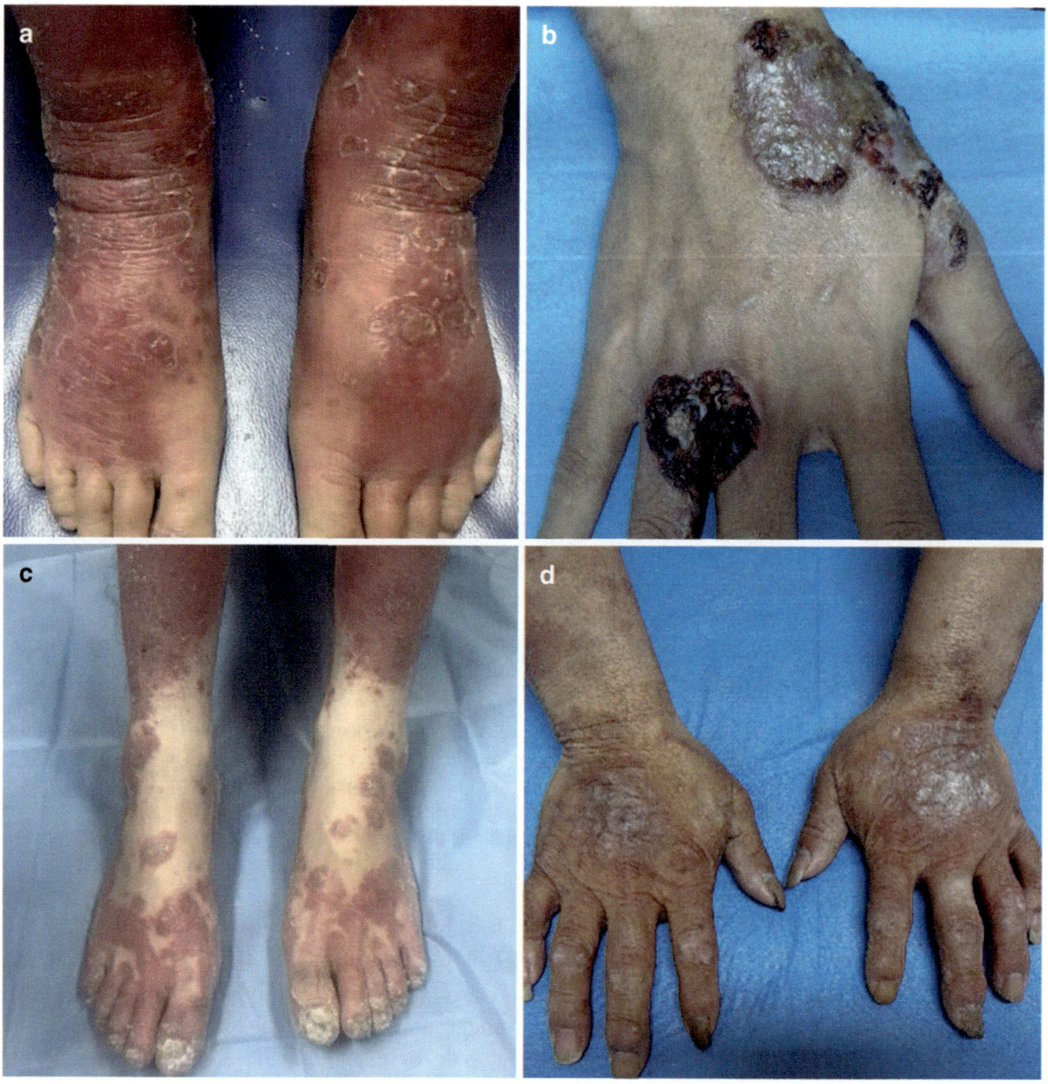

Fig. 6.19 Visual appearance of various types of psoriasis. (**a**) Visual observation of psoriasis vulgaris shows red papules on the lower extremities and dorsum of the feet, covered with silvery scales. (**b**) Visual observation of pustular psoriasis shows dark red papules on the dorsum of the hands covered with scales and pustules. (**c**) Visual observation of erythrodermic psoriasis shows large erythema and desquamation of the lower extremities skin. (**d**) Visual observation of psoriatic arthritis shows red papules on both deformed hands

6.3.1.3 Erythrodermic Psoriasis

It is rare and severe. It is often caused by the use of strong irritant drugs in the advanced stage of psoriasis vulgaris or long-term massive use of glucocorticoids, fast dose reduction, or sudden discontinuation. It appears as massive erythema, swelling, and desquamation of the skin all over the body surface. Some patients have systemic symptoms such as fever and chills, and so on (Fig. 6.19C).

6.3.1.4 Arthropathic Psoriasis

Arthropathic psoriasis is an inflammatory arthropathy associated with psoriasis, is also known as psoriatic arthritis (PsA). It occurs at any age and the peak age is between 30 and 50 years old. There is no significant difference in the incidence between male and female. Patients have symptoms such as pain, stiffness, and deformity of the joints (Fig. 6.19D).

6.3.2 Ultrasound Manifestation

6.3.2.1 Psoriasis Vulgaris

On gray-scale ultrasound, lesions in progressive, stationary, and degenerative phases are located in epidermis. It shows thick and linear hyperechogenic surface with posterior acoustic shadowing. The shadowing indicates hyperkeratosis and hypokeratosis of stratum corneum. Various degrees of thickening of the stratum spinosum are observed in the epidermis, showing a hypoechoic band. The dermis is thickened with increased echogenicity (Fig. 6.20).

6.3.3 Pustular Psoriasis and Erythrodermic Psoriasis

Gray-scale ultrasound findings are similar for the two types. Both types also show relative thick and hyperechoic stratum corneum, however, there is no posterior acoustic shadowing. In addition, the echogenicity of dermis is decreased. An extremely hypoechoic band between the stratum corneum and dermis is present (Fig. 6.20).

6.3.3.1 Psoriatic Arthropathy (PsA)

For PsA, enthesitis (also known as terminal disease) is the most basic clinical symptom. The enthesitis refers to inflammation of ligaments, tendons, joint capsules, and other insertions into the bone, which can cause bone destruction and new bone formation. As the disease progresses, PsA leads to serious complications such as joint stiffness and deformation (Fig. 6.21).

PsA also involves synovium and tendons, leading to synovial hyperplasia, tenosynovitis (or peritendinitis), and tendinopathy.

Gray-scale ultrasound of synovial hyperplasia usually shows hypoechogenic or hyperechogenic lesion in the joint (Fig. 6.22A). Color Doppler ultrasound or power Doppler ultrasound show rich blood flow signals in the active phase of PsA (Fig. 6.22B).

Tenosynovitis is characterized by thickening and decreased echogenicity of tendon sheath. In the phase of active PsA, color Doppler ultrasound shows rich blood flow signals in and around the tendon sheath (Fig. 6.23).

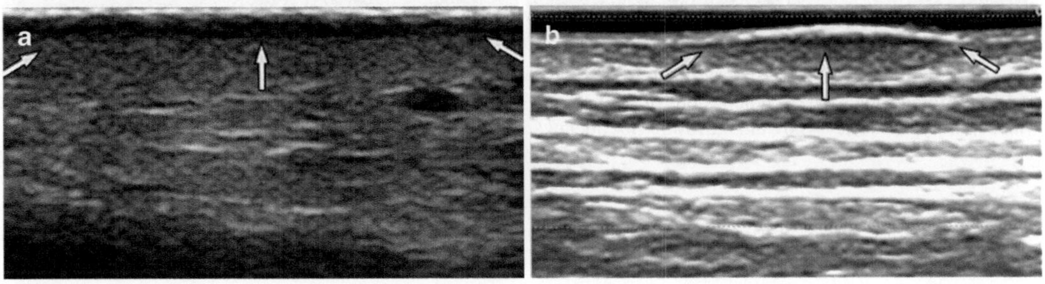

Fig. 6.20 Psoriasis. (**a**) On gray-scale ultrasound, psoriasis vulgaris shows that the epidermis and dermis are thickened, and a hypoechoic band (arrows) is visible between the hyperechoic stratum corneum and dermis (Frequency: 22 MHz). (**b**) On gray-scale ultrasound, pustular psoriasis shows that the stratum corneum is thickened slightly. A hypoechoic band (arrows) is visible between the stratum corneum and dermis (Frequency: 22 MHz)

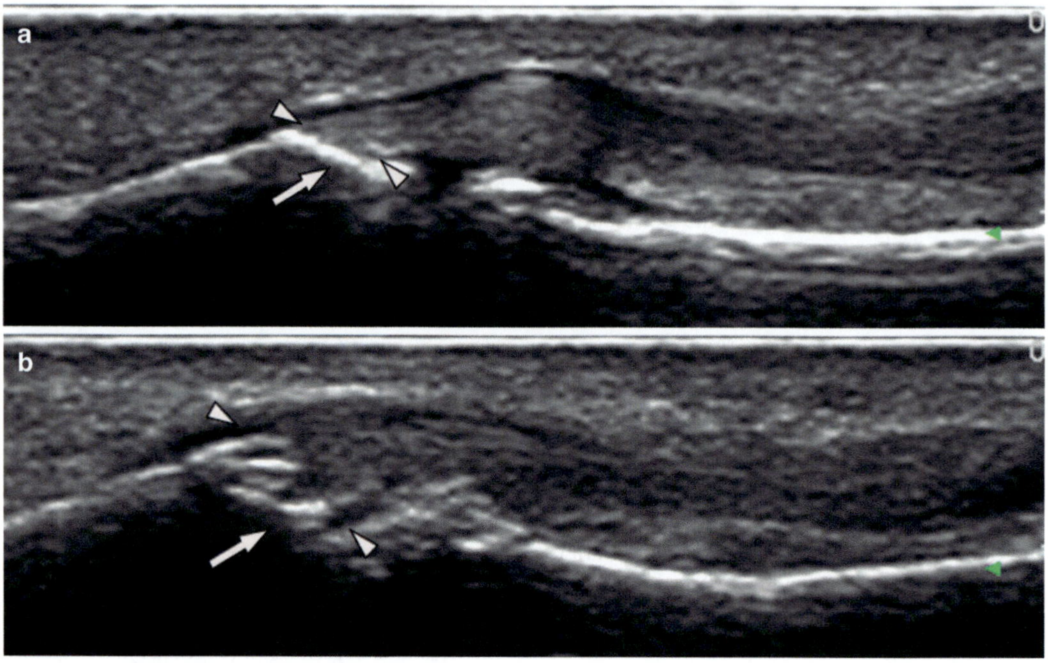

Fig. 6.21 Arthropathic psoriasis: enthesitis of tendon. (**a**) Gray-scale ultrasound shows the distal attachment point of flexor tendon (△) in normal joint. The bone cortex is smooth (arrow) (Frequency: 22 MHz). (**b**) Gray-scale ultrasound shows that the distal attachment point of the flexor tendon becomes hypoechoic, thickened, blunt, and the normal fibrous structure is absent (△). Bone cortex is rough and uneven at the attachment (arrow) (Frequency: 22 MHz)

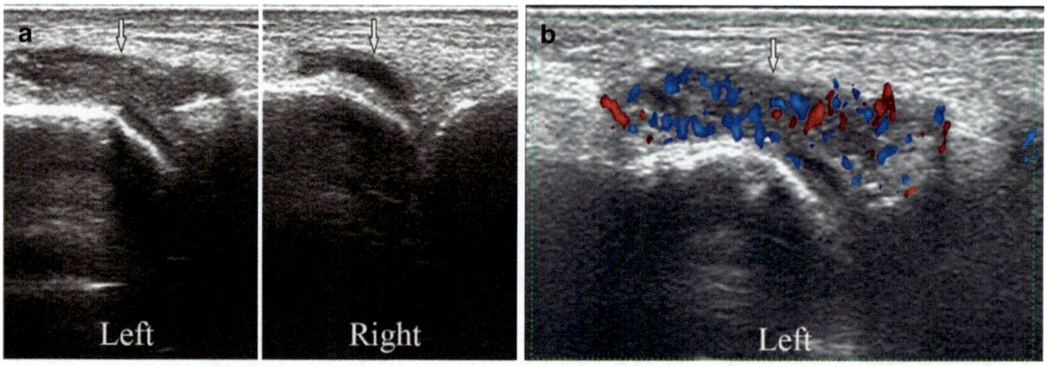

Fig. 6.22 Arthropathic psoriasis: synovitis. (**a**) Gray-scale ultrasound shows hypoechoic lesions in joint space, which are hyperplastic synovium (arrows) (Frequency: 22 MHz). (**b**) Color Doppler ultrasound shows rich blood flow signals in the lesion (arrows) (Frequency: 22 MHz)

On gray-scale ultrasound, tendon sheath effusion shows dilatation of the tendon sheath with an anechoic area. There are no blood flow signals in the effusion on color Doppler ultrasound (Fig. 6.24A). Tendinitis shows thickened and hypoechoic tendons without internal tearing (Fig. 6.24B).

6.3.4 Differential Diagnosis

6.3.4.1 Seborrheic Dermatitis

The disease is common in adults and newborns, and lesions often begin to appear on the scalp and gradually spread downward. It often occurs in sweaty and hairy sites. The initial lesion appears

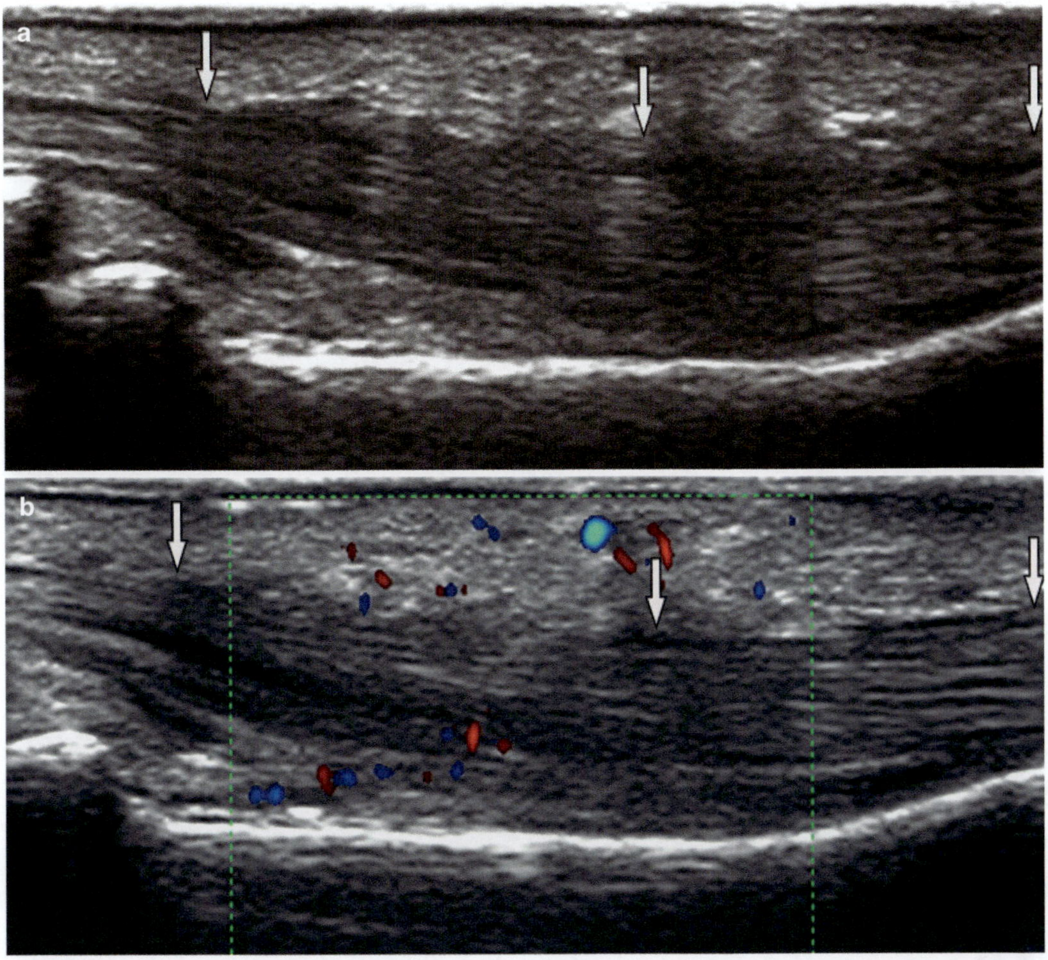

Fig. 6.23 Arthropathic psoriasis: tenosynovitis. (**a**) Gray-scale ultrasound shows the tendon sheath of the flexor tendon is thickened and hypoechogenic (arrows) (Frequency: 22 MHz). (**b**) Color Doppler ultrasound shows rich blood flow signals in and around the tendon sheath (arrows) (Frequency: 22 MHz)

as a small red papule around the hair follicles. Gradually, the lesion fuses into red patch and is covered by greasy scales or scabs. It is accompanied by various degrees of pruritus. It is difficult to differentiate them by ultrasound. Clinical manifestations are helpful to differentiate the two entities.

6.3.4.2 Gouty Arthritis

Gouty arthritis often involves the first metatarsophalangeal joint. Patients often have a history of hyperuricemia. Patients often present with severe joint pain and dyskinesia in the acute phase. On gray-scale ultrasound, characteristic features are multiple punctate crystals, double-contour sign (a hyperechoic irregular line formed by monosodium urate crystals in hyaline cartilage and a parallel hyperechoic line formed by the cortical bone), and tophi. However, PsA often accompanies with the skin lesion of psoriasis and enthesitis of tendon is the typical feature.

6.3.4.3 Rheumatoid Arthritis (RA)

Similar to PsA, all of them involve the small joints, but rheumatoid factor often is positive in RA. On ultrasound, synovitis is the characteristic feature. However, patients with PsA often have a history of psoriasis, and rheumatoid factor is often negative. Enthesitis is the typical feature of PsA.

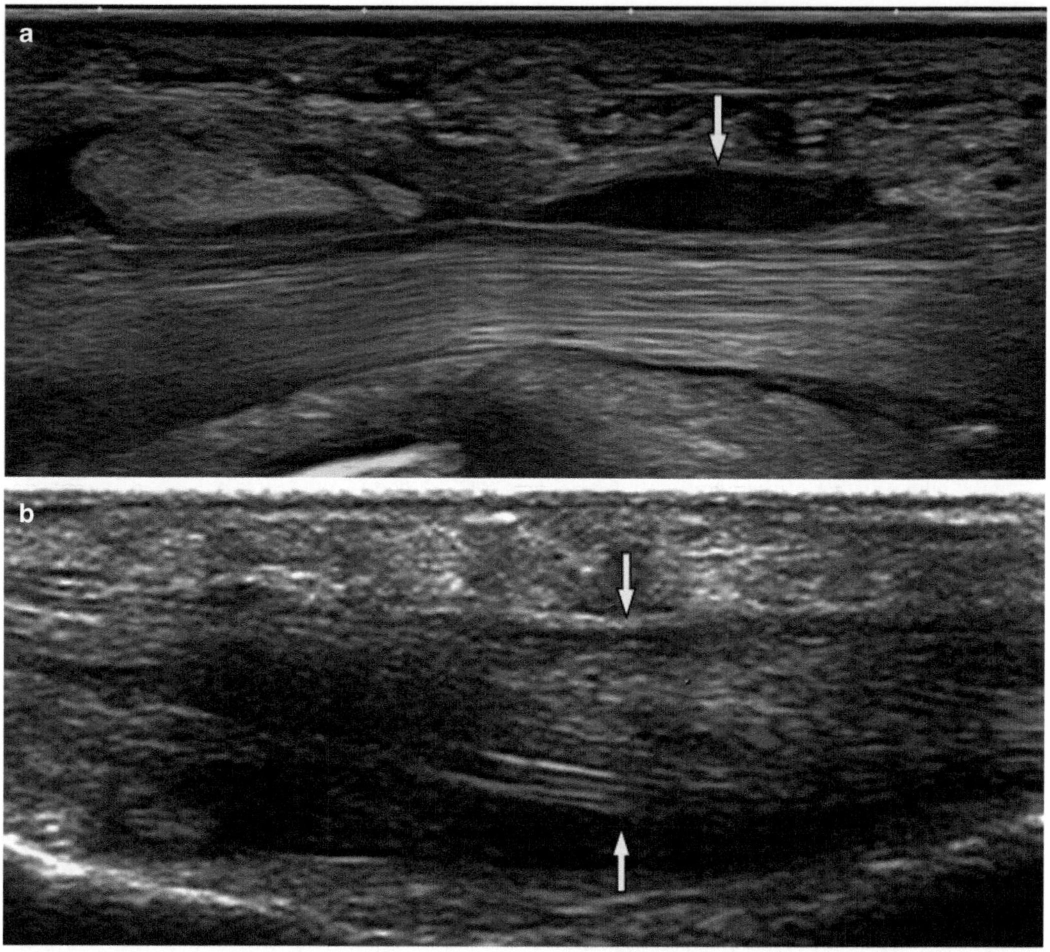

Fig. 6.24 Arthropathic psoriasis: tendon effusion and tendinitis. (**a**) Gray-scale ultrasound shows an anechoic area in tendon sheath (arrow), with good ultrasound transmission (Frequency: 22 MHz). (**b**) Gray-scale ultrasound shows local thickening and hypoechogenicity of the flexor tendon (arrows) (Frequency: 22 MHz)

6.3.5 Diagnosis Clues

1. Visual appearance shows that skin changes of psoriasis are predominantly erythema and scales. Patients with PsA often have pain, swelling, tenderness, stiffness, and dyskinesia of the joints.
2. Ultrasound findings vary in different types of psoriasis. Among them, PsA is characterized by enthesitis. Non-specific arthritic findings such as synovitis, tenosynovitis, and joint effusion are also visible.

Key Points

- Psoriasis is a chronic inflammatory skin disease. The disease has a long disease duration and is prone to recur. This disease is common in young adults.
- Ultrasound findings vary in different types of psoriasis.
- Arthropathic psoriasis is characterized by enthesitis.

6.4 Gouty Arthritis

6.4.1 Clinical Manifestation and Pathology

Gout is caused by prolonged hyperuricemia which leads to the formation of monosodium urate (MSU) crystals that accumulate in joints and other tissues. It is the most common form of inflammatory arthritis in adults. Although hyperuricemia is required for the development of gout, only 20% of patients with hyperuricemia will develop into gout. Studies suggested that the reason why hyperuricemia do not develop into gout was that the mechanism is initiated in the body to induce crystal autolysis, which blocks gout flares.

Recently, with the improvement of living standards and changes in dietary patterns, the incidence of gout is increasing. The incidence of gout in China is about 1.1%. Men are more likely to develop into gout than women. There are four phases in its progression: asymptomatic hyperuricemic phase, acute gout phase, intercritical phase, and chronic tophaceous gout.

In the asymptomatic hyperuricemic phase, patients only present with elevated serum uric acid without any clinical symptoms. The acute phase is characterized by sudden severe joint pain, accompanied with skin redness and swelling. Patients present with great difficulty walking or inability to use the affected joint. Most of gout involve a single joint, which can be relieved spontaneously in about 1 week. During the intercritical phase, the patient's symptoms of redness, swelling, and pain are significantly relieved. In the chronic tophaceous gout, patients with shorter disease duration are asymptomatic. And patients with longer disease duration will have bone erosion and tophi, resulting in joint deformation, which will affect the function of joints and the quality of life (Fig. 6.25).

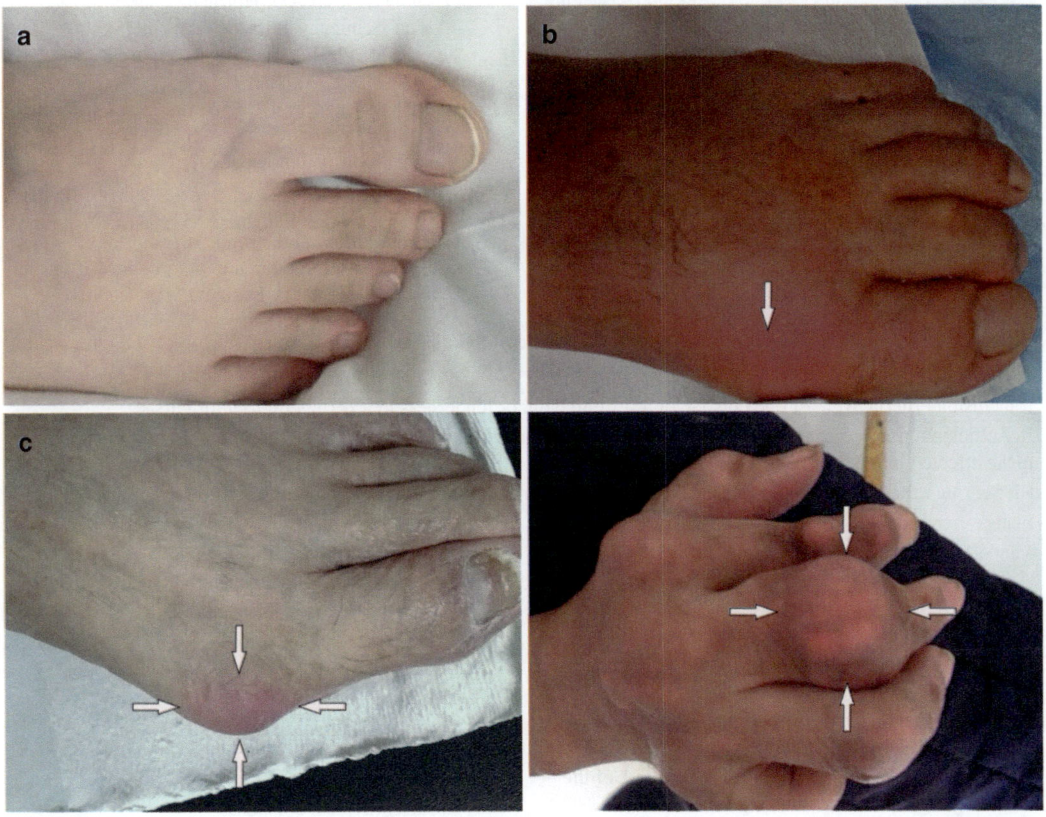

Fig. 6.25 Visual appearance of gout at different phases. (**a**) In the asymptomatic hyperuricemic phase, the appearance of the first metatarsophalangeal joint is normal. (**b**) In the acute phase, the skin at the first metatarsophalangeal joint is red and swollen (arrow). (**c**) In the intercritical phase, the skin at the first metatarsophalangeal joint is slightly red and not swollen (arrows). (**d**) In the chronic tophaceous gout, tophi are visible in interphalangeal joints, resulting in joint deformation (arrows)

The first metatarsophalangeal joint is most frequently affected by gout, followed by the midfoot joint, ankle joint, knee joint, metacarpophalangeal joint, and interphalangeal joint.

The gold standard for the diagnosis of gout is the presence of monosodium urate crystals in the joint or bursa (i.e., in synovial fluid) or tophi (Fig. 6.26). However, it is not often used in clinical practice because of invasion and difficulty with aspiration of joints and/or examination of the sample under polarizing microscopy. At present, the classification criteria for gout established by the American College of Rheumatology/European League Against Rheumatism in 2015 are clinically used, which includes clinical manifestations, laboratory tests, and imaging examinations. The classification criteria for gout uses a scoring system, and the threshold score for diagnosing gout was ≥8 (Table 6.1).

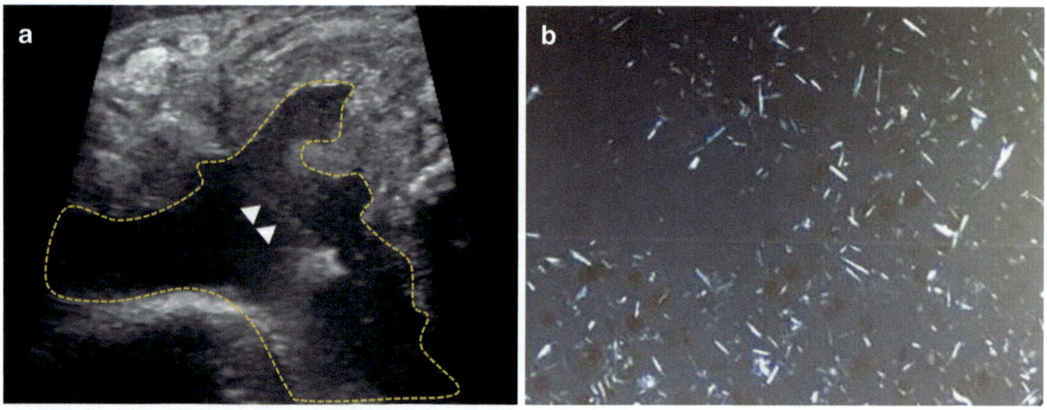

Fig. 6.26 The gold standard for diagnosis of gout. (**a**) Gray-scale ultrasound shows anechoic effusion (dotted line) and linear hyperechogenicity (needle of syringe) (△) in the cavity of metatarsophalangeal joint (Frequency: 15 MHz). (**b**) Needle-like urate crystals are observed under polarizing microscopy

Table 6.1 2015 Gout Classification Criteria of the American College of Rheumatology/European League Against Rheumatism

I. Inclusion criteria: At least one episode of swelling, pain, or tenderness in a peripheral joint or bursae		
II. Sufficient criteria (if met, patients can diagnosed as gout without the criteria below): Presence of MSU crystals in the affected joint or bursa or tophi		
III. Scoring criteria (used when sufficient criteria are not met)		
Items	Categories	Score
Joint affected during symptom episode	Ankle or midfoot (without involvement the first metatarsophalangeal joint)	1
	The first metatarsophalangeal joint is involved	2
Characteristics of symptom episode • Redness of the affected joint • Can't bear touch or pressure to affected joint • Difficulty in walking or inability to use affected joint	One characteristic	1
	Two characteristics	2
	Three characteristics	3
Time course of episode of symptoms: At least 2 of the following regardless of treatment • Time to maximal pain within 24 h • Symptoms resolve within 14 days • Complete resolution between symptomatic episodes	One typical episode	1
	Recurrent typical episodes	2

Table 6.1 (continued)

Clinical evidence of tophi (draining or chalk-like subcutaneous nodule under transparent skin, often with overlying vascularity, located in typical locations: joints, ears, olecranon bursae, finger pads, tendons)	Present	4
Serum urate level	< 4 mg/dl (0.24 mmol/L)	−4
	4 to 6 mg/dl (0.24 to 0.36 mmol/L)	0
	6 to 8 mg/dl (0.36 to 0.48 mmol/L)	2
	8 to 10 mg/dl (0.48 to 0.60 mmol/L)	3
	≥ 10 mg/dl (0.60 mmol/L)	4
Previous synovial fluid analysis of a symptomatic joint or bursa	MUS negative	−2
Imaging evidence of urate deposition in symptomatic (ever) joint or bursa: ultrasound evidence of double-contour sign or DECT demonstrating urate deposition	Present (any)	4
Imaging evidence of gout-related joint damage: conventional radiography of the hands and/or feet demonstrates at least 1 erosion	Present	4

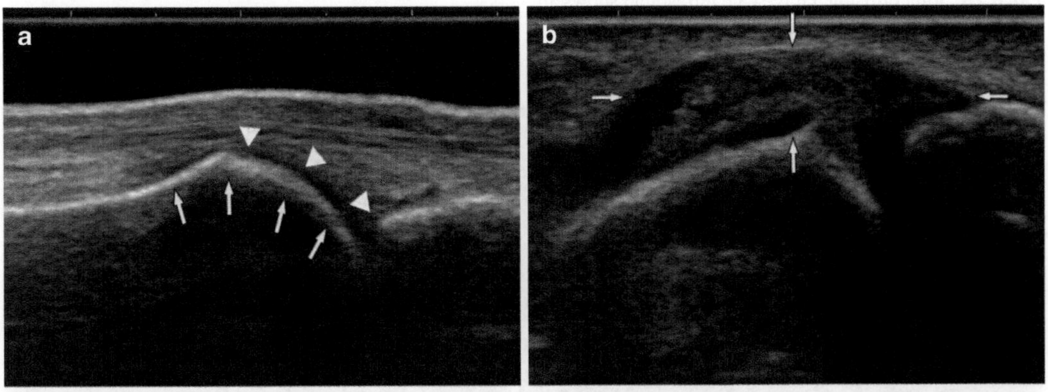

Fig. 6.27 Normal joint and synovial hyperplasia. (**a**) Gray-scale ultrasound shows that normal cortical bone (arrows) is hyperechogenic, smooth, and continuous on the first metatarsophalangeal joint, and cartilage is the anechoic line on the surface of cortical bone (▽) (Frequency: 15 MHz). (**b**) Gray-scale ultrasound shows that synovial hyperplasia is characterized by a heterogeneous hypoechoic structure in the joint (arrows) (Frequency: 15 MHz)

6.4.2 High-Frequency Ultrasound

6.4.2.1 Gray-Scale Ultrasound

In patients with a short disease duration, the following ultrasound features are found at the affected joint:

1. Synovial hyperplasia, which is characterized by heterogeneous hypoechogenic structure in the joints in the acute phase, and increased echogenecity in the intercritical and chronic phases (Fig. 6.27).
2. Joint effusion, which is characterized by anechogenic areas in the joint cavity (Fig. 6.28).
3. Crystals, defined as hyperechoic spots (smaller than 1 mm in diameter) located in the synovium, joint effusion, subcutaneous tissue, or tendons, which can appear as "snowstorm sign" (Fig. 6.29).
4. "Double-contour sign" (DCS), which consists of a hyperechoic irregular line formed by MSU crystals in hyaline cartilage and a parallel hyperechoic line formed by the cortical bone (independent of the scanning angle of

the ultrasound transducer). Among those features, DCS shows the highest specificity for diagnosing gout (Fig. 6.30).

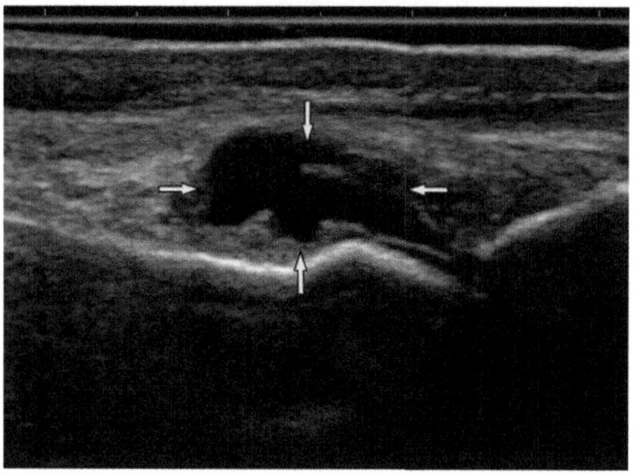

Fig. 6.28 Joint effusion. Gray-scale ultrasound shows an anechoic structure (arrows) in the joint cavity (Frequency: 15 MHz)

In addition to the above features, patients with longer disease duration can also appear the following ultrasound features:

1. Bone erosion, defined as interruption of the bone cortical margin that could be detected in two perpendicular planes (Fig. 6.31).
2. Tophi, characterized by a circumscribed, hypoechoic to hyperechoic, heterogeneous structure with occasional posterior acoustic shadowing, and a small anechoic rim (Fig. 6.32).

6.4.2.2 Color Doppler Ultrasound

Gout in acute phase shows rich blood flow signals in the synovium, gout in the intercritical phase shows rare blood flow signals, and there are no blood flow signals in the synovium of chronic gout (Fig. 6.33).

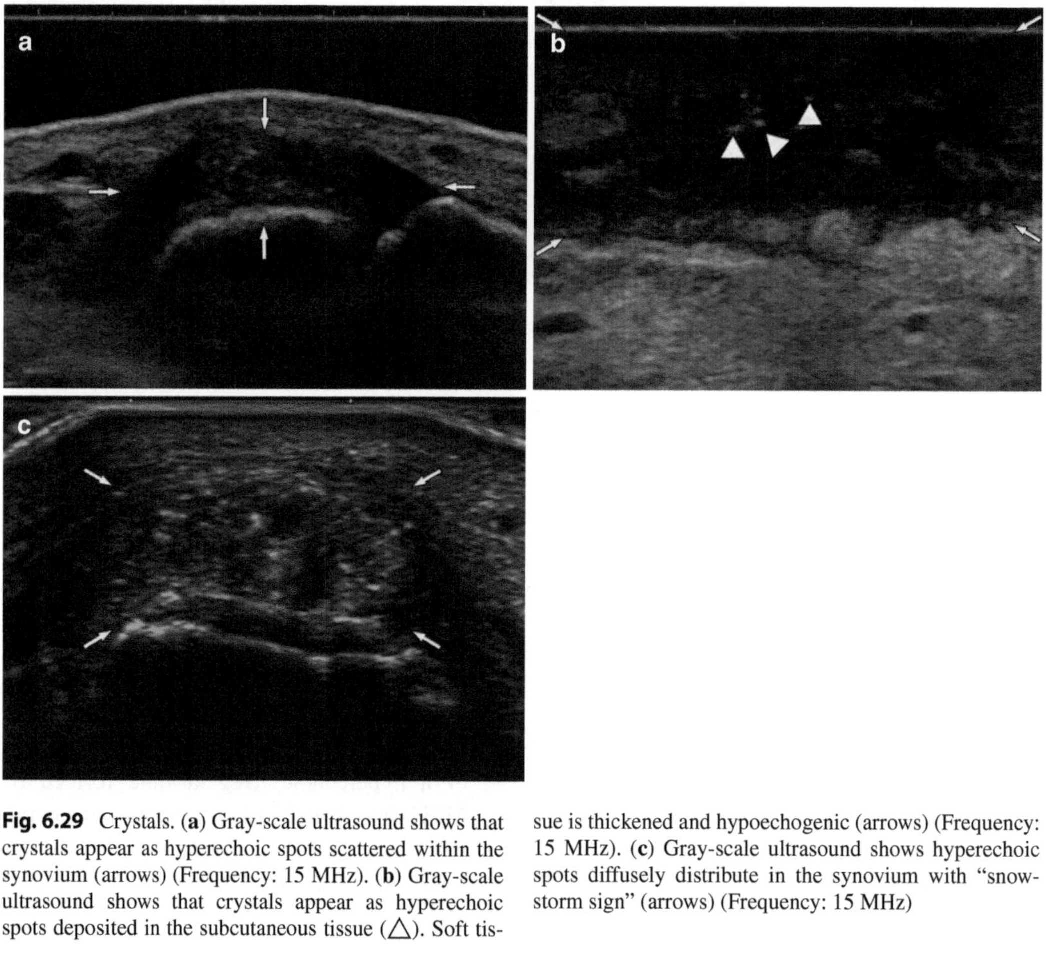

Fig. 6.29 Crystals. (**a**) Gray-scale ultrasound shows that crystals appear as hyperechoic spots scattered within the synovium (arrows) (Frequency: 15 MHz). (**b**) Gray-scale ultrasound shows that crystals appear as hyperechoic spots deposited in the subcutaneous tissue (△). Soft tissue is thickened and hypoechogenic (arrows) (Frequency: 15 MHz). (**c**) Gray-scale ultrasound shows hyperechoic spots diffusely distribute in the synovium with "snowstorm sign" (arrows) (Frequency: 15 MHz)

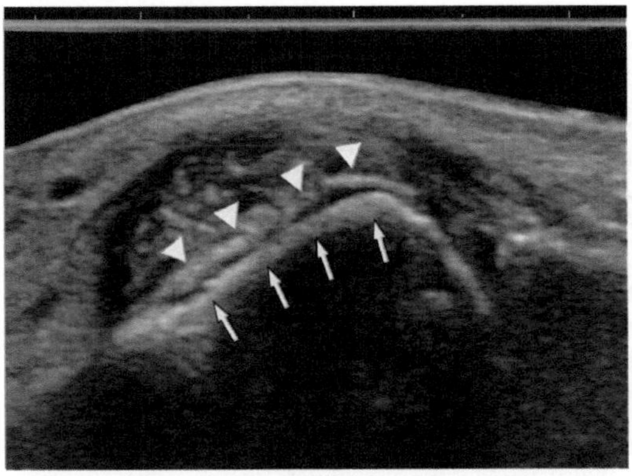

Fig. 6.30 DCS. Gray-scale ultrasound shows hyperechogenic line formed by crystal deposition on the cartilage surface (▽) and a parallel hyperechogenic line formed by cortical bone (arrows) (Frequency: 15 MHz)

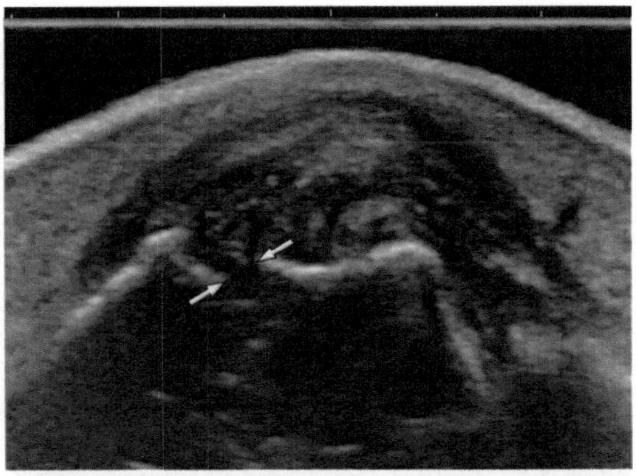

Fig. 6.31 Bone erosion. Gray-scale ultrasound shows the disruption of cortical bone (arrows) (Frequency: 15 MHz)

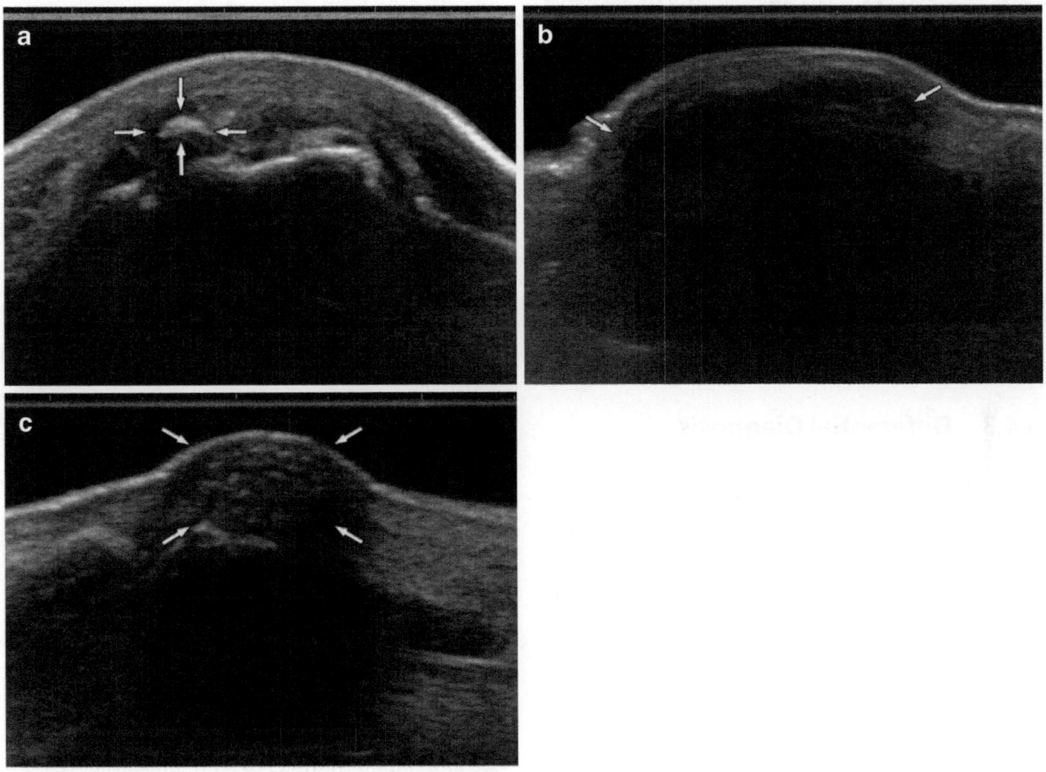

Fig. 6.32 Tophi. (**a**) Gray-scale ultrasound shows a mass-like hyperechogenic structure (arrows) in the synovium without posterior acoustic shadowing (Frequency: 15 MHz). (**b**) Gray-scale ultrasound shows a patchy hyperechogenic structure (arrows) in the subcutaneous tissue with a wide posterior acoustic shadowing (Frequency: 15 MHz). (**c**) Gray-scale ultrasound shows an oval hypoechoic structure (arrows) in the subcutaneous tissue with multiple hyperechogenic spots (Frequency: 15 MHz)

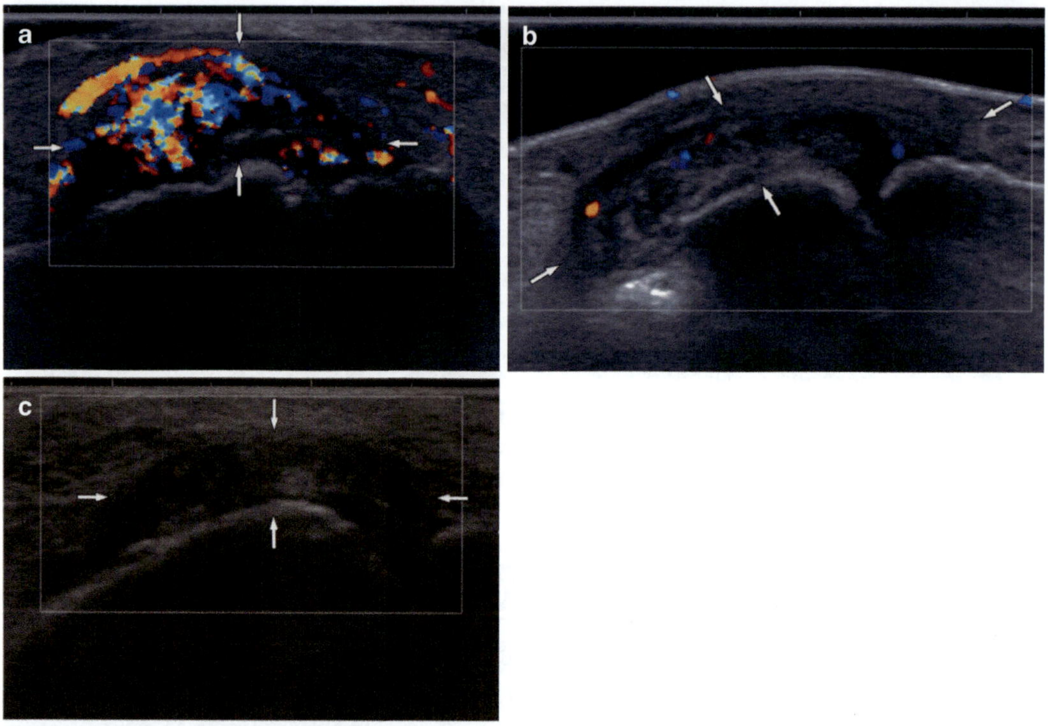

Fig. 6.33 Color Doppler flow images at different phases of gout. (**a**) Color Doppler ultrasound shows rich blood flow signals (arrows) in the synovium in the acute phase of gout (Frequency: 15 MHz). (**b**) Color Doppler ultrasound shows rare blood flow signals (arrows) in the synovium in the intercritical phase of gout (Frequency: 15 MHz). (**c**) Color Doppler ultrasound shows no blood flow signals (arrows) in the synovium in the chronic gout (Frequency: 15 MHz)

6.4.3 Differential Diagnosis

6.4.3.1 RA

RA is an autoimmune disease with symmetrical polyarthritis (hand and foot joints). Clinically, RA is common in women and its clinical manifestations include morning stiffness, swelling of joints, and night pain. Anti-cyclic citrullinated peptide antibodies or rheumatoid factor often is positive. The main pathological change is synovitis. While gout often affects a single joint, the characteristic site is the first metatarsophalangeal joint. In addition, most patients have associated hyperuricemia.

On gray-scale ultrasound, RA is characterized by synovitis. Bone erosion occurs with the progression of the disease. In gout, crystals are visible in most affected joints, and specific features of DCS and tophi are visible in some cases. Clinical manifestations, laboratory examinations, and ultrasound features are helpful to differentiate the two entities.

6.4.3.2 Osteoarthritis

Osteoarthritis is a chronic degenerative disease that occurs in middle-aged and elderly people. It is characterized by gradually increasing joint damage and degeneration. Clinical manifestations of osteoarthritis include joint pain, stiffness, and limited flexion and extension. The symptoms of patients with osteoarthritis often last for months or even years. However, patients with gout are often accompanied with sudden pain, which can be relieved spontaneously in about 1 week.

On gray-scale ultrasound, osteoarthritis shows thinning or disappearance of cartilage, joint effusion, and osteophyte formation. However, crystals, DCS, and tophi are visible in gout.

6.4.4 Diagnosis Clues

1. The characteristic site of gout is the first metatarsophalangeal joint, often affecting one joint.
2. Patients are often accompanied with hyperuricemia. Patients with acute flares of gout manifested as sudden severe pain of the affected joint with skin redness and swelling.
3. Ultrasound features of gout include synovitis, joint effusion, crystals, DCS, bone erosion, and tophi. Among them, DCS, tophi and "snowstorm sign" show high specificity for diagnosing gout.

6.4.5 Clinical Significance

Ultrasound is an important modality for the diagnosis of gout. In 2015, the American College of Rheumatology/European League Against Rheumatism classification criteria for gout demonstrated the value of DCS on ultrasound for the diagnosis of gout. In addition, studies have showed that tophi and "snowstorm sign" on ultrasound can also increase the diagnostic performance of gout. Sensitivity and specificity of ultrasound features reported in previous studies are shown in Table 6.2.

Our previous study found that color Doppler flow signals were richer in the acute phase of gout than in the intercritical phase, and the stiffness of the synovium in the intercritical phase was significantly higher than that in the acute phase of gout on two-dimensional SWE. Color Doppler ultrasound and two-dimensional SWE could be used to differentiate the phases of gout.

Table 6.2 Sensitivity and specificity of ultrasound features in gout

Ultrasound features	Sensitivity	Specificity
DCS	0.72 ~ 0.91	0.68 ~ 0.83
Tophi	0.34 ~ 0.87	0.38 ~ 0.96
Snowstorm sign	0.23 ~ 0.42	0.85 ~ 0.94

Key Points

- Gouty arthritis occurs on the joint and is characterized by severe pain with skin redness and swelling, most commonly affecting the first metatarsophalangeal joint.
- Hyperuricemia is the basis of its pathogenesis.
- Specific ultrasound features are "double contour sign" tophi, and "snowstorm sign".

6.5 Summary

High-frequency ultrasound is valuable in assessing non-tumor skin lesions, such as morphea, hidradenitis suppurativa, foreign bodies, cellulitis, odontogenic cutaneous fistula and psoriasis. In recent years, conventional B-mode ultrasound findings, blood flow assessment, and stiffness measurement have also been used in clinical practice.

Firstly, high-frequency ultrasound is valuable in the diagnosis of non-neoplastic skin diseases, such as foreign bodies and odontogenic cutaneous fistula. Ultrasound is recommended for patients with suspected odontogenic cutaneous fistula and foreign bodies. The diagnosis helps to choose appropriate management for patients.

Secondly, high-frequency ultrasound is valuable in evaluating the effect during disease treatment. Ultrasound is used to assess the dermal changes during the treatment of morphea by measuring dermal thickness and observe the boundary and internal microcysts in hidradenitis suppurativa before surgery. Some scholars used color Doppler ultrasound to assess the activity of morphea and found that vascular density can reflect the activity of the disease. SWE has been used to quantitatively assess the skin stiffness of morphea at different stages. And shear wave velocity can more sensitively reflect physiological changes of skin disease than skin thickness measurement.

Key Points

- High-frequency ultrasound is valuable in diagnosis and evaluating the treatment effect of non-tumor diseases of the skin.
- SWE can quantitatively evaluate the tissue stiffness, providing a new method for evaluation of non-tumor diseases of the skin.

Suggested Reading

1. Sexology Group. Chinese Society of Dermatology and Venereology, STD Subcommittee of Chinese Dermatologist Association, guidelines for the diagnosis and treatment of Condyloma Acuminatum (2014) [J] (in Chinese). Chinese J Dermatol. 2014;47(8):598–9.
2. Wortsman X, Wortsman J. Clinical usefulness of variable-frequency ultrasound in localized lesions of the skin [J]. J Am Acad Dermatol. 2010;62(2):247–56.
3. Kleinerman R, Whang TB, Bard RL, et al. Ultrasound in dermatology: principles and applications [J]. J Am Acad Dermatol. 2012;67(3):478–87.
4. Bhatta AK, Keyal U, Liu Y. Application of high frequency ultrasound in dermatology [J]. Discov Med. 2018;26(145):237–42.
5. Zhang LJ, Guerrero-Juarez CF, Hata T, et al. Dermal adipocytes protect against invasive staphylococcus aureus skin infection [J]. Science. 2015;347(6217):67–71.
6. Subramaniam S, Bober J, Chao J, et al. Point-of-care ultrasound for diagnosis of abscess in skin and soft tissue infections [J]. Acad Emerg Med. 2016;23(11):1298–306.
7. Sterling JC, Gibbs S, Haque Hussain SS, et al. British Association of Dermatologist' guidelines for the management of cutaneous warts 2014 [J]. Br J Dermatol. 2014;171(4):696–712.
8. Michalek IM, Loring B, John SM. A systematic review of worldwide epidemiology of psoriasis [J]. J Eur Acad Dermatol Venereol. 2017;31(2):205–12.
9. Zabotti A, Bandinelli F, Batticciotto A, et al. Musculoskeletal ultrasonography for psoriatic arthritis and psoriasis patients: a systematic literature review [J]. Rheumatology. 2017;56(9):1518–32.
10. Acquacalda E, Albert C, Montaudie H, et al. Ultrasound study of entheses in psoriasis patients with or without musculoskeletal symptoms: a prospective study [J]. Joint Bone Spine. 2015;82(4):267–71.
11. Blankenship RB, Baker T. Imaging modalities in wounds and superficial skin infections [J]. Emerg Med Clin North Am. 2007;25(1):223–34.
12. Kreuter A, Gambichler T, Breuckmann F, et al. Pulsed high-dose corticosteroids combined with low-dose methotrexate in severe localized scleroderma [J]. Arch Dermatol. 2005;141(7):847–52.
13. Wortsman X, Jemec GB. Real-time compound imaging ultrasound of hidradenitis suppurativa [J]. Dermatol Surg. 2007;33(11):1340–2.
14. El-Zawahry MB, Abdel EEHM, Abd-El-Rahman RS, et al. Ultrasound biomicroscopy in the diagnosis of skin diseases [J]. Eur J Dermatol. 2007;17(6):469–75.
15. Chen HC, Kadono T, Mimura Y, et al. High-frequency ultrasound as a useful device in the preliminary differentiation of lichen sclerosuset atrophicus from morphea [J]. J Dermatol. 2004;31(7):556–9.
16. Wortsman X, Wortsman J, Sazunic I, et al. Activity assessment in morphea using color Doppler ultrasound [J]. J Am Acad Dermatol. 2011;65(5):942–8.
17. Yang Y, Yan F, Wang L, et al. Quantification of skin stiffness in patients with systemic sclerosis using real-time shear wave elastography: a preliminary study [J]. Clin Exp Rheumatol. 2018;36(Suppl 113(4)):118–25.
18. Yang Y, Qiu L, Wang L, et al. Quantitative assessment of skin stiffness using ultrasound shear wave elastography in systemic sclerosis [J]. Ultrasound Med Biol. 2019;45(4):902–12.
19. Wortsman X. Sonography of dermatologic emergencies [J]. J Ultrasound Med. 2017;36(9):1905–14.
20. Meister P, Bückmann FW, Konrad E. Nodular fasciitis (analysis of 100 cases and review of the literature) [J]. Pathol Res Pract. 1978;162(2):133–65.
21. Lee KJ, Jin W, Kim GY, et al. Sonographic features of superficial-type nodular fasciitis in the musculoskeletal system [J]. J Ultrasound Med. 2015;34(8):1465–71.
22. Nikolaidis P, Gabriel HA, Lamba AR, et al. Sonographic appearance of nodular fasciitis [J]. J Ultrasound Med. 2006;25(2):281–5.
23. Kim ST, Kim HJ, Park SW, et al. Nodular fasciitis in the head and neck: CT and MR imaging findings [J]. AJNR Am J Neuroradiol. 2005; 26(10):2617–23.
24. Filotico R, Mastrandrea V. Cutaneous lupus erythematosus: clinico-pathologic correlation. [J]. G Ital Dermatol Venereol. 2018;153(2):216–29.
25. Naredo E, Uson J, Jimrnez-Palop M. et al. Ultrasound-detected musculoskeletal urate crystal deposition: which joints and what findings should be assessed for diagnosing gout? [J]. Ann Rheum Dis. 2014;73(8):1522–8.
26. Glazebrook KN. Guimaraes LS, Murthy NS, et al. Identification of intraarticular and periarticular uric acid crystals with dual-energy CT: initial evaluation [J]. Radiology. 2011;261(2):516–24.
27. Wang Q, Guo LH, Li XL, et al. Differentiating the acute phase of gout from the intercritical phase with ultrasound and quantitative shear wave elastography [J]. Eur Radiol. 2018;28(12):5316–27.
28. Richette P, Doherty M, Pascual E, et al. 2018 updated European league against rheumatism evidence-based recommendations for the diagnosis of gout [J]. Ann Rheum Dis. 2020;79(1):31–8.
29. Denton CP, Khanna D. Systemic sclerosis [J]. Lancet (London, England). 2017, 390(10103):1685–99.
30. Li H, Furst DE, Yang L, et al. High-frequency ultrasound of the skin in systemic sclerosis: an exploratory study to examine correlation with disease activity and to define the minimally detectable difference [J]. Arthritis Res Ther. 2018;20(1):181.
31. Yang Y, Yan F, Qiu L, et al. Quantification of skin stiffness in patients with systemic sclerosis using real-time shear wave elastography: a preliminary study [J]. Clin Exp Rheumatol. 2018;36(4):S118–25.
32. Muro Y, Sugiura K, Akiyama M. Cutaneous manifestations in dermatomyositis: key clinical and serological features-a comprehensive review [J]. Clin Rev Allergy Immunol. 2016;51(3):293–302.

33. Malattia C, Damasio MB, Pederzoli S, et al. Whole-body MRI in the assessment of disease activity in juvenile dermatomyositis [J]. Ann Rheum Dis. 2014;73(6):1083–90.
34. Tian J, Liang G, Qi W, et al. Odontogenic cutaneous sinus tract associated with a mandibular second molar having a rare distolingual root: a case report [J]. Head Face Med. 2015;11:13.
35. Gupta R, Hasselgren G. Prevalence of odontogenic sinus tracts in patients referred for endodontic therapy [J]. J Endod. 2003;29(12):798–800.
36. Sheehan DJ, Potter BJ, Davis LS. Cutaneous draining sinus tract of odontogenic origin: unusual presentation of a challenging diagnosis [J]. South Med J. 2005;98(2):250–2.

Skin Aging and Plastic Surgery

7

Xiao-Long Li, Le-Hang Guo, Jia-Xin Li,
Hui-Xiong Xu, Wei-Wei Ren, Dan-Dan Shan,
Yun-Chao Chen, and Zi-Tong Chen

7.1 Skin Aging

The skin gradually ages under the interaction of internal and external factors, resulting in changes in appearance as well as decline and disorder of physiological functions. Skin aging does not cause dysfunction, but it can cause a series of psychological problems such as anxiety. In the aging process of skin, the external environment of promoting factors is particularly important, especially solar radiation (ultraviolet, infrared, or visible light) exposure.

Although skin aging is irreversible, external protection and various scientific interventions play a role in delaying the aging process. Therefore, the monitoring and assessment of skin aging are vital for clinicians. Ultrasound is one of the techniques to assess skin aging.

Studies have showed that the total thickness of the skin remains constant until the age of 70 years, after which it gradually decreases. On ultrasound, "subepidermal low echoic band (SLEB)" and "hyperechoic dermis" changes with age are the characteristic ultrasound findings of skin aging. SLEB gradually becomes thicker, and it is more obvious on the exposed side of the sun. The thickness of SLEB is 0 mm in infants and accounts for 75% of the thickness of whole skin layers in the elderly, which corresponding to the papillary dermis pathologically. Contrastly, the thickness of hyperechoic dermis gradually decreases with age and pathologically corresponds to the reticular dermis (Fig. 7.1).

However, it should be pointed out that even the resolution of high-frequency ultrasound is close to 20 μm, it is still not enough to clearly

X.-L. Li (✉) · W.-W. Ren · D.-D. Shan · Z.-T. Chen
Department of Medical Ultrasound, Shanghai Tenth People's Hospital, Ultrasound Research and Education Institute, School of Medicine, Tongji University, Shanghai, China

L.-H. Guo
Department of Medical Ultrasound, Shanghai Skin Disease Hospital, Ultrasound Research and Education Institute, School of Medicine, Tongji University, Shanghai, China

J.-X. Li
Department of Dermatologic Surgery, Shanghai Skin Disease Hospital, School of Medicine, Tongji University, Shanghai, China

H.-X. Xu
Department of Medical Ultrasound, Shanghai Tenth People's Hospital, Ultrasound Research and Education Institute, School of Medicine, Tongji University, Shanghai, China

Department of Medical Ultrasound, Shanghai Skin Disease Hospital, Ultrasound Research and Education Institute, School of Medicine, Tongji University, Shanghai, China

Y.-C. Chen
Department of Medical Ultrasound, Xiang'an Hospital, Xiamen University, Fujian, China

H. Xu et al. (eds.), *Diagnostic Ultrasound in Dermatology*,
https://doi.org/10.1007/978-981-16-7345-0_7

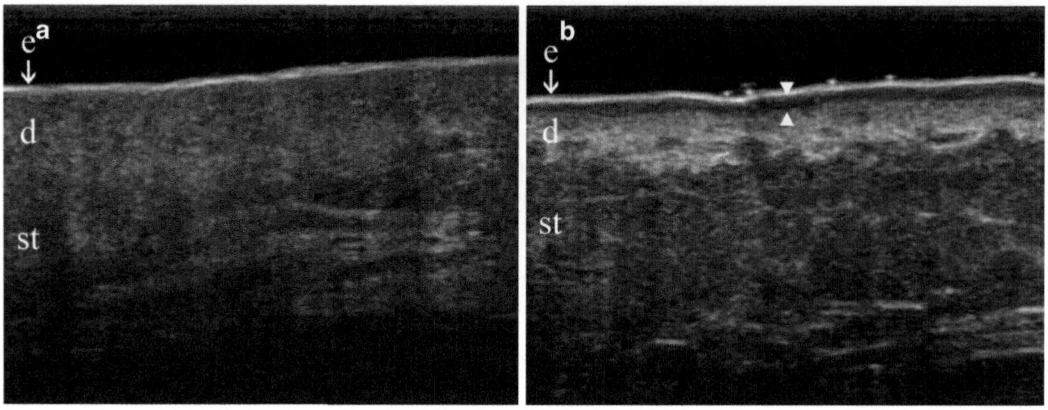

Fig. 7.1 Changes of epidermis and dermis in the elderly and child. (**a**) Ultrasound of normal skin in the face of a 2-year-old child. The SLEB is absent. (**b**) Ultrasound of normal skin in the face of a 70-year-old man. The SLEB is obviously visible (△). The dermis shows increased echogenicity, and the thickness is decreased (e indicates the epidermis, d indicates the dermis, st indicates the subcutaneous tissue)

show the microstructural changes of aging skin besides the above ultrasound findings.

Key Points
- On ultrasound, "SLEB" and "hyperechoic dermis" changes with age are the characteristic ultrasound findings of skin aging.
- Ultrasound is one of the techniques to assess skin aging.

7.2 Plastic Surgery

With the development and popularization of high-frequency ultrasound and focused ultrasound, ultrasound has been gradually widely used by plastic surgeons. It plays an important role in cosmetic and reconstructive surgery. Clinical applications of ultrasound include imaging and treatment. Literatures showed that in plastic and cosmetic surgery fields, ultrasound was well-established in breast (18.15%) (Figs. 7.2 and 7.3), head and neck (10.23%), microsurgery and reconstruction (21.80%), skin (17.50%), liposuction for weight reduction (28.38%), and others (4.96%).

In the head and neck surgeries, ultrasound is used to display the muscles, arterioles, nerves, and bony structures, as well as the measurement of skin thickness before and after treatment. It provides a safe and accurate preoperative plan and intraoperative guidance for surgery. Focused ultrasound has a satisfactory esthetic effect in wrinkle reduction and skin tightness, which has become an important application field of ultrasound therapy.

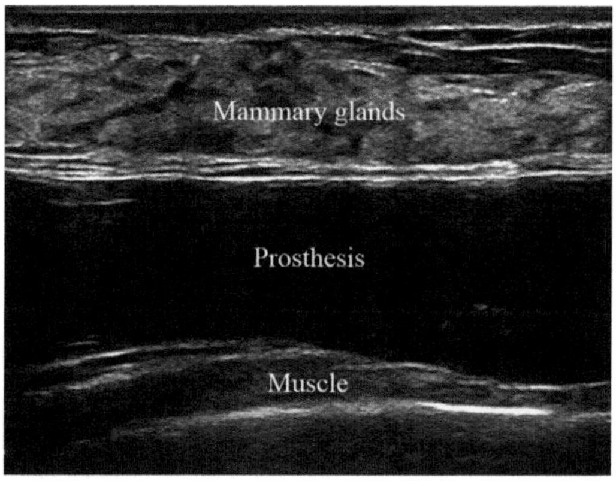

Fig. 7.2 Ultrasound of breast prosthesis. Gray-scale ultrasound shows anechoic prosthesis between mammary glands and muscle

In terms of microsurgery, ultrasound is mainly used to assess the vessels. Preoperative identification and localization of key vessels supplying the transplanted flap aims to avoid the damage of the blood vessels and block of the blood vessels selectively. It is also used to monitor the flap recovery to assess the efficacy after the surgery. In addition, the application of contrast-enhanced ultrasound in this field is prominent, which shows higher sensitivity and negative predictive value

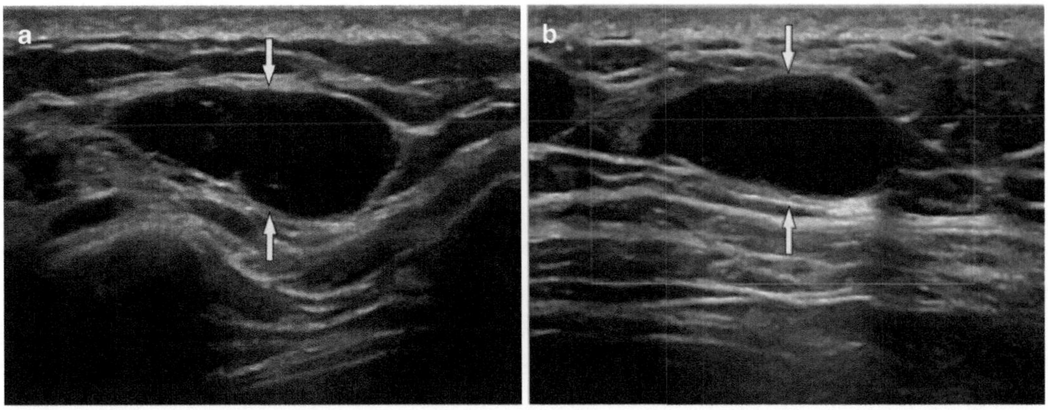

Fig. 7.3 Leakage of breast prosthesis. (**a**) Gray-scale ultrasound shows anechoic prosthesis (arrows) in mammary glands. (**b**) Color Doppler ultrasound shows no blood flow signals in the prosthesis (arrows)

than color Doppler ultrasound, and has great advantages in evaluating the course, patency of flap blood vessels, and fat perfusion.

Due to the rapid development of economy, people have a higher pursuit of body shape, and the demand of liposuction is very huge. In this context, ultrasound-guided liposuction has greatly improved the safety of the procedure, as well as reduced the operation time and the pain it brings.

In terms of treatment, ultrasound is used to promote the production of new collagen and the recovery of skin and subcutaneous tissue. The principle is that the thermal effect of high-frequency focused ultrasound leads to the breakage of hydrogen bond of molecules in the target area, effectively stimulates and promotes collagen production, so as to improve the elasticity and tightness of skin. In addition, ultrasound wave, as a kind of energy, has the properties of focusing, tissue penetration, and energy deposition, which can destroy and emulsify fat. Compared with traditional liposuction technology, ultrasound-assisted liposuction can remove fat more safely and efficiently.

In summary, ultrasound has dual functions of diagnosis and treatment in the field of cosmetic and plastic surgery. With the assistance of ultrasound, preoperative plan is more accurate, the surgical process is accelerated, the incidence of complications is reduced, and the patients' satisfaction is effectively improved. It should be pointed out that although the reduction of relevant equipment costs is conducive to the promotion of technology, it results in abuse and inappropriate operation to some extent. Therefore, in the process of developing ultrasound, it is necessary to always emphasize the importance of quality control and standardized operation. Only in this way, mankind will truly benefit from the development of the technology.

Key Point

- Ultrasound technology has dual functions of diagnosis and treatment in the field of cosmetic plastic surgery and medical treatment.

Suggested Reading

1. Szymańska E, Nowicki A, Mlosek K, et al. Skin imaging with high frequency ultrasound -preliminary results [J]. Eur J Ultrasound. 2000;12(1):9–16.
2. Kumagai K, Koike H, Nagaoka R, et al. High-resolution ultrasound imaging of human skin in vivo by using three-dimensional ultrasound microscopy [J]. Ultrasound Med Biol. 2012;38(10):1833–8.
3. Newton VL, Mcconnell JC, Hibbert SA, et al. Skin ageing: molecular pathology, dermal remodeling and the imaging revolution [J]. G Ital Dermatol Venereol. 2015;150(6):665–74.
4. Shung KK. High frequency ultrasonic imaging [J]. J Med Ultrasound. 2009;17(1):25–30.
5. Steinmetz P. Bedside ultrasound. Montreal [M]. Canada: A-line Press; 2013.
6. Miller DL, Smith NB, Bailey MR, et al. Overview of therapeutic ultrasound applications and safety considerations [J]. J Ultrasound Med. 2012;31:623–34.

8 Future Development

Le-Hang Guo, Hui-Xiong Xu, Qian Cheng,
Yun-Chao Chen, and Zi-Tong Chen

8.1 New Diagnosis and Treatment Mode

Traditionally, the diagnosis of skin diseases mainly is based on the visual appearance (including dermoscopy) and invasive skin biopsy. However, there lacks a simple and economical diagnostic modality between the above two methods. On the one hand, this modality can accurately screen suspicious high-risk cases, and on the other hand, it can avoid unnecessary biopsy of low-risk cases. In order to achieve the above purposes, we propose to embed high-frequency ultrasound in the traditional procedure to establish a new diagnosis and treatment modality of skin diseases (Fig. 8.1).

8.2 Future Prospects

Ultrasound has developed rapidly under the promotion of medical bioengineering technology, which is expected to revolutionize the work pattern of the whole non-invasive skin diagnosis.

8.2.1 I. Ultrafast Ultrasound Localization Microscopy for Deep Super-Resolution Imaging

At present, there are bottlenecks in the resolution of ultrasound imaging. The main reason is the phenomenon of "diffraction" in ultrasound which makes ultrasound imaging technology restricted to the balance of resolution and penetration for a long time, and the imaging resolution continues to stay at the submillimeter level. For the fine skin structures, such as sweat glands, hair follicles, peripheral nerves, and other skin appendages, the resolution of high-frequency ultrasound is still necessary to be further improved. At the same time, there is a great challenge in blood flow imaging at high frequency.

L.-H. Guo (✉)
Department of Medical Ultrasound, Shanghai Skin Disease Hospital, Ultrasound Research and Education Institute, School of Medicine, Tongji University, Shanghai, China

H.-X. Xu
Department of Medical Ultrasound, Shanghai Skin Disease Hospital, Ultrasound Research and Education Institute, School of Medicine, Tongji University, Shanghai, China

Z.-T. Chen
Department of Medical Ultrasound, Shanghai Tenth People's Hospital, Ultrasound Research and Education Institute, School of Medicine, Tongji University, Shanghai, China

Q. Cheng
School of Physics Science and Engineering, Tongji University, Shanghai, China

Y.-C. Chen
Department of Medical Ultrasound, Xiang'an Hospital, Xiamen University, Fujian, China

H. Xu et al. (eds.), *Diagnostic Ultrasound in Dermatology*,
https://doi.org/10.1007/978-981-16-7345-0_8

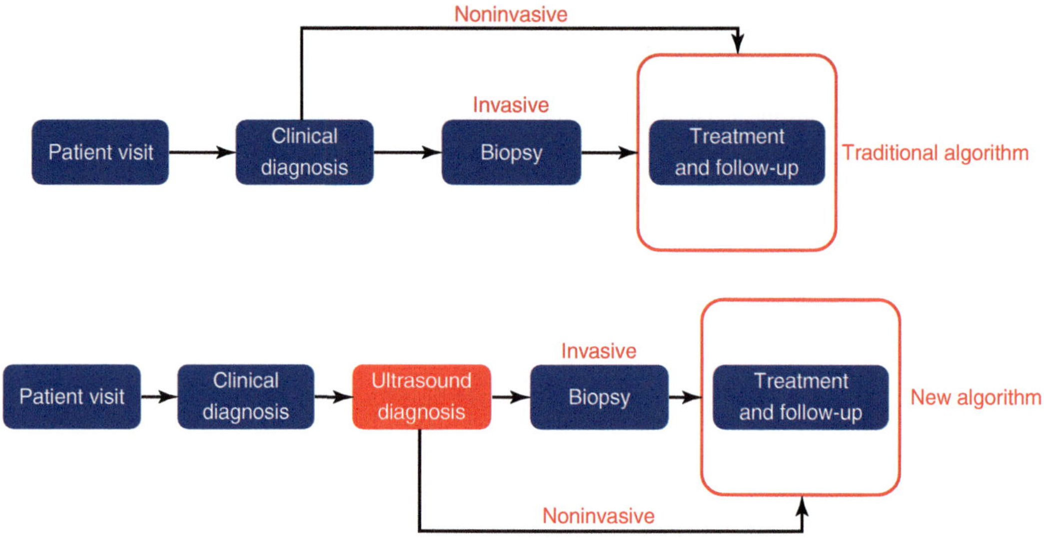

Fig. 8.1 High-frequency ultrasound is expected to change the diagnosis and treatment algorithm of skin diseases

It has been shown that the emerging ultrafast ultrasound localization microscope can be used both for structural imaging and hemodynamic quantification of rodent cerebral microvessels (less than 10 μm in diameter) more than 10 mm below the tissue surface. This technique is originally designed to achieve super-resolution imaging of tiny blood vessels on a microscale. The principle is to perform ultrasound imaging at ultrafast frame rates (more than 500 frames/s) by intravenous injection of inert gas microbubbles, capturing the transient signal decorrelation, thus providing a method similar to optical localization microscopy. The above research results lay the foundation for the clinical application of non-invasive microscopic imaging based on ultrasound. Ultrafast ultrasound localization microscopy breaks through the limitation of diffraction. Super resolution is conducive to clearly displaying the subtle structure of the skin, and has the dual-modality imaging ability of structure and perfusion, providing valuable information for clinical practice. In addition, this technique provides high frame rates and is easy to be popularized in clinical practice. Therefore, ultrafast ultrasound localization microscopy is considered to have great potential in the field of dermatology.

8.2.2 II. Stretchable Ultrasound Transducer

The surface of the human body is not absolutely flat and shows varying degrees of curvature. Some areas such as joints and facial areas have irregular contours. However, the existing ultrasound transducer is rigid structures. The contact surface of the high-frequency ultrasound transducer and the skin is straight. The rigid transducer can influence ultrasound imaging. Firstly, it will flatten the elevated lesion, affecting the evaluation of the morphology and size of the lesion. Secondly, the transducer cannot conform to the lesions located in the elevated or depressed sites, such as the nasal bridge, nasolabial fold, hip groove, auricle, and other parts, resulting in poor imaging quality.

At present, some research reported a stretchable ultrasound transducer that can conform to and detect nonplanar complex surfaces. The transducer consists of a 10 × 10 array of piezoelectric transducers that exploit an "island-bridge" layout with multilayer electrodes, encapsulated by thin and compliant silicone elastomers. The transducer connected by an island-bridge structured matrix. Each island hosts a rigid element. The wavy bridges can unfold to accommodate the externally applied strain, with limited strain in the components themselves. Therefore, the lesions will be maximally matched with the stretchable transducer. The above design will greatly improve the imaging quality of skin ultrasound in the future.

8.2.3 III. Automatic Scanning with the Aid of AI

Ultrasound examination of skin diseases is currently completed manually, but this working mode has two drawbacks: firstly, the location of skin diseases is superficial and sensitive to pressure, so it is required that the operator should keep the transducer in a state of "contact without compression" on the lesion surface. However, in the process of examination, it is difficult to maintain the above state and the operator often presses inadvertently; secondly, the view of high-frequency ultrasound transducer is generally narrow, but the skin lesion sometimes is extensive. Therefore, it is required to cover all areas of the lesions. The process is cumbersome and time-consuming.

Automatic scanning with the aid of AI is expected to achieve intelligent mechanical holding and programmed scanning. The pressure feedback device can provide accurate mechanical state of body surface and further help to control the transducer through dynamic calibration and movement trajectory matching. In this way, the transducer can be always kept in an ideal state of "contact without pressure" in the longitudinal direction.

At the same time, through visual recognition and intelligent path planning technology, the boundary of the lesion can be automatically identified. Based on this, the trace of the transducer in the transverse direction can be managed reasonably, and point-by-point scanning can also be achieved. Automatic scanning with the aid of AI may replace the scanning method of repeated scanning manually. The implementation of the above technology will liberate labor and improve examination efficiency and image quality.

8.2.4 IV. Progress of Skin Photoacoustic Imaging

The progression of many skin diseases is related to the content and distribution of hemoglobin, collagen, lipids, and other molecules. These chemical components are difficult to be detected in ultrasound imaging, but can be easily detected in photoacoustic imaging (PAI). The technology can be used as a supplementary examination method of ultrasound in clinical practice.

In the past 20 years, PAI has been developed rapidly. It is a new biomedical imaging technology that uses pulsed laser as acoustic excitation source to excite tissue, resulting in the generation of a wide-band ultrasound wave, then reconstructing the photoacoustic images. Based on the differences in light absorption and thermal elastic properties of biological tissues, physicochemical information can be visualized.

Since various molecules in tissues carry a large number of carbon, hydrogen, oxygen, nitrogen, phosphorus, and other elements, the resonance frequencies of molecular bonds between these elements are mostly located in the visible light and infrared bands. Therefore, many biological molecules, such as oxygenated hemoglobin, deoxyhemoglobin, phospholipids, collagen, and water have different wavelength-dependent optical absorption properties. When pulsed lasers of different wavelengths are used to irradiate biological tissues, molecules in the tissues will absorb lasers of different wavelengths to generate ultrasound, and the information of these molecules can be visualized by image reconstruction or spectrum analysis.

First, PAI has a natural advantage in identifying vessels. In the near infrared (NIR) bands, the light absorption rate of hemoglobin is higher than other molecules. Therefore, PAI has a high specificity for visualizing hemoglobin and has great potential in the diagnosis of vascular malformations. A photoacoustic research team of Tongji University has successfully applied PAI technology to preliminary clinical trials for the diagnosis and follow-up of port wine stain (PWS). Its theory

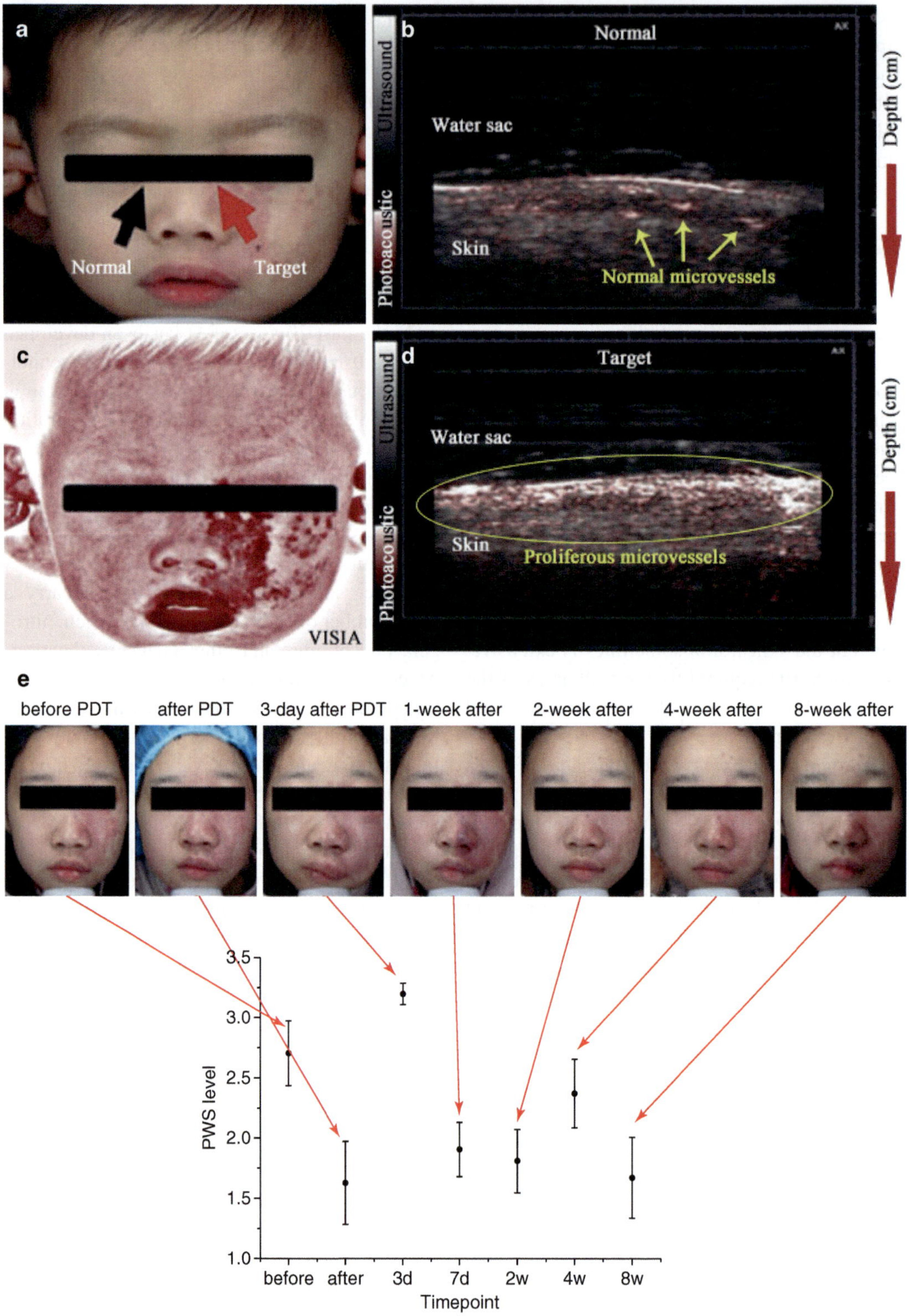

Fig. 8.2 Application of PAI in PWS. (**a**) Visual appearance of patient A with PWS. (**b**) Ultrasound (gray-scale) and photoacoustic (pseudocolor) fusion imaging of the healthy side for patient A. (**c**) VISIA figure of face for patient A. (**d**) Ultrasound (gray-scale) and photoacoustic (pseudocolor) fusion imaging of the erythematous side for patient A. (**e**) Photoacoustic quantification assessment curve of PWS vascular proliferation levels before and after PDT for patient B

and clinical trial results are published by Springer Press in the book of *LED-based Biomedical Photoacoustic Imaging: From Bench to Bedside*. The results of the follow-up in patients with PWS showed that photoacoustic successfully imaged the proliferation of subcutaneous microvessels, and provided quantitative data like skin thickness and microvascular density of PWS. Therefore, physicians can better select the treatment plan (Fig. 8.2).

In the range of light penetration depth, this technique can also assist physicians to evaluate many other skin diseases associated with vascular malformations or telangiectasia, such as AK, BD, superficial BCC, SCC, and EMPD, as well as some inflammatory skin diseases, such as psoriasis.

Secondly, in addition to hemoglobin, PAI is also sensitive to phospholipids, collagen, melanin, water, and other molecules. Therefore, this technology has great potential in early diagnosis and efficacy monitoring of tumors.

Key Points

- High-frequency ultrasound is valuable for the clinical diagnosis and treatment of skin diseases.
- Newly ultrasound technology is expected to change the traditional medical pattern of skin diseases.
- PAI can evaluate vascular malformations and telangiectasia within light penetration depth. It is expected to play a role in diagnosis and follow-up of skin diseases.

Suggested Reading

1. Xu HX, Guo LH. Application of high frequency ultrasound in diagnosis of skin diseases [J] (in Chinese). Oncol Imaging. 2019;28(5):289–95.
2. National Clinical Research Center for Skin and Immune Diseases. Expert consensus on high-frequency skin ultrasound diagnosis of common skin diseases [J] (in Chinese). Chinese J Frontiers Med Sci (Electronic Version). 2019;11(8):23–8.
3. Errico C, Pierre J, Pezet S, et al. Ultrafast ultrasound localization microscopy for deep super-resolution vascular imaging [J]. Nature. 2015;527(7579):499–502.
4. Kim YJ, Seo JH, Kim HR, et al. Development of a control algorithm for the ultrasound scanning robot (NCCUSR) using ultrasound image and force feedback [J]. Int J Med Robot. 2017;13(2).
5. Hu H, Zhu X, Wang C, et al. Stretchable ultrasonic transducer arrays for three-dimensional imaging on complex surfaces[J]. Sci Adv, 2018, 4(3): eaar3979.
6. Wang X, Pang Y, Xie X, et al. Non-invasive laser-induced photoacoustic tomography for structural and functional in vivo imaging of the brain [J]. Nat Biotechnol. 2003;21(7):803–6.
7. Mallidi S, Luke GP, Emelianov S. Photoacoustic imaging in cancer detection, diagnosis, and treatment guidance [J]. Trends Biotech. 2011;29(5):213–21.
8. Huang S, Qin Y, Chen Y, et al. Interstitial assessment of aggressive prostate cancer by physiochemical photoacoustics: an ex vivo study with intact human prostates [J]. Med Phys. 2018;45(9):4125–32.

Appendix

Appendix A: Template of Reports for Skin Ultrasound

Hospital LOGO

Skin Ultrasound Report of × × Hospital

(Please tick "√" in the "☐" and fill in the corresponding text at the horizontal line and space)

Outpatient/Inpatient No.: ________________

Patient Name:	Patient Age:	Patient Gender:	Ward:
Clinical Diagnosis:	Doctor in charge:	Date of Application:	Ultrasound device:

Lesion site: ________________

Ultrasound findings

Size:	Diameter: ☐ Size measurement _____× _____; ☐ Thickness of _____mm; ☐ distance from body surface _____mm.
Involvement level:	☐ Epidermis ☐ Dermis ☐ Subcutaneous soft tissue ☐ Deep structures (bone, muscle, fascia, etc.)
Echogenicity:	☐ Hypoechogenic ☐ Isoechogenic ☐ Hyperechogenic ☐ Anechogenic ☐ High echogenic ☐ Solid ☐ Cystic ☐ Mixture of solid and cystic ☐ Homogeneous ☐ Heterogeneous
Growth pattern:	☐ Crawling ☐ Nodular ☐ Regular ☐ Irregular
Surface features:	Surface morphology: ☐ Elevated ☐ Wrinkled ☐ Depressed ☐ Flat Abnormal keratosis: ☐ Yes ☐ None
Bottom features:	Bottom morphology: ☐ Flat ☐ Convex ☐ Irregular The boundary: ☐ ill-defined ☐ well-defined
Demarcation line:	☐ Epidermal/dermal junction ☐ Dermal/subcutaneous soft tissue junction Relation to the above demarcation line: ☐ Far away ☐ Contact ☐ Breakthrough
Special signs:	____
Blood flow signals:	☐ No ☐ Rare ☐ Rich ☐ Presence of thick nutrient vessels
Lymph node status:	Site_____, Diameter _____×_____, longest diameter/ shortest diameter > or < 2, Corticomedullary demarcation ☐ Clear ☐ Unclear ☐ Disappeared Lymphatic hilum ☐ Clear ☐ Unclear ☐ Disappeared Blood flow signals ☐ Portal ☐ Periphery ☐ Irregular

Impression/Conclusion/Diagnosis

Examining Doctor: Recording person: Checker: Date:

H. Xu et al. (eds.), *Diagnostic Ultrasound in Dermatology*,
https://doi.org/10.1007/978-981-16-7345-0

Appendix B: Template of Application Form for Skin Ultrasound

Hospital LOGO

Application Form for Skin Ultrasound of × × Hospital

(Please tick "√" in the "☐")

Outpatient/Inpatient No.: ____________

Name		Gender	☐ M ☐ F	Age		Department		Doctor in charge	

Medical history:

Clinical Diagnosis:

History of infectious diseases: ☐ None ☐ Yes, Disease condition _______

Skin ultrasound

☐ Superficial mass or skin lesion

Site: 1. 2. 3.

____

☐ Lymph node

Site: ☐ Neck

☐ Axilla

☐ Inguen

☐ Other parts ____

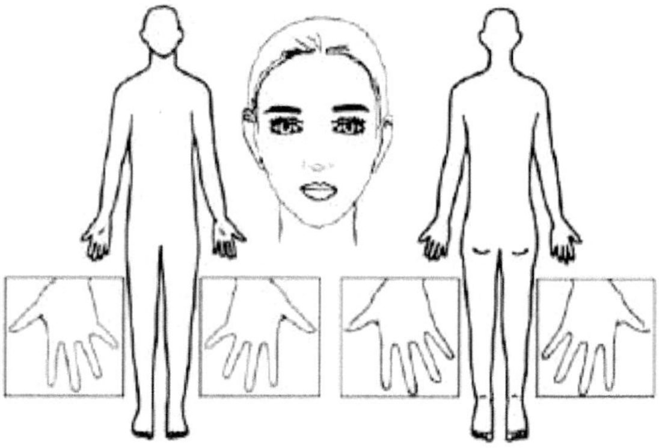

Joint Ultrasound

Joint site: ☐ Hand joints (wrist and distal hand joints)

☐ Foot joints (ankle and distal foot joints)

☐ Elbow joints ☐ Shoulder joints ☐ Knee joints ☐ Other _______

Points

1. Examination time: × × × ×.
2. Examination place: × × × ×.
3. Time of receipt of report: 5~10 minutes after examination

GPSR Compliance

The European Union's (EU) General Product Safety Regulation (GPSR) is a set of rules that requires consumer products to be safe and our obligations to ensure this.

If you have any concerns about our products, you can contact us on ProductSafety@springernature.com

In case Publisher is established outside the EU, the EU authorized representative is:

Springer Nature Customer Service Center GmbH
Europaplatz 3
69115 Heidelberg, Germany

Batch number: 10731385

Printed by Printforce, the Netherlands